Presented

with the compliments of

Allen & Hanburys Limited

Greenford, Middlesex

England

Steroids in Asthma:

A Reappraisal in the Light of Inhalation Therapy

Steroids in Asthma:
A Reappraisal in the Light of Inhalation Therapy

guest editor
T.J.H. Clark

editorial advisory group

G.K. Crompton
Simon Godfrey
Ian Gregg
M.C.F. Pain
Margaret Turner-Warwick
M. Henry Williams

ADIS Press

Auckland • New York • London • Sydney • Hong Kong • Tokyo • Mexico

Steroids in Asthma:
A Reappraisal in the Light of Inhalation Therapy

National Library of New Zealand

Steroids in asthma

Bibliography
Includes index
ISBN 0-86471-002-X

1. Asthma - Chemotherapy
2. Steroid drugs
I. Clark, T.J.H. (Timothy John Hayes)

616.2'38061

First printing

ADIS Press
15 Rawene Road, Birkenhead, Auckland 10, New Zealand

Printed in Hong Kong by Dai Nippon Printing Co. (HK) Ltd

list of contributors

R.N. Brogden
Scientific Editor, Australasian Drug Information Services, Auckland, New Zealand

P. Sherwood Burge
Consultant Physician, Solihull Hospital, West Midlands, England

G.M. Cochrane
Consultant Physician, New Cross Hospital, London SE14, England

G.K. Crompton
Consultant Physician, Northern General Hospital, Edinburgh, Scotland

Trevor Gebbie
Consultant Physician, Wellington Clinical School of Medicine, Wellington Hospital, New Zealand

G.J. Gibson
Consultant Physician, Regional Cardiothoracic Centre, Freeman Hospital, Newcastle-upon-Tyne, England

A.B. Kay
Professor of Clinical Immunology, Cardiothoracic Institute, University of London, England

S.P. Newman
Senior Physicist, Department of Thoracic Medicine, Royal Free Hospital, London, NW3, England

M.C.F. Pain
Director of Thoracic Medicine, Royal Melbourne Hospital, Victoria 3050, Australia

J. Morrison Smith
Consultant Physician, Penyraber, Fishguard, Wales

Jonathan Webb
Consultant Physician, Brook General Hospital, London, SE18, England

J.D. Wilson
Associate Professor in Immunology, School of Medicine, University of Auckland, New Zealand

foreword

There is little doubt that many asthmatic patients have benefited from the introduction of corticosteroids, but appreciation of this benefit has been tempered by worries about side effects. Thus early enthusiasm was followed by an almost excessive aversion to corticosteroid treatment because of the systemic side effects experienced by some patients with asthma. In the process, it is often forgotten that systemic side effects of consequence to patients come from long term administration and not the short course of treatment which is so often essential to prevent an asthmatic attack evolving into a severe one which may be life threatening. This has led to many patients being denied the benefits of a short intensive course of corticosteroids and this in turn may have contributed to some asthma fatalities. The publicity given to the unwanted systemic effects has also obscured the fact that many asthmatic patients benefit from only a relatively small regular dose of corticosteroid which can substantially improve their way of life without much risk of side effect. These considerations have led to a reluctance to prescribe corticosteroids by many clinicians and this has been paralleled by a similar hesitation by patients who take this treatment.

The introduction of inhaled corticosteroid treatment in the United Kingdom in 1972 has substantially changed the situation as patients now have the opportunity of taking effective corticosteroid treatment regularly with very little risk of unwanted side effect. This means that the majority of patients whose asthma is inadequately controlled by other treatments can now be treated either by a short course of systemic corticosteroids to deal with an acute attack, or the regular use of inhaled corticosteroids to suppress asthma.

When inhaled corticosteroids were first introduced there were continuing fears about the use of corticosteroids in general and further worries that inhaled treatment might carry with it its own topical disadvantages. After 10 years those fears and worries have largely abated. We now have a much better understanding of their use which has also enabled us to obtain a better perspective about the role of corticosteroids in general.

It is for these reasons that when the publishers approached me to ask if I would be Guest Editor of this venture I readily agreed. I did so in part because the time was ripe for this reappraisal but also because I hoped that the views expressed by the authors of this book would reinforce my own belief that inhaled corticosteroids are still being used too infrequently, to the detriment of patient care. In my view, the baleful reputation of systemic corticosteroids has cast too long a shadow over the treatment of asthma inappropriately limiting the more widespread use of inhaled corticosteroids. I hope this book will better illuminate the subject by providing sufficient information for the reader to appreciate the arguments in favour of the view that inhaled corticosteroid treatment has a more widespread application in the treatment of asthma than originally conceived for systemic corticosteroids. The reader will be able to judge for himself if this personal view is echoed by others and whether it has substance as we have been able to assemble a distinguished group of authors to review the position.

My main role as Guest Editor was to advise on the choice of authors and the editorial advisory group and we have been very lucky to obtain the support of so many able colleagues in producing this book and editing it. In this reappraisal of corticosteroid treatment, we have taken a reasonably broad view of the subject so that treatment can be seen in the context of asthma itself. It has also been necessary to review other treatments of asthma as the role of corticosteroids must be evaluated in the context of overall management. I hope this approach will enable the reader to acquire a better grasp of asthma therapy in general and corticosteroid treatment in particular.

This book would not have been possible without the willing cooperation of the authors as well as the hard work of the publishers. On behalf of the Editorial Advisory Group I would like to thank all those involved in the production of this book which marks the successful completion of the first decade of use of inhaled corticosteroid treatment. We all hope the book will guide the clinician into a better and more discriminating use of corticosteroid treatment over the next 10 years.

T.J.H. Clark
November 11, 1982

list of contents

Chapter I

Asthma: The Dimension of the Problem

J.D. Wilson

Asthma is one of the classic diseases recognised by Hippocrates over 2,000 years ago, yet today it is still frequently misdiagnosed and under-treated. Despite its venerable ancestry asthma has been considered a significant health problem only in the latter half of the 20th century. Before that its morbidity was overshadowed by infectious diseases and malnutrition while its mortality was all but denied.

By most criteria asthma, in developed countries at least, is now a major health problem affecting from 2 to 20% of the population. Asthma inadequately treated can be personally one of the most disabling and disruptive illnesses, resulting in lost schooling, absences from work, major alterations in lifestyle, prolonged morbidity and significant mortality. In terms of the cost of drugs and the provision of hospital and community medical care control of asthma has become one of the most expensive items in the health services bill for many countries.

The last 20 to 30 years have seen growing understanding of the pathophysiology of the disease and a treasure trove of effective antiasthma medication which has transformed the lives of many patients previously restricted in their activities by their respiratory symptoms. Improved skills in intensive care medicine have reduced, almost to zero, the hazards of severe acute asthma in hospital.

Despite these major clinical advances, hospital admissions for asthma continue to rise; a significant proportion of patients are either not diagnosed or not treated; many patients, despite chronic disease, are inadequately treated, while deaths from asthma far from disappearing have become more frequent in some countries (Jackson et al., 1982). The large range of drugs now available has brought its own problems in terms of more complicated therapeutic regimens which can confuse patients, or which may be inappropriately tailored for individual patients.

It is consequently an opportune time to re-evaluate the role of one of the most valuable of the recent medications for asthma - inhaled steroids - for their appropriate use can simplify and improve the treatment of asthma leading to reduced morbidity and mortality.

What is Asthma?

The simplest descriptive definition of asthma remains the most satisfactory and the most convenient in the absence of a clear unifying concept of its pathogenesis.

'Asthma is a disease characterised by wide variations over short periods of time in resistance to airflow in intrapulmonary airways' (Scadding, 1977).

This definition has its limitations and is usually qualified in different ways. Few clinicians for example, would label a patient who has had a single episode of wheeze as having asthma; but they are likely to do so if wheezing episodes become recurrent, although how many recurrences are needed to constitute asthma is a variable and very individual clinical decision. The definition implies objective measurement of airways resistance, and demonstrable reversibility of obstruction of at least 15 to 20% is considered necessary to sustain the diagnosis of asthma.

There are diagnostic difficulties in separating asthma from bronchitis (see table 11.2). In children the term wheezy bronchitis has long been used where cough and sputum predominate over wheeze. McNicol and Williams (1973) in a longitudinal study of a randomly selected group of children with recurrent wheeze, some of whom had been labelled as having asthma and others as having wheezy bronchitis, concluded that all children had the same disease - asthma. Many patients with chronic bronchitis have some reversible component of their airways obstruction.

Epidemiology

How Common is Asthma?

Epidemiological studies to establish the prevalence of asthma in different communities face some methodological problems. The disease has periods of remission so symptoms and signs may not be present when the patients are interviewed. Most surveys have not included airflow measurements, for logistic reasons, so estimates of prevalence are usually based on questionnaires about wheeze and the conclusions of past medical consultations. One study which did evaluate bronchial airways function in patients with presumed asthma, found 62% had significant airways obstruction on the day of testing, but in 38%, it was normal (McQueen et al., 1979).

While wheeze may be taken by some as an indication of asthma, particularly if it is recurrent, is associated with dyspnoea, or is exercise-induced, the occasional wheezy episode may be discounted or considered evidence of transient bronchial hyper-reactivity commonly occurring following some forms of viral bronchitis (Empey et al., 1976). Such difficulties with interpretation explain some of the differences in prevalence between studies in different countries.

Prevalence can be determined as point prevalence - having asthma at the time of the study, or as cumulative prevalence - ever having asthma at any time. Cumulative prevalence is the more commonly used.

Gregg (1977) summarised data which showed differences in childhood asthma prevalence in different countries: 0.7 to 2.0% in Scandinavia, 2.0 to 5.1% in the United Kingdom and the United States, and 5.4 to 7.4% in Australia and New Zealand. Figures as low as 0.2% have been reported in rural India. When wheeze and/or wheezy bronchitis are considered, the prevalence is much higher at 9.9 to 24.9% in the United Kingdom, 7.1 to 30% in the United States and 16.1 to 33% in Australia and New Zealand. For adults the asthma prevalence has been reported as 1.1 to 2.3% in Scandinavia, 2.0 to 5.4% in the United Kingdom and 4.1 to 9.9% in the United States.

A recent, detailed longitudinal study conducted over a 4-year period in Tuscon, Arizona, examined asthma prevalence at different ages in a non-Mexican white population (Dodge and Burrows, 1980). Conservatively they considered an individual had asthma if so diagnosed by their doctor and found the point prevalence of asthma to be 6.6% of the community as a whole, the highest rates being found in children - up to 10% - then decreasing in the late teens but increasing again in the twenties. When wheeze, either with infection or otherwise, was considered the prevalence rose to over 30% in most age groups. 1.4% of their community developed medically diagnosed asthma for the first time during the 4 years of the study.

Few other chronic diseases affect so many of the population for so long.

Racial and Environmental Differences in Prevalence

Racial and environmental differences in asthma prevalence are difficult to contrast or to compare because of methodological differences between studies but some general conclusions can be drawn. Asthma, compared with its prevalence in developed countries, is rare in Papua New Guinea Highlanders, in certain North American Indian tribes, in Eskimos (Gregg, 1977) and villagers in the Gambia (Godfrey, 1975). But there is evidence that when members of these low asthma regions move to urban areas asthma becomes more common (Godfrey, 1975).

The most detailed information on the influence of environment on the prevalence of asthma comes from the Tokelau Islanders, many of whom moved to New Zealand in 1966 after a hurricane devastated their island. Waite et al. (1980) examined 1160 children of Tokelau descent born in New Zealand and 706 children born, and still living, in the parent island. Asthma was significantly more prevalent in the New Zealand residents, 25.3% compared with the island children, 11.0% (p < 0.001). The environmental factors which are associated with increased asthma prevalence may include allergens such as dust mites, pollens and fungi but this has not been established.

Natural History of Asthma

The prevalence rate at different ages suggests little change in the overall frequency of asthma throughout life. McQueen et al. (1979) found the asthma point prevalence was about 4% throughout all age groups while Dodge and Burrows (1980) found a point prevalence of 6% for most ages, although the highest frequency was found in children. As asthma can develop at any age these data could obscure loss of asthma by some age groups and the development of the disease by others. Longitudinal studies are needed to determine the true natural history of asthma.

Asthma most commonly first appears in childhood. Of children with asthma the majority lose their symptoms around adolescence. Rackemann and Edwards (1952) found 71% of asthmatic children were symptom-free at 20 years. Blair (1977) followed a series of asthmatic children to the age of 20 years and found 52% were then completely symptom-free, while 21% suffered continuing asthma. However, in a further 22% the disease remitted in adolescence but then recurred after a symptom-free period of several years.

Comparable conclusions came from a very detailed survey in Melbourne of a randomly-selected group of wheezy children followed to the age of 21 years (Martin et al., 1980). Over half the children with infrequent wheeze lost their symptoms by early adult life. However, only 20% of those with frequent childhood wheezing became wheeze-free, although half had a considerable reduction in their symptoms at 21 years. Of those who wheezed frequently at the age of 14 one quarter had more severe disease when they were 21.

Although most wheezy children will have fewer respiratory symptoms after adolescence, in some the wheeze will return, while few of the children with severe asthma can expect to be asthma-free in adult life.

The Adverse Consequences of Chronic Asthma

Morbidity

Childhood asthma, if severe or poorly controlled, presents the child with a number of potential hazards. Growth may be retarded, both from the disease and from its treatment if continuous systemic steroids have to be used, although most of the loss is recovered by adult life. Schooling is frequently disrupted in the poorly controlled asthmatic and increasing morbidity results from nights of broken sleep. The lifestyle of many asthmatic patients can be disrupted by an inability to participate in sports and other activities. Martin et al. (1982) found that one third of their large group of asthmatic patients were missing substantial time from work and were restricting their sports activity. The personalities of many asthmatics may be permanently altered by over-protective parents, and by the stresses of chronic illness.

Some physical deformities such as kyphosis, barrel chest and Harrison's sulcus may develop in asthmatic children. The most severe cases of asthma, if unrelieved, can deteriorate to become respiratory cripples.

Many patients when their asthmatic symptoms are misinterpreted as recurrent infection receive antibiotic therapy which has little impact on their recovery and their symptoms persist for lack of specific therapy. Some patients seek alternative occupations because of their respiratory symptoms - either because they have limitations in their exercise tolerance or because they develop specific occupational-induced asthma. High risk industries include metal smelting, plastics, and baking (see Chapter V).

In contrast to most other chronic diseases, patients with moderate to severe asthma can anticipate some years of disruption to sleep, lifestyle, schooling and work if they are not well treated. However, if the correct diagnosis is made, appropriate antiasthma therapy is administered competently, and the patients helped to understand the nature of their disease and its treatment, much of the morbidity from asthma can be avoided.

Mortality

Traditionally asthma was considered to be a non-lethal disease as Osler's dictum, that asthmatic patients pant into old age, reflects. The 'epidemic' of fatal asthma in the middle to late 1960s demolished this concept and drew attention to the real possibility of death from asthma, not just in older patients whose final attack had continued over some days, but also in younger asthmatics during apparently short, severe asthmatic attacks (Fraser et al., 1971).

Initially this epidemic in the United Kingdom, Australia, Norway and then in New Zealand was interpreted as a consequence of the toxic effects of new bronchodilator aerosols, in particular isoprenaline forte, used to excess. Although there was no epidemic in countries that had not introduced the new medication at that time the question has not been answered to the satisfaction of all (Stolley and Schinner, 1978) and the current view of most authorities is that patients dying from asthma had placed undue reliance on their inhalers instead of seeking urgent medical help when their symptoms were not responding (Editorial, 1979). In particular most patients who died did not not receive corticosteroids during their final attack (Speizer et al., 1968).

A number of studies have since addressed the problem of fatal asthma. A fatal attack may have persisted unremitting for days or may have been perceived for only a few minutes or hours before death. The great majority of patients die outside hospital (Macdonald et al., 1976). Factors which might identify at-risk patients include severe asthma, previous hospital admissions, recent discharge from hospital, recent withdrawal of steroids, wide swings in peak expiratory flow rates, a history of sudden catastrophic asthma attacks, lack of a crisis plan to cope with emergencies and lack of prophylactic medication such as steroids (Ormerod and Stableforth, 1980; Crompton et al., 1979).

A more recent 'epidemic' of fatal asthma has occurred in New Zealand with a death rate in the 5 to 34 age group rising from 1.4/100,000 in 1975 to 4.1/100,000 in 1979 (Jackson et al., 1982). When this is contrasted with the general impression of some United States authorities that .. 'on a world-wide basis the diagnosis of asthma as a cause of death in most age groups is below 2/1,000,000 people' .. (Speizer, 1978), it emphasises the need for constant vigilance to detect changing patterns in the morbidity and mortality of asthma, and to reverse any complacency regarding the adequacy of medical management. Although no definite conclusions can be drawn about the causes of these recent findings, suboptimal use of maintenance treatment and, in particular, the lack of systemic steroids during final attacks have been suggested as possible contributing factors (Wilson et al., 1981; Sutherland and Wilson, 1981).

From all studies on fatal asthma one feature stands out. Few asthmatics die when their therapy is adequate and when their education about their disease and its management is satisfactory. Above all, few fatalities have occurred in patients who are using steroids systemically or by inhalation (Speizer et al., 1968; Grant, 1982; Ormerod and Stableforth, 1980), but protection is not absolute.

Changing Treatment Patterns

Until the 20th century little specific therapy was available for treating asthma other than anticholinergics in various forms, such as stramonium cigarettes. Some had achieved spectacular success with their patients by removing them from irritant or allergic materials but generally this was the luck of the empiricist. Immunotherapy to desensitise asthmatic patients against real or presumed allergens was widely practised from 1920 onwards, and still is, although careful studies in recent times have found little benefit from this approach (Lichtenstein, 1978).

Bronchodilators

Adrenaline, initially extracted from adrenal glands and then synthesised, was the first regularly used drug with bronchodilator qualities and was followed by ephedrine and the methylxanthines in the 1930s. Ahlquist's distinction of sympathetic receptors into α and β, the former mediating constriction of smooth muscle of blood vessels, bladder and sphincters of the gastrointestinal tract, and the latter stimulating the heart, producing vasodilatation, bronchodilatation and skeletal muscle tremor, provided the pharmacological charter for the development of more selective bronchodilator drugs (Ahlquist, 1948). Isoprenaline (isoproterenol) was among the first non-selective β-agonists, since supplanted by the more selective β_2-agonists which, with their reduction in β_1 activity had less cardiac effects while retaining the β_2 effects of bronchodilatation and skeletal muscle tremor.

Bronchodilators and other antiasthmatic drugs are discussed fully in Chapter VI.

Corticosteroids

Systemic corticosteroids arrived with a fanfare as the most effective antiasthma agent of all but the sounds were quickly muted when the side effects of high dose and long term steroid therapy became apparent. However, steroids rapidly demonstrated their capacity to reverse the previously irreversible asthma attack and have become central drugs for asthma management. Corticosteroids, as will be seen later in this book, have a role both in aborting acute asthma attacks and in preventing and damping down recurring attacks. Self-administration of steroids by mouth, or intravenous steroid therapy in hospital, is widely used to shorten periods of intense bronchoconstriction which have responded poorly to bronchodilators (Collins et al., 1975). Many patients have profoundly reduced their morbidity from asthma by this means. See Chapter VII.

The second major value of corticosteroids is in the long term prophylactic therapy of asthma, preferably by inhalation. Because of concern over the possibility of steroid side effects, widespread adoption of this method of asthma management proceeded relatively slowly. However, experience has shown inhaled steroids can bring control of asthma to the majority of patients for whom intermittent bronchodilator therapy is inadequate, without troublesome side effects, and that their concomitant use in the minority of patients requiring prednisolone prophylaxis enables at least some reduction in the systemic steroid requirement.

There is no doubt that the morbidity of asthma is likely to be significantly reduced with the more widespread use of inhaled corticosteroids. It is possible that the resulting higher expectations of both the asthmatic patient and his doctor will bring about a reduction in mortality also.

The New Technology

Improvements in intensive inpatient care of acute asthma have kept pace with the pharmacological advances. Hospital admission of patients implies severe asthma unresponsive to the usual treatments and a battery of measures to reverse acute respiratory obstruction is available; as death from acute asthma is rare in specialist respiratory units, these measures are obviously highly successful (Hersch et al., 1977).

In acute severe asthma aminophylline, β-agonists and steroids can be delivered intravenously by injection, conventional infusion or by continuous infusion pump. Nebulisers and devices for intermittent positive pressure breathing have been shown to be highly effective ways of administering bronchodilators (Webber et al., 1982). Oxygen is a mandatory component of therapy in the early stages. Arterial blood gas monitoring charts the severity of the metabolic changes consequent on the obstruction and warns of additional intravenous measures which may be needed (p.39). In extreme circumstances intubation and mechanical ventilation may be necessary despite its hazard. Rarely this is required repeatedly in patients who suffer anaphylactic-like asthma (Crompton et al., 1979). Bronchial lavage is now rarely practised though some clinicians find it may reverse a patient's trend towards irreversible asthma (Greening, 1982).

Self-referral

A growing trend in the management of severe asthma has been that of self-referral to hospital (p.111). By this approach, pioneered by the Edinburgh Emergency Asthma Admission Service, patients can, when they experience a failing response to medication, admit themselves directly to hospital bypassing their general practitioner and avoiding unnecessary delays. The value of this approach lies in the strong suggestion that asthma fatalities are reduced among at risk patients (Crompton et al., 1979).

Is Asthma Underdiagnosed and Undertreated?

Some of the difficulties of answering this question stem from the problems of defining asthma unless objective criteria are used. A survey analysed a group of 34 cases of asthma in children selected randomly from one hospital paediatric outpatients department in London, and from a similar clinic at Newcastle-on-Tyne (Speight, 1978). The results showed a major shortfall in making an unequivocal diagnosis of asthma. Only 2 of the 34 families had been told that their child had asthma and only 6 of the 32 general practitioner referral letters mentioned asthma. Wheezing, wheezy bronchitis, and bronchospasm were mentioned in 11 and in 12, only infection or bronchitis; 3 cases were referred as cardiac problems with exertional dyspnoea. Despite this alarming lack of a diagnosis of asthma nearly half the children had missed at least 6 weeks of school in the previous 12 months, and many while attending school had been excluded from sports because of respiratory symptoms. Asthmatic attacks in some had been severe enough to warrant hospital admission.

Some of the diagnostic difficulties arise from differences in terminology or a misplaced concern about using the term asthma as it may frighten some patients or parents. Anderson et al. (1981), in a survey of 284 9-year-old wheezy children found about one third of those with broken sleep or disturbed activity from respiratory symptoms had received no antiasthma therapy in the previous month. Use of appropriate medication was much more common when the diagnosis of asthma had been made, but only half of the children most affected were labelled as asthmatic. Comparable results were found by Sears et al., (1982) in 7-year-old children. When the diagnosis was bronchitis with wheeze only 4 of 106 children were treated with bronchodilator therapy, while 16 of the 36 with asthma were receiving these drugs.

Stellman et al. (1982), in a group of 70 asthmatics newly referred to a hospital outpatient clinic, found that in one third the diagnosis of asthma had not been considered. On presentation 9% were using inhaled steroids. After formal assessment inhaled steroids were felt to be necessary for 40%. McQueen et al. (1979), found in a community survey that less than 50% of asthmatics had bronchodilator therapy, and less than 16% had prophylactic medication in the form of sodium cromoglycate or steroid.

Martin et al. (1982) studying a group of 336 21-year-olds, who had been followed since the age of 7 when they had had recurrent wheeze, found that the patients' knowledge about their asthma was poor, particularly among those with less troublesome symptoms.

Half of the patients with frequent episodic asthma and one third with persistent asthma did not regard excess use of bronchodilator aerosols as potentially dangerous, and certainly not as an indication to seek further medical help. Over three-quarters of those with frequent episodic asthma and 40% of those with persistent asthma were not receiving adequate treatment. One third of those with persistent asthma were missing substantial time from work because of respiratory disease, and a similar proportion were restricting sporting activities. Disturbingly, the incidence of smoking was high in all asthma groups.

In a recent study of the circumstances leading to 90 deaths from asthma, a panel from the British Thoracic Association (BTA Study, 1982) judged drug treatment in the month before the fatal attack as satisfactory in only 35 of the 90 and, in the panel's view, general supervision and management in the last year of life was thought satisfactory in only 3 of the 90 patients.

How Should We Manage Asthma?

The management of asthma is now at the crossroads. Despite exciting pharmacological and technological advances a significant proportion of asthma patients remain undiagnosed, many with continuing symptoms are still inadequately treated, and the fatality rate is not falling. The stage has clearly been reached where the major challenge is not the discovery of new antiasthma drugs but the more effective use of the treatments already available.

Patient Education

As with diabetes, the other long term disease where treatment dosage is commonly regulated by the patient, care must be taken to ensure that patients with asthma clearly understand what their drugs can and cannot do, and how they are to be used. Crompton (1982) has recently summarised the problems some patients continue to have with pressurised aerosols despite their receiving detailed instructions and demonstrations of how to use them correctly. Too often continuing morbidity results from a patient's lack of understanding about the differences between a bronchodilator drug and prophylactic drugs such as inhaled steroids or sodium cromoglycate (p.178; Appendix 1).

Crisis Plan

In all analyses of death from asthma it is clear that many patients do not know what to do when their usual medication is becoming ineffective. They delayed too long before seeking further medical help. This problem is central to the management of asthma and all patients should be provided with a crisis plan emphasising the warning signals which indicate professional medical help is required.

Designing Individual Treatments for Individual Patients

Too frequently most asthmatic patients in a clinic or a practice receive identical therapy. Yet one of the most valuable developments in recent years has been the provision of different delivery formulations of drugs to suit different conditions e.g. β-sympathomimetic agents can be provided as short- or long-acting tablets, in a syrup, by metered dose inhalers, by inhaled powders for the poorly coordinated patient, or by various nebuliser systems. When care is taken to choose the formulation appropriate, not only to the severity of the patient's disease, but also to their skills in coordination or comprehension of their treatment schedule then therapeutic failures and inadequacies of compliance can usually be forestalled.

Frequently the decision to introduce prophylactic therapy is delayed for too long and the patient suffers the consequence of repeated *ad hoc* treatments for acute asthma from different emergency doctors. A 1 to 2 month clinical trial of an inhaled steroid usually is sufficient to convince both patient and the clinician of its substantial advantages in terms of well-being and ease of disease management.

Emergency Self Referral

For the most severe attacks of acute asthma delay in reaching hospital may be the final contributor to the patient's death. The experience of the Edinburgh Emergency Asthma Admission Service where patients take themselves directly to hospital if their treatment fails provides a convincing argument for the widespread adoption of this practice.

Corticosteroids

The study of Stellman et al. (1982) who found only 6 of 70 asthmatic patients referred to a hospital clinic were using inhaled steroids, is disturbing. If management of these patients' asthma had been proving sufficiently difficult for specialist referral to seem necessary why had inhaled steroids not been administered before? The clinic certainly felt that at least 40% of them should have been on steroids. This question is difficult to answer but there is possibly a carry over of concern about the dangers of long term corticosteroid therapy, incorrectly equating systemic with inhaled treatment, and despite the unchallengable evidence of the safety of these agents over many years of continued use (p.181,201).

Even more alarming is the finding of Ormerod and Stableforth in 1980 and Wilson et al., (1981) that the majority of patients dying of their disease were not receiving corticosteroids during their final attack. One of the definitive conclusions of the 1960s epidemic of fatal asthma was that under-use of corticosteroids was a major predisposing factor.

In Conclusion

In the light of the continuing morbidity of asthma, usually from underdiagnosis and undertreatment, and of too frequent asthma fatalities, there is a compelling case for the much wider use of antiasthma drugs. The contribution that corticosteroids, especially their prophylactic use by inhalation, can make is not yet fully appreciated or employed.

References

Ahlquist, R.P.: A study of the adrenotropic receptors. American Journal of Physiology 153: 586 (1948).

Anderson, H.R.; Bailey, P. and West, S.: Trends in the hospital care of acute childhood asthma 1970-8: a regional study. British Medical Journal 281: 1191 (1980).

Anderson, H.R.; Bailey, P.A.; Cooper, J.S. and Palmer, J.C.: Influence of morbidity, illness label, and social, family, and health service factors on drug treatment of childhood asthma. Lancet 2: 1030 (1981).

Arnold, A.G.; Lane, D.J. and Zapata, E.: The speed of onset and severity of acute severe asthma. British Journal of Diseases of the Chest 76: 157 (1982).

Blair, H.: Natural history of childhood asthma. Archives of Disease in Childhood 52: 613 (1977).

British Thoracic Association: Death from asthma in two regions of England. British Medical Journal 285: 1251 (1982).

Collins, J.V.; Clark, T.J.M.; Braru, D. and Townsend, J.: The use of corticosteroids in the treatment of acute asthma. Quarterly Journal of Medicine 44: 259 (1975).

Crompton, G.K.: Problems patients have using pressurized aerosol inhalers. European Journal of Respiratory Diseases 63 (Suppl. 119): 101 (1982).

Crompton, G.K.; Grant, I.W.B. and Bloomfield, P.: Edinburgh Emergency Asthma Admission Service: a report on 10 years' experience. British Medical Journal 2: 1199 (1979).

Dodge, R.R. and Burrows, B.: The prevalence and incidence of asthma and asthma-like symptoms in a general population sample. American Review of Respiratory Disease 122: 567 (1980).

Editorial: Fatal asthma. Lancet 2: 337 (1979).

Empey, D.W.; Laitene, L.A.; Jacobs, L.; Gold, W.M. and Nadel, J.A.: Mechanisms of bronchial hyperreactivity in normal subjects after upper respiratory tract infections. American Review of Respiratory Disease 113: 131 (1976).

Fraser, P.M.; Speizer, F.E.; Waters, S.D.M.; Doll, R. and Mann, M.W.: The circumstances preceding death from asthma in young people in 1968-1969. British Journal of Diseases of the Chest 65: 71 (1971).

Godfrey, R.C.: Asthma and IgE levels in rural and urban communities of the Gambia. Clinical Allergy 5: 201 (1975).

Grant, I.W.B.: Are corticosteroids necessary in the treatment of severe acute asthma? British Journal of Diseases of the Chest 76: 125 (1982).

Greening, A.P.: Bronchoalveolar lavage. British Medical Journal 284: 1896 (1982).

Gregg, I.: Epidemiology in asthma; in Clark and Godfrey (Eds) Asthma, p. 214 (Chapman and Hart, London 1977).

Hersch, M.R.; Clark, T.J.H. and Branthwaite, M.A.: Asthma analysis of sudden deaths and ventilatory arrests in hospital. British Medical Journal 1: 808 (1977).

Jackson, R.T.; Beaglehole, R.; Rea, H.H. and Sutherland, D.C.: Asthma mortality: A new epidemic in New Zealand. British Medical Journal 285: 771 (1982).

Lichtenstein, L.M.: An evaluation of the role of immunotherapy in asthma. American Review of Respiratory Diseases 117: 191 (1978).

Martin, A.J.; McLennan, L.; Landau, L.I. and Phelan, P.D.: The natural history of childhood asthma to adult life. British Medical Journal 28: 1397 (1980).

Martin, A.J.; Landau, L.I. and Phelan, P.D.: Asthma from childhood at age 21: the patient and his disease. British Medical Journal 284: 380 (1982).

Macdonald, J.B.; Seaton, A. and Williams, D.A.: Asthma deaths in Cardiff 1963-74: 90 deaths outside hospital. British Medical Journal 1: 1493 (1976).

McNicol, K.N. and Williams, H.B.: Spectrum of asthma in children. 1 Clinical and physiological components. British Medical Journal 4: (1973).

McQueen, F.; Holdaway, M.D. and Sears, M.R.: A study of asthma in a Dunedin suburban area. New Zealand Medical Journal 89: 335 (1979).

Ormerod, L.P. and Stableforth, D.E.: Asthma mortality in Birmingham 1975-7: 53 Deaths. British Medical Journal 1: 687 (1980).

Rackemann, F.M. and Edwards, M.C.: Asthma in children: a follow-up study of 688 patients after an interval of 20 years. New England Journal of Medicine 246: 815 (1952).

Scadding, J.G.: Definition and clinical categories of asthma; in Clark and Godfrey (Eds) Asthma, p.1 (Chapman and Hall, London, 1977).

Sears, M.R.; Jones, D.T.; Silva, P.A.; Simpson, A. and Williams, S.M.: Asthma in seven year old children: a report from the Dunedin Multi-disciplinary Child Development Study. New Zealand Medical Journal 95: 533 (1982).

Speight, A.N.P.: Is childhood asthma being underdiagnosed and undertreated? British Medical Journal 2: 331 (1978).

Speizer, F.E.: Epidemiological aspects of asthma. Triangle 17: 117 (1978).

Speizer, F.E.; Doll, R.; Heaf, P. and Strang, L.B.: Investigations into use of drugs preceding death from asthma. British Medical Journal 1: 339 (1968).

Stanhope, J.M.; Rees, R.O. and Mangan, A.J.: Asthma and wheeze in New Zealand adolescents. New Zealand Medical Journal 90: 279 (1979).

Stellman, J.L.; Spicer, J.E. and Cayton, R.M.: Morbidity from chronic asthma. Thorax 37: 218 (1982).

Stolley, P.D. and Schinner, R.: Association between asthma mortality and isoproterenol aerosols: a review. Preventive Medicine 7: 519 (1978).

Sutherland, D.C. and Wilson, J.D.: Theophylline, beta-agonists and fatal asthma. Lancet 2: 988 (1981).

Waite, D.A.; Eyles, E.F.; Tonkin, S.L. and O'Donnell, T.U.: Asthma prevalence in Tokelauan children in two environments. Clinical Allergy 10: 71 (1980).

Webber, B.A.; Collins, J.V. and Branthwaite, M.A.: Severe acute asthma: a comparison of three methods of inhaling salbutamol. British Journal of Diseases of the Chest 76: (1982).

Wilson, J.D.; Sutherland, D.C. and Thomas, A.C.: Has the change to beta-agonists combined with oral theophylline increased cases of fatal asthma? Lancet 1: 1235 (1981).

Chapter II

Pathophysiology and Clinical Correlates of Asthma

G. J. Gibson

To the pathologist the term 'asthma' conveys a picture of more or less specific structural abnormalities in the bronchial lumen and wall. On the other hand the physiologist may have a more general concept of 'variable airways obstruction'; he may also wish to include 'bronchial hyper-reactivity' in his definition and some would wish this to be formally demonstrated before the label 'asthma' is attached to an individual patient. To the experienced clinician the diagnosis is often straightforward; he may well subscribe to the standard functional definition – but he will also use other information such as age of onset, pattern of symptoms, the presence of commonly associated conditions such as rhinitis, the presence of sputum or blood eosinophilia, positive skin tests etc., to support his diagnosis in an individual patient. Reconciling these viewpoints is not difficult in the typical young patient with episodic wheezing and easily demonstrable variable airflow obstruction, but in many patients the diagnosis is not so easy, the distinction between 'asthma' and 'chronic obstructive airway (lung) disease' may be blurred and sometimes variability of airway narrowing may only become apparent when treatment appropriate for asthma is given to a patient with apparently 'irreversible' airways obstruction.

The definition of asthma has occupied the attention of many eminent committees but the results have generally been less than satisfactory. No single figure can be put on the amount of variability necessary to sustain the diagnosis – a patient whose FEV_1 rises from 1.5L to 2.5L after being given a bronchodilator clearly has asthma, but what of a patient whose FEV_1 improves by a similar proportional amount from 0.3 to 0.5L? The emphasis is rightly on 'variability' rather than 'reversibility' of airways obstruction. Complete reversibility is probably rare and the majority of asthmatic subjects in clinical remission have some functional abnormality; the more sensitive the test applied, the more often such abnormalities are found. On the other hand completely 'irreversible' airways obstruction is also rare and the great majority of patients with 'chronic obstructive airways disease' show a meas-

---

Glossary

D_LC0	Diffusing capacity of carbon monoxide
FEV_1	Forced expiratory volume in 1 second
FRC	Functional residual capacity
PEF	Peak expiratory flow
PV	Pressure-volume
TLC	Total lung capacity
V_A	Alveolar volume
VC	Vital capacity
$\dot{V}/\dot{Q}$:	Ventilation: perfusion

ureable small improvement after a bronchodilator. 'Variable' and 'persistent' airflow obstruction are therefore preferable to 'reversible' and 'irreversible'. Whether the more 'variable' and the more 'persistent' groups of patients form two distinct populations or represent a continuous distribution is a matter of considerable doubt; also many patients with a past history of typical asthma develop severe persistent airflow obstruction after many years. Whether this can be prevented by more aggressive treatment to iron out the variability in the early stages remains a major unanswered question.

Morbid Anatomy

There are four main sources of information on the pathological changes in the lungs in asthma. First, and most obviously, data from patients who die with asthma, secondly autopsy information from patients who happen to be asthmatic but who die of other causes, thirdly bronchial biopsies in asthmatics in remission and fourthly experimental models of asthma in animals.

Autopsy Findings in Asthma Deaths

The findings at autopsy in patients who have died of severe asthma are well known (Dunnill, 1971): to the naked eye the lungs appear over-distended and they fail to deflate when the chest is opened; the cut surface shows characteristic 'mucous plugs' occluding medium sized airways (fig. 2.1).

The plugs are grey in colour, glistening and very tenacious and it requires little imagination to realise their implications for

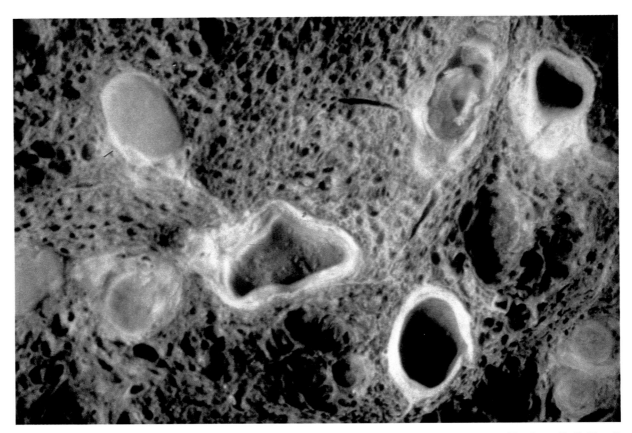

Fig. 2.1. Mucous plugging of several airways in the lung of a patient who died of asthma. (By courtesy of Professor B. E. Heard).

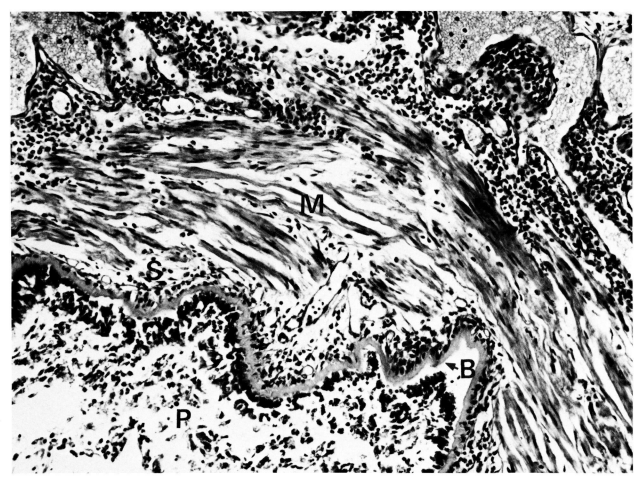

Fig. 2.2. Postmortem bronchus from a case of severe asthma. The lumen contains a mucous plug (P) mixed with eosinophils and desquamated epithelium. There is pronounced muscle hypertrophy and hyperplasia of the smooth muscle (M). The submucosa (S) is infiltrated by inflammatory cells, most of which are eosinophils. The basement membrane (B) is thickened. H & E x 48. (By courtesy of Dr. T. Ashcroft).

pulmonary gas exchange or to understand the failure of bronchodilator drugs to achieve the desired therapeutic effect in such lungs. The plugs are composed of cells (epithelial cells and eosinophils), mucous and serous elements, the last probably resulting from exudation through an abnormally permeable inflamed epithelium. The contents of the plugs correspond to those of expectorated Curschmann spirals, Creola bodies (clusters of epithelial cells) and Charcot-Leyden crystals (derived from eosinophils). Effective clearance of the plugs is inhibited not only by their tenacity, but also in many cases by damage to, or actual shedding of, the bronchial epithelium which grossly interferes with the normal clearance mechanisms of ciliary action. Histologically, segments of the mucosa may appear completely denuded with areas of regeneration, oedema may be prominent and submucosal inflammation severe, with an infiltrate in which eosinophils are abundant (fig. 2.2). Other noteworthy features are apparent thickening of the basement membrane of the bronchial epithelium, hypertrophy of the mucous glands and hypertrophy of bronchial smooth muscle. The increase in smooth muscle appears to be relatively specific for asthma and patients dying of 'chronic bronchitis' with no asthmatic features show little or no increase.

Findings in Non-asthma
Deaths and on Biopsy

Patients who have died of asthma comprise the ultimate selected group and the relevance of these autopsy findings to everyday asthma may therefore be questionable. But a similar bronchial exudate is found in the lungs of asthmatic patients in apparent remission who die of other causes and oedema and narrowing of large bronchi can be readily demonstrated bronchoscopically *in vivo* during acute bronchial challenge. Similar histological changes, but of lesser degree, are also recognisable in biopsy specimens and a regular finding is the deposition of fibrillar collagen immediately beneath the true basement membrane. The significance of this is uncertain.

Animal Models of Asthma

Models of asthma have been developed in experimental animals, particularly to study immunological mechanisms. The animals are naturally or artificially sensitised to specific antigens to which they are subsequently exposed by inhalation. Antigen-antibody interaction on the surface of mast cells stimulates release of the mediators of the asthmatic attack. Most of the bronchial mast cells are, however, not on the mucosal surface but in the submucosa adjacent to blood vessels and neural ganglia; it has been suggested that the antigen binds to the small proportion of sensitised mast cells in the bronchial lumen or on the surface and then their access to submucosal mast cells is enhanced by increased permeability of the epithelium, with loosening of the normal 'tight junctions' between cells so that the reaction is amplified (Hogg, 1978). None of the animal models of asthma is ideal and, although the pattern of response may resemble acute allergen challenge in atopic asthmatics, it may have little relevance to clinical asthma, since patients with 'intrinsic' asthma have no demonstrable immunological sensitivity and 'extrinsic' asthmatics respond not only to specific allergens but also to nonspecific stimuli.

Bronchial Hyper-reactivity

Both physiologists and clinicians agree that a feature common (and perhaps fundamental) to patients with asthma is an increased reactivity of the airways to a variety of nonspecific stimuli. This hyper-reactivity may be demonstrated using chemical agents which mimic the effects of the parasympathetic nervous system (methacholine), substances which are released naturally from mast cells (histamine) or exogenous irritants (sulphur dioxide, citric acid); similar effects are also produced by cooling and drying of the bronchial epithelium by breathing cold dry air at rest or on exercise. The clinical correlates of this nonspecific bronchial hyper-reactivity include the common symptoms of wheezing after exercise, on going outdoors in cold weather or on exposure to irritant particulate matter such as tobacco smoke. The physiologist sees the same phenomenon in asthmatic patients whose FEV_1 declines with repeated measurements and in whom forced expiratory manoeuvres provoke coughing.

Underlying Mechanisms

The underlying mechanism remains uncertain (Boushey et al., 1980). Among the hypotheses are an abnormality of the bronchial smooth muscle itself, abnormal autonomic neural control of the airways and increased permeability of, or damage to, the bronchial epithelium.

An Anatomical Hypothesis

The increased bulk of smooth muscle in asthmatic airways has already been alluded to: this may be an important fundamental abnormality or may act as an amplifier of other mechanisms of bronchial hyper-reactivity, since a more powerful contraction in response to a given stimulus would account for many of the observations. Studies of the physiology of asthmatic bronchial smooth muscle are only in their infancy but they offer interesting prospects for unravelling the nature of the hyper-reactive airway.

An Adrenergic Hypothesis

The autonomic control of airway calibre has been more fully studied, but many questions remain unanswered. Bronchial hyper-reactivity has been attributed to disorders of the cholinergic or adrenergic systems and the more recently discovered purinergic system is a third candidate. Bronchial smooth muscle tone in both normal and asthmatic subjects is importantly influenced by the activity of the parasympathetic nervous system; the vagus nerve carries both efferent stimuli to the muscle and afferent information from sensory irritant receptors in the airways, whose stimulation provokes bronchoconstriction via a reflex arc. Bronchial smooth muscle also has adrenoceptors; α-receptors, which are constrictor, are few and of doubtful significance – hence the very weak therapeutic effect of α-blocking drugs; β-receptors, which are dilator, are much more important. They are stimulated naturally by circulating catecholamines and their discovery has been of great benefit to patients with asthma, and to pharmaceutical industrial research as a target for drugs. Despite the presence of adrenoceptors, there is no good evidence for a direct adrenergic nerve supply to human bronchial smooth muscle. The sympathetic nerves in the airways are distributed mainly to small vessels and also to autonomic ganglia where their activity may modulate the degree of parasympathetic tone. In the normal subject both β-sympathomimetic drugs and parasympathetic antagonists produce measurable bronchodilatation. Presumably both act by antagonising a small degree of resting parasympathetic tone. In unstressed normal subjects there is no significant adrenergic tone and β-blocking drugs have no effect. Under the influence of stress, however, a bronchoconstrictor effect may appear, presumably resulting from antagonism of the effects of catecholamines. Szentivanyi (1968) suggested that a state of partial β-blockade may underlie the asthmatic state. There is evidence from various tissues that adrenoceptor function in asthmatic patients may be abnormal with reduced responses of β-receptors and increased α-effects. In many cases this may have resulted from therapy with β-agonist drugs and it has proved remarkably difficult to demonstrate a reduced response of *bronchial* β-receptors in asthma. The failure of a therapeutic effect in severe asthma is more likely to be due to mechanical factors (as illustrated in figure 2.1) than to impaired sensitivity of β-receptors. A telling piece of evidence against Szentivanyi's hypothesis is that treatment with a β-blocking drug does not make normal subjects asthmatic. Also if a state of natural partial β-blockade already existed in asthmatic subjects it would be unlikely that introduction of an exogenous β-blocker would have a large effect – yet the greatly increased sensitivity of asthmatic patients to β-blockers is well known and suggests that their bronchial β-receptors normally maintain a high level of activity.

A Cholinergic Hypothesis

If not the adrenergic system, then is the cholinergic system at fault? A popular hypothesis to account for bronchial hyper-reactivity invokes increased activity of the parasympathetic nervous system, possibly by a reflex initiated by stimulation of vagally innervated irritant receptors. Important supporting evidence comes from the state of bronchial hyper-reactivity which occurs in normal subjects after viral bronchial infections or which can be induced by exposure to various noxious gases such as ozone, nitrogen dioxide and sulphur dioxide or to some agents incriminated as causes of occupational asthma. These effects are largely abolished by anticholinergic drugs (atropine or ipratropium) and are probably a result of sensitisation or greater exposure of irritant receptors consequent on epithelial damage. This form of bronchial hyper-reactivity does not necessarily have the same mechanism as the hyper-reactivity of asthma since it is less intense and more transient and presumably is not associated with the smooth muscle hypertrophy which characterises asthma.

The effects of cholinergic blockade in asthma are variable. In acute challenge with antigen both in sensitised dogs and in allergic asthmatic patients some studies have shown complete inhibition while others have shown either no protection or only an effect compatible with the degree of bronchodilatation produced. The evidence on the mechanism of histamine provocation is also conflicting: histamine has a direct constrictor effect on smooth muscle but also is known to stimulate irritant receptors and may have an indirect effect via a cholinergic reflex. A final verdict on the role of the parasympathetic nervous system is not possible – it seems likely to be relevant to the transient acquired hyper-reactivity of normal subjects described above and probably to some patients with asthma but whether it represents a major fundamental abnormality responsible for clinical asthma remains uncertain.

Other Hypotheses

Intriguing prospects have been opened up by the description (Richardson and Beland, 1976) of the non-adrenergic inhibitory or 'purinergic' nerve supply to the airways. Abnormalities of similar nerves in the embryologically related gastrointestinal tract have been associated with defective smooth muscle function in Hirschsprung's disease – but whether similar nerves supplying the bronchi may be relevant to asthma remains to be determined.

Another potential contributor to bronchial hyper-reactivity in asthma is an abnormal permeability of the bronchial epithelium, allowing greater access of noxious agents to irritant receptors or to the smooth muscle itself. In the acquired transient form of hyper-reactivity, such as after viral infections, this mechanism seems likely to be important and is supported by the pathological evidence in severe asthma. In asthma in remission, however, the evidence is not convincing; increased epithelial permeability cannot be the sole determinant of hyper-reactivity as it is demonstrable with agents such as histamine when given by the intravenous route as well as by inhalation.

Tests of Bronchial Reactivity

A major problem which in practice confounds the interpretation of tests of bronchial reactivity, is the level of baseline pre-challenge airway function. If we were simply measuring the length of a strip of smooth muscle, the assessment of its response would be simple. But, because of the normal stimulus-response relationship, the magnitude of that response would depend on the resting muscle fibre length (fig. 2.3). The resistance of an airway bears an inverse fourth power relationship to its diameter, so that as the airway narrows a progressively greater change in resistance is expected for a given change in muscle length (which is directly proportional to diameter – fig. 2.3). For both of these reasons an apparently greater bronchial reactivity would *a priori* be expected for the same stimulus if the subject started with increased smooth muscle tone and therefore with an abnormally high airways resistance. The overall airways resistance represents a complex sum of the resistances of individual airways arranged both in series and in parallel, and how much more complex interpretation becomes when the index of airway calibre is not the 'pure' measurement of resistance but the FEV_1. This is easier to perform (and indeed may give more clinically relevant information) but it does not bear a simple quantitative relationship to airway dimensions. Perhaps with all these theoretical objections it is surprising that simple tests of bronchial reactivity convey any useful information. With cautious interpretation, however, much can be learned.

Chemical Challenge

Of the chemical stimuli used to assess bronchial reactivity, histamine and methacholine are the most commonly used; the former has the advantage of rapid metabolism so that graded increasing doses may be given in quick succession. To assess the response either the airways resistance measured plethysmographically or the FEV_1 may be used; the former avoids the potential problem that a full inspiration may itself affect the degree of bronchoconstriction, but in practice FEV_1 is suitable for most purposes. The most popular index of bronchial reactivity is the PC_{20}, the concentration of histamine which provokes a fall in FEV_1 of 20% below the control level (Cockcroft et al., 1977). [If specific airways conductance is measured a larger proportional fall such as 35 or 40% may be used as the end point.] Two main techniques of inhaling the solution of histamine acid phosphate have been proposed – either 2 minutes of tidal breathing via a nebuliser (Cockcroft et al., 1977) or 5 full inspirations from a specially designed dosimeter (Chai et al., 1975) but they give similar values for PC_{20} (Ryan et al., 1981).

The theoretical reasons already considered suggest that the more severe the airways obstruction, the lower the PC_{20} will be and the consensus of studies in patients with established airways obstruction indicates this is the case. In comparing the results of repeat tests in an individual it is therefore essential to check that the pre-challenge level of airway function is similar on the different occasions. For the clinical diagnosis of asthma the most useful discriminatory role of nonspecific inhalation challenge is in the patient with relatively normal pre-challenge function.

The level of reactivity in asthmatic patients may vary from time to time with the level of persisting airway narrowing, but it has also been shown in allergic patients that following allergen exposure there may be an increased nonspecific reactivity, demonstrated by histamine or methacholine challenge, which persists for hours or days with little or no difference in baseline airway function (Cockcroft et al., 1977). This may underlie the well recognised prolonged or recurrent asthmatic attacks which sometimes follow 'late' asthmatic responses and may be of particular relevance to certain types of occupational asthma.

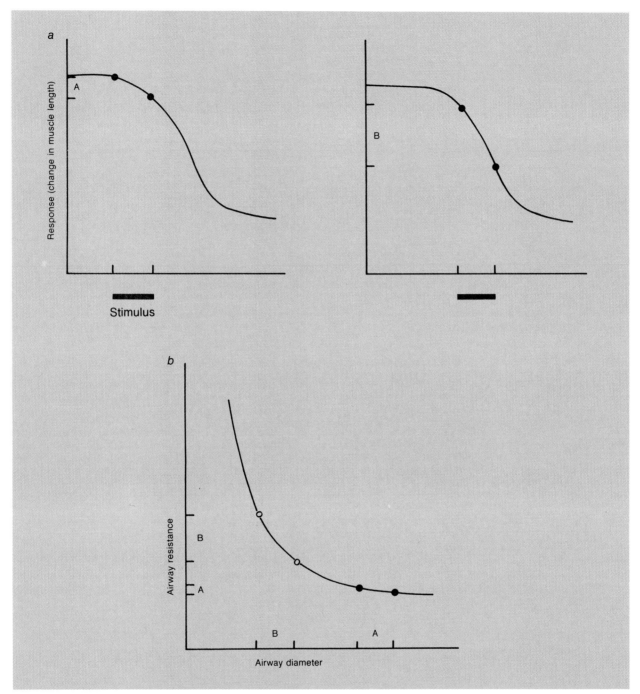

Fig. 2.3. Possible effects of geometrical factors on indices of bronchial reactivity. *a)* Schematic stimulus-response relationship of bronchial smooth muscle: at normal resting muscle length (left hand diagram) a given stimulus produces a small response, A, but if the muscle is already partly contracted (right hand diagram) the same stimulus produces a much larger response, B, because of the shape of the stimulus-response curve (after Benson [1975]). *b)* Relationship between airway diameter (i.e. a function of muscle length) and resistance: when resting airway dimensions are normal and resistance is low, a given reduction in diameter A, produces a much smaller increase in airways resistance than if the airway is already narrowed before the stimulus is applied, B.

Exercise Challenge

The other form of challenge test popular for identifying and sometimes assessing treatment of asthma is exercise. The elegant studies of McFadden and colleagues (Strauss et al., 1978) on respiratory heat exchange during exercise have demonstrated that a stimulus to the development of exercise induced asthma (EIA) is cooling and drying of the airway mucosa as inspired air is warmed and humidified. This is a further manifestation of bronchial hyper-reactivity: in normal subjects exercise does not provoke broncho-constriction although it may be demonstrated with much greater degrees of respiratory heat exchange during hyperventilation of sub-freezing air. These studies have added to our knowledge of the stimulus to asthma following exercise without further elucidating the exact mechanism of bronchial hyper-reactivity. The findings are also consistent with certain features which patients themselves often recognise, for example the adverse effects of exercise at cold ambient temperature and the relative freedom from attacks in the warm humid atmosphere of the swimming pool. Most studies of exercise-induced asthma have concentrated on asthmatic children, for the simple reason that a high proportion of the maximum oxygen uptake is necessary to provoke a reaction and most unfit adult asthmatics are incapable of maintaining the necessary work rate. A period of 6 to 8 minutes at about 75% of capacity is optimal and this implies a heart rate in young subjects exceeding 160 beats per minute (Anderson et al., 1975). Characteristically during exercise there is slight bronchodilatation but then within 5 or 10 minutes of ceasing exercise, progressive bronchoconstriction develops, with a nadir of airway function 10 to 20 minutes after exercise and progressive improvement thereafter. A refractory period of about 2 hours follows, during which the bronchoconstrictor response of a further exercise test is attenuated or abolished. If the first period of exercise can be maintained for longer than 6 to 8 minutes, no significant airway narrowing may be demonstrable and many asthmatics recognise their ability to 'run through' attacks in this way or to avoid EIA by a 'warm up' period of exercise. It has been suggested that the refractory period is consistent with exhaustion and resynthesis of bronchoconstrictor mediators but the evidence for release of mediators during exercise induced asthma is controversial and the fact that a similar refractory period does not occur after asthma due to hyperventilation of cold air is evidence against this mechanism. An alternative explanation for the protective effect of exercise against further EIA is a build-up of circulating catecholamines. Pretreatment with bronchodilator drugs or cromoglycate attenuates or prevents EIA. Single pre-exercise exposures to oral or inhaled steroids have no effect but with more prolonged administration as maintenance treatment there may be some diminution of the response to exercise, perhaps reflecting better overall symptomatic control (p.201).

The discovery of the stimulus causing EIA has led to the development of alternative challenge techniques during isocapnic hyperventilation at rest of inspired air which is dry and cold. These have the advantage of greater applicability to the asthmatic population as a whole, since they can also be used in patients unable to perform the exercise necessary to provoke asthma.

Mechanical Function of the Lungs

Lung Volumes

Asthma is primarily a disease of the airways but changes are also seen in the mechanical behaviour of the lungs. The total lung capacity (TLC) measured by plethysmography is usually greater than normal in asthmatic patients with significant airflow obstruction but, as with other causes of airway narrowing, it may be markedly underestimated by the inert gas dilution technique. On the other hand there is some evidence that the plethysmographic method may overestimate TLC during an attack. The large increases, which may be measured acutely, seem unlikely to be all artefactual and in some cases the change in TLC is also clearly demonstrable by radiography. As in other forms of airflow obstruction the vital capacity (VC) is often decreased, depending on the degree of airway narrowing, and residual volume is correspondingly high. Functional residual capacity (FRC) is also characteristically increased.

Lung Distensibility

Alterations in the pressure-volume (PV) curve of the lungs are such that at any absolute lung volume, the recoil pressure of the lungs is less than normal (fig. 2.4). The mechanism is not clear but similar changes have been demonstrated acutely in dogs breathing through an artificial resistance. Unlike in emphysema, the static compliance of the lungs is not increased compared to normal but the shift of the PV curve implies that the compliance is measured over a tidal breathing range well above normal volumes (fig. 2.4). The rise in FRC may be thought of as a useful adaptation to compensate for the loss of elastic lung recoil and for the airway narrowing, since lung recoil pressure is an important determinant of airway calibre and it increases as lung volume increases. The

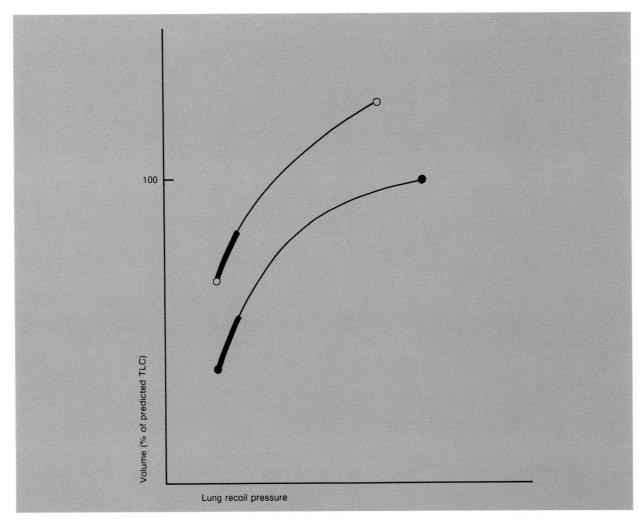

Fig. 2.4. Static expiratory pressure volume curves plotted between TLC and FRC for a normal subject (solid circles) and a patient with asthma (open circles). Note that TLC is above normal in the asthmatic and lung recoil pressure is less than normal but the static compliance measured over the approximate tidal breathing range (thickened lines) is similar in the two subjects.

position of FRC is not, however, determined solely by the lungs, but also by the passive elastic properties of the chest wall. TLC also is dependent on the function of both the lungs and chest wall – it is normally determined by a balance between the recoil of the respiratory system and the power of the inspiratory muscles. The considerable abnormalities of both of these volumes in many patients with asthma therefore imply major changes also in the passive and active mechanical performance of the chest wall and its muscles, which seem capable of accommodating rapidly to a varying severity of airflow obstruction.

Airway Narrowing

The reduction of lung recoil pressure probably makes some contribution to the abnormally high airways resistance and low maximum flow in asthma, but undoubtedly the major factor is structural narrowing of individual airways or loss of parallel airways by complete occlusion of some. The relative roles of smooth muscle contraction, oedema and airway secretions are usually impossible to quantitate. Tests of airway function show only the characteristic pattern of diffuse intrathoracic airways obstruction with no specific features other than variability. Thus maximum expiratory flows (including peak flow), are reduced more than maximum inspiratory flows, the FEV_1/VC ratio is reduced, airways conductance is low and resistance correspondingly high. In relation to lung recoil pressure, maximum flow and airways conductance are reduced implying 'intrinsic' narrowing of the airways rather than loss of support by surrounding lung as the major mechanism of reduction of airflow.

Relation of Airflow to Lung Volume

The limitations imposed by airway narrowing are graphically represented by the maximum flow volume curve, a refinement of simple spirometry which relates flow to volume rather than volume to time (fig. 2.5). As asthma worsens, maximum flows fall and, as discussed above, lung volumes usually increase; this implies that the inspiratory muscles are working at progressively higher lung volumes where their mechanical advantage becomes less. At these increased volumes the lung may become less compliant, so that the inspiratory muscles expend more energy in overcoming elastic forces. Gradual attenuation of the 'available' expiratory flow reserve leads to the situation where maximum expiratory flow is developed at rest and the patient is breathing 'on the maximum flow volume curve' (fig. 2.5). The only courses then available if alveolar ventilation is becoming compromised are to increase the frequency of breathing or to increase FRC further. Both impose additional demands on the *inspiratory* muscles, even though the obstruction to airflow is predominantly *expiratory*. It is therefore not surprising that many patients find greater discomfort during breathing in than when breathing out. The limitations to maximum flow also emphasise the mechanical constraints on the breathing pattern: because of the very poor expiratory flows which can be generated low in the vital capacity (fig. 2.5), encouraging such patients to prolong expiration further is a fruitless exercise and the most mechanically efficient breathing pattern to adopt is one with rapid frequency and relatively small tidal volume. This is, however, not efficient in terms of gas exchange because each breath has to flush out an irreducible dead space and therefore a relatively greater proportion of the total ventilation is wasted on

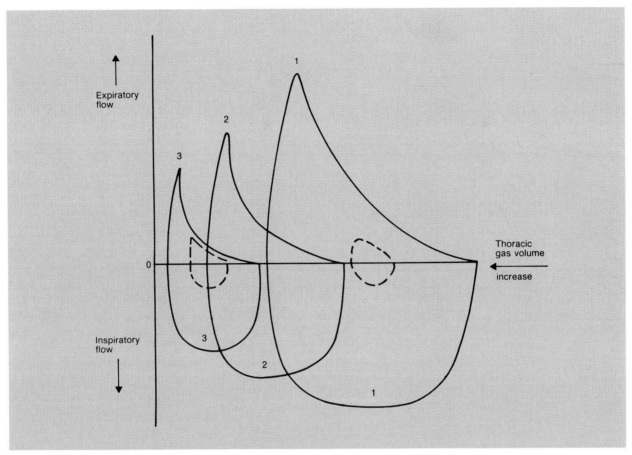

Fig. 2.5. Schematic maximum flow volume curves (solid lines) as asthma worsens. The abscissa records absolute thoracic gas volume to take account of the increasing TLC as asthma worsens. With mild airways obstruction (curve 1) the flows during a tidal breath (broken lines) are much less than the maximum achievable at the same lung volume. As airways obstruction worsens all maximum flows are reduced and in the most severe situation illustrated (curve 3) maximum flow is developed during tidal expiration.

dead space. The main obstruction to airflow is expiratory because dynamic airway narrowing during expiration exacerbates the structural abnormalities. During inspiration the negative extra bronchial intrathoracic pressure acts to maintain airway patency, but structural narrowing is still present so maximum inspiratory flow is also reduced, albeit much less severely impaired than expiratory flow. In severe asthma the clearly visible exhaustion of the patient is accompanied by physiologically demonstrable fatigue of the respiratory muscles. Once this develops the compensatory mechanisms may break down and ventilatory failure rapidly ensues.

Relationship of Symptoms to Narrowing

The approximate relationships between symptoms and the severity of airway narrowing is illustrated in figure 2.6. Most severe attacks of asthma do not develop 'out of the blue' but against a background of poor control and unstable airway function. The level of airway narrowing at which symptoms are noticeable depends very much on the patient's psyche, expectations and level of activity and also on the degree of variability and rapidity with which asthma develops. There may be a world of difference between the 'chronic asthmatic' well adjusted to an FEV_1 of 1.5L and the patient whose usual airway function is close to normal but who becomes markedly distressed in an attack when his FEV_1 falls from say 4L to 1.5L. The presence or absence of wheezing is a notoriously unreliable guide to the severity of airways obstruction – very wheezy asthmatics sometimes have surprisingly good function and, on the other hand, the 'silent' chest in a severe attack has an ominous reputation. There is no substitute for attempting a measurement of airway function and even in severe asthma most patients can produce a valid FEV_1. If this proves impossible other physical signs such as the ability to talk or the heart rate are more reliable as guides to severity than are the presence, quality or intensity of wheezes (see p.37).

Site of Airway Obstruction

In an established asthmatic attack there is generalised narrowing of intrathoracic airways and all indices of airway function are abnormal. In milder asthma the predominant site of narrowing

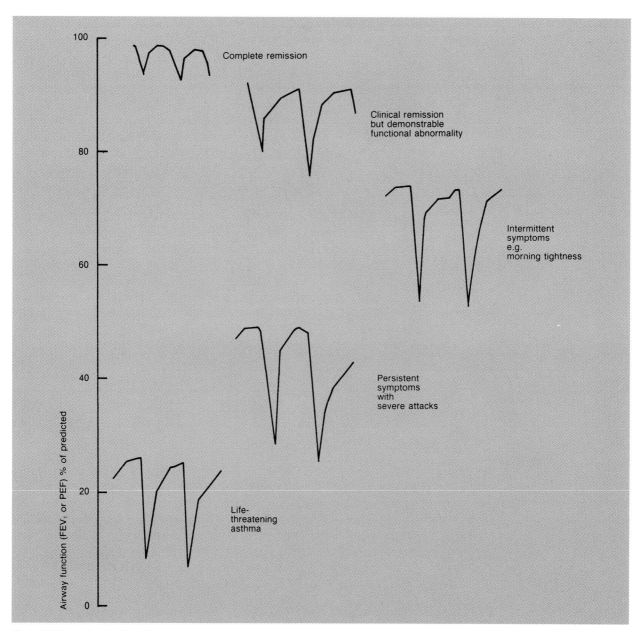

Fig. 2.6. Schematic relationship between degree of airways obstruction and clinical features. Patients admitted to hospital with severe asthma usually have values for FEV_1 or PEF less than 20% of predicted.

may vary between individuals. Probably the majority of asthmatics in clinical remission have abnormal function even when simple measurements such as FEV_1 and PEF are within normal limits. The demonstration of these abnormalities may require more subtle tests which reflect changes in the smaller airways – perhaps small mucous plugs, as the few relevant pathological studies would suggest. When the effects of an acute antigen challenge are directly observed bronchoscopically, narrowing of much larger airways is easily seen and the changes are then probably diffuse. Attempts have been made to locate the main site of airway narrowing by comparing maximum flow volume curves breathing air and a mixture of helium and oxygen. Helium, which has a low density, increases flow when it is predominantly turbulent and hence dependent on gas density. Helium would therefore be expected to increase maximum flow if the site of flow limitation were in larger airways. By this means it has been possible to show that in some patients it is predominantly the larger airways which determine maximum flow but in others the site of limitation is more peripheral (Antic and Macklem, 1976). This conclusion cannot, however, necessarily be translated into the exact site of airway narrowing: a major effect of increased narrowing of the smaller airways is to make the central airways more susceptible to dynamic forces, so that the sites of maximum bronchoconstriction and of flow limitation are not necessarily the same. It has recently been suggested that a part of the airway more proximal still, i.e. larynx and trachea, may be an important site of narrowing in some patients (Lisboa et al., 1980). Location of the major site of narrowing in individual patients might be clinically relevant if different drugs had their main effects at different sites in the airway but there is no evidence that this is so in asthma.

Variability of Airway Function

The hallmark of asthmatic airway narrowing is its variability. In many patients this may be apparent as a large improvement in FEV_1 or PEF after a single dose of a bronchodilator aerosol. Such a response is diagnostic, but failure to demonstrate it should not be taken as evidence against asthma. A small response may be seen either because the asthma is 'too good' i.e. function is virtually normal, or 'too bad' where for mechanical, or other reasons, the drug does not adequately penetrate the bronchial tree or cannot induce a response. It is usually between these extremes that the largest responses can be demonstrated (fig. 2.7). Nonetheless, even if the pre-bronchodilator function is within normal limits, patients with a history of asthma may be distinguished by larger than average responses (Lorber et al., 1978). Because of accompanying increases in VC after bronchodilator, reliance should not be placed on the ratio FEV_1/VC (which is extremely valuable for demonstrating the *presence* of airways obstruction) for indicating the magnitude of any *improvement* in airways obstruction. Occasionally the ratio may fall, especially in severe asthma where the VC may be limited by the patient's inability to sustain the expiration and this aspect may improve relatively more after a bronchodilator than does the FEV_1. Occasional patients have been described in whom the FEV_1 and maximum flow rates fell after bronchodilator while a rise in airways conductance (i.e. lower resistance) implied bronchodilatation. Theoretically this would be possible if smooth muscle relaxation rendered the airway less rigid and therefore more susceptible to dynamic expiratory compression i.e. to squeezing by the high intrathoracic pressures developed during a forced expiratory manoeuvre. Since airways conductance is measured at low flow and with minimal effort it more closely reflects the unstressed calibre of the airway. In practice this paradoxical finding is sufficiently rare to be ignored.

As emphasised earlier, it is variability rather than reversibility of airway narrowing which is important and it is here that home monitoring of simple tests such as PEF comes into its own (see Chapter III). In the author's view the FEV_1 is the single most useful and reliable clinical estimate of airway narrowing and should be the measurement of choice in the hospital ward, outpatient clinic or doctor's surgery. The PEF gives less specific information; it is, however, extremely useful in practice to have the patient make regular measurements of PEF at home or at his place of work. It is worth 'calibrating' the PEF against the FEV_1 when both measurements are available to get a better 'feel' for the overall severity of asthma. Not infrequently a patient seen in an outpatient clinic with virtually normal function complains of severe nocturnal or early morning symptoms. It is all too easy to dismiss these symptoms or treat them as left ventricular failure unless measurements are made at the appropriate time. For diagnostic purposes a bronchial challenge test is informative but for the assessment of se-

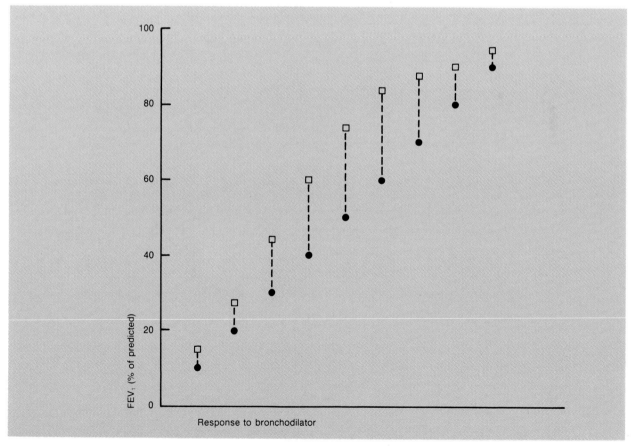

Fig.2.7. Schematic relationship between FEV_1 and acute response to bronchodilator. When airway function is close to normal the increase is likely to be relatively small because of the 'ceiling' effect; similarly small increases are seen with very poor airway function when the obstruction is usually due mainly to inflammatory changes and mucous plugging rather than to bronchoconstriction.

verity there is no substitute for a measurement at the time of symptoms. A peak flow record such as that illustrated in figure 2.8 is diagnostic of asthma and also shows the characteristic 'early morning dip'. Diurnal variation of airway function is seen in normal subjects and that occurring in asthma may be regarded as an exaggeration of the normal, observed more in some patients than others. The exact mechanism is not clear but diurnal rhythms of adrenal cortical and medullary function, slowing of mucociliary clearance during sleep and waning effects of drugs may all play a part.

Prognosis

Once an asthmatic, always an asthmatic? Many children 'grow out' of their troublesome symptoms but admit in later life that colds make them wheeze, they may have persistently abnormal 'sensitive' tests of airway function and may have demonstrably increased bronchial reactivity. By and large those who have the most troublesome asthma in childhood continue to show the most severe symptoms and persistent functional abnormalities in adult life (Martin et al., 1980).

Gas Exchange Function

In the presence of significant generalised airways obstruction the distribution of ventilation is uneven. This may be demonstrated by simple tests of overall function such as following the concentration of expired nitrogen during a slow expiration after a full inspiration of pure oxygen. At a cruder regional level gross

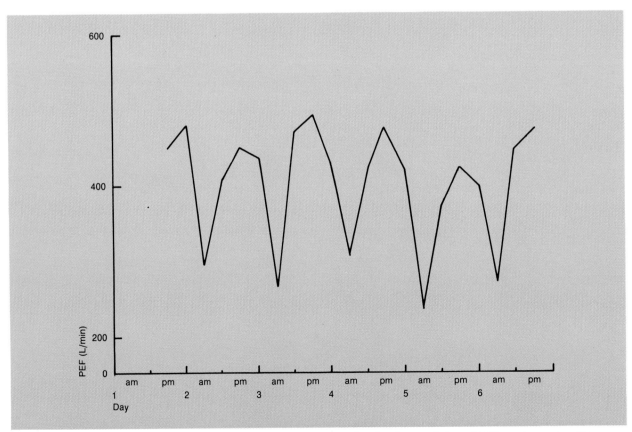

Fig. 2.8. Record of PEF measured 6 hourly in an asthmatic patient, showing the characteristic variability and morning dip.

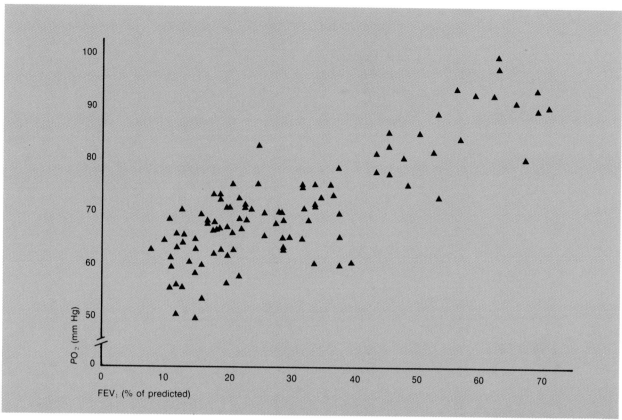

Fig. 2.9. Relation of arterial PO_2 to FEV_1 in 101 patients with asthma studied by McFadden and Lyons (1968). Note that the PaO_2 is usually well preserved (above 60 mmHg) until airflow obstruction is very severe. (Reproduced with the publishers' permission).

irregularities of the distribution of ventilation are visible by radioisotope scanning and the large defects which are seen are accompanied by similar defects of perfusion; the latter is usually attributed to local vasoconstriction stimulated by the reduced local PO_2 resulting from poor regional ventilation. Despite this apparent matching of ventilation and perfusion at a macroscopic level, there is undoubted ventilation/perfusion ($\dot{V}/\dot{Q}$) mismatching in smaller lung units within lung regions. This disturbance of $\dot{V}/\dot{Q}$ matching at a local level has been elegantly demonstrated by the inert gas technique of Wagner and colleagues even in relatively mild asthma (Wagner et al., 1978); it is this 'microscopic' abnormality of gas exchange which is responsible for the development of a widened alveolar-arterial PO_2 difference and a fall in PaO_2. Their study suggested that there may be two populations of alveoli in mild asthma – one with relatively normal gas exchange and the other with a grossly reduced ventilation/perfusion ratio. The effect of the latter is to lower the PaO_2 and they may represent alveoli distal to obstructed small airways which retain very slow ventilation via collateral channels. They are not completely unventilated as the 'anatomical' shunt demonstrable by breathing pure oxygen is not increased in asthma.

By and large the PaO_2 is fairly well maintained until asthma becomes very severe: McFadden and Lyons (1968) studied the arterial blood gases in a large number of patients with asthma of varying severity and showed a clear linear relationship between

PaO_2 and FEV_1 (fig. 2.9). The important message from these data is that even mild degrees of hypoxaemia should be taken seriously, as a PaO_2 below 60mm Hg (8 kPa) i.e. a saturation of haemoglobin with oxygen of 90%, usually implies very severe airways obstruction. The tendency for PaO_2 to fall may be partly compensated by an increased cardiac output so that the mixed venous blood perfusing the lungs is relatively better oxygenated than if the cardiac output were normal. It is easy when dealing with patients with chronic airways obstruction to become blasé about such levels of PaO_2, but the implications in asthma, where the PaO_2 has fallen acutely from normal values are very different from chronic obstructive airways disease, where events happen much more slowly and compensatory adaptations have time to develop (indeed many such patients 'in remission' have values of PaO_2 of 60mm Hg or below). A similar contrast is apparent if values of $PaCO_2$ are compared (fig. 2.10); mild or moderate asthma is typically accompanied by increased ventilation and a low arterial PCO_2. Hypercapnia is an ominous finding and even a normal $PaCO_2$ may indicate that the patient is in transition between the low value of a moderate attack and a high $PaCO_2$ which may herald a fatal attack. Elevation of $PaCO_2$ in this situation essentially reflects suffocation of the patient as eloquently illustrated by the severe mucous plugging found at autopsy (fig. 2.1). Clinically the patient with severe asthma appears increasingly exhausted, becomes unable to

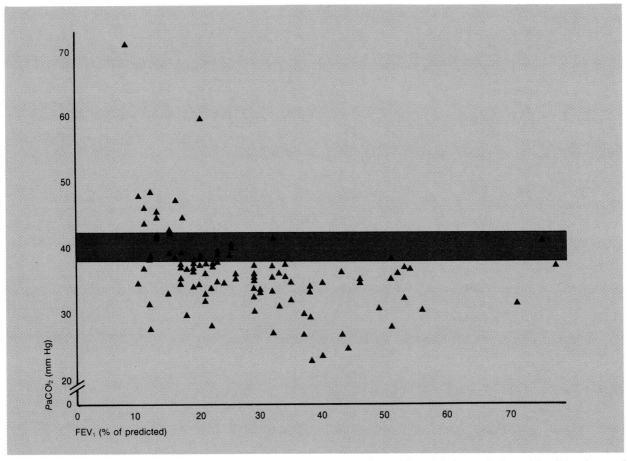

Fig. 2.10. Relation of arterial PCO_2 to FEV_1 in same patients as illustrated in figure 2.9. $PaCO_2$ is usually low with mild asthma and hypercapnia develops only when airflow obstruction is very severe. (Reproduced with the publishers' permission).

speak complete sentences and usually has a pronounced tachycardia; marked pulsus paradoxus may be detectable on palpatation. The total ventilation may remain abnormally high even in the presence of CO_2 retention – but the majority is wasted or 'dead-space' ventilation because of the grossly inefficient gas exchange and the effective or alveolar ventilation becomes progressively less.

A further simple measurement of pulmonary function which is often useful in the assessment of patients with airways obstruction is the diffusing capacity for carbon monoxide (D_LCO). This is rarely measurable in an acute asthmatic attack but it is characteristic of the more stable patient with asthma that the D_LCO measured by the single breath technique is well preserved. In particular CO uptake per litre of ventilated lung (diffusion coefficient, KCO or D_L/V_A) provides a useful index for distinguishing between airways obstruction related to asthma and to emphysema, where the value is reduced. The steady state D_LCO has less discriminatory value because it is more affected by ventilation/perfusion mismatching and it tends to be impaired in all forms of airflow obstruction. Much interest, and some controversy, has been aroused by reports that the single breath D_LCO may often be elevated in asthma. Some of the discrepancies in the literature are possibly related to methodology and the results may depend on whether the alveolar volume (V_A) used in the calculation is estimated simultaneously during the breath hold or by a separate multibreath helium dilution technique. The measurement of D_LCO derived from the latter will be higher in the presence of significant airflow obstruction and may overestimate the total diffusing capacity of the lungs by assuming that all the alveoli can function as well as the better ventilated areas. The KCO is the same by either method and is more consistently elevated in asthma, possibly because the better ventilated alveoli are also the better perfused and their capillaries contain a disproportionate amount of the total pulmonary capillary blood volume.

Ventilatory Control

Unlike the situation in patients with chronic airflow obstruction, there is usually no controversy about a possible central defect of respiratory control in asthma. One look at a patient with severe asthma suffices to show that the 'drive to breathe' is increased rather than decreased and when CO_2 retention occurs this is a consequence of very severely disordered mechanical function. This does not, however, mean that the ventilatory response to CO_2 will be normal since, as with any cause of airflow obstruction, ventilation is a poor index of the neural drive to breathe. Nor does it mean that uncontrolled oxygen or sedatives are safe. Quite the contrary, as the frequent association of sedation with deterioration and death in severe asthma shows. Also, in the presence of established or incipient CO_2 retention from any cause, a high inspired oxygen concentration may lead to worsening hypercapnia either by an inhibitory effect on the chemoreceptors or, perhaps more likely, via its effects on the pulmonary vasculature and gas exchange. Within the normal population there is considerable variation of respiratory chemosensitivity and Rebuck and Read (1971) showed that patients who developed CO_2 retention during an acute asthmatic attack had lower than average ventilatory responses to

CO_2 in remission. Thus the subject's innate chemosensitivity may be an important determinant of his response to the insult of a severe asthmatic attack.

In Conclusion

This attempt to integrate many of the physiological, pathological and clinical features of asthma has of necessity been sketchy because of limitations of space and even larger limitations of knowledge. Certain points bear re-emphasis. Our present working definition of asthma as variable airflow obstruction is unsatisfactory but until a more specific definition(s) in terms of aetiology or pathogenesis is possible it has to serve as the lowest common denominator. It is instructive to note what the definition omits:

1) There is no universally applicable arbitrary level of 'variability'

2) There is no absolute means of distinguishing between 'asthmatics' (many of whom are also 'bronchitic') and 'bronchitics' (some of whom are 'asthmatic')

3) It makes no reference to 'allergy' - indeed the emphasis of immunological mechanisms of asthma has declined in recent years as recognition of nonspecific hyper-reactivity has increased

4) Also, it makes no reference to psychopathology and practicing chest physicians are usually impressed with the psychological stability of the majority of their asthmatic patients rather than with the frequency of 'nervous' or 'psychosomatic' asthma.

Asthma is one of the most challenging but at the same time most satisfactory conditions for the physician to manage. Much has been learned in recent years and many unsolved questions remain but, more disappointingly, much of the knowledge gained is not being logically applied. Of the outstanding questions, those related to aetiology are the most obvious: is bronchial hyper-reactivity synonymous with 'asthma' as recognised by physiologists, pathologists and clinicians? If so, what is its mechanism or mechanisms? In relation to pathophysiology, what is the main cause of airway narrowing in the acute episode? What causes the long term, apparently non-reversible, airway narrowing seen in some patients but not in others? How are the changes in lung distensibility and chest wall function produced? In relation to therapy, how important is it in chronic treatment to maintain optimal airway function? Would this prevent or reduce long term damage?

While awaiting the answers to these questions there are several areas where clinical management could be improved by greater awareness and alertness on the part of both the patient and doctor. Failure of recognition of asthma by non-specialists remains depressingly common – all too often the patient is dismissed as a 'bronchitic' and once such a label is attached the shutters come down on further thought or attempts at appropriate therapy. Even if asthma is recognised, its severity may not be; this is seen in two main contexts: in the outpatient who wakes wheezing every night but who when seen in surgery or clinic is symptom free; and secondly, in the casualty department or hospital ward where emergency treatment of the severe attack produces some relief but the severity of persisting airway narrowing is not recognised because no measurements are made and too much reliance is placed on auscultation for wheezes. Finally it is important to re-emphasise that the severe attack usually develops against a background of poor control and it is during these earlier stages that recognition and appropriate therapeutic intervention are vital. Only rarely is the role of respiratory function testing in asthma to perform a battery of complex investigations in a laboratory; much more valuable are simple measurements which can be performed frequently and, more importantly, at the time the patient is symptomatic.

References

Anderson, S.D.; Silverman, M.; Konig, P. and Godfrey, S.: Exercise induced asthma. British Journal of Diseases of the Chest 69: 1 (1975).

Antic, R. and Macklem, P.T.: The influence of clinical factors on the site of airway obstruction in asthma. American Review of Respiratory Disease 114: 851 (1976).

Benson M.K.: Bronchial hyperreactivity. British Journal of Diseases of the Chest 69: 227 (1975).

Boushey, H.A.; Holtzman, M.J.; Sheller, J.R. and Nadel, J.A.: Bronchial hyperreactivity. American Review of Respiratory Disease 121: 389 (1980).

Chai, H.; Farr, R.S.; Froehlich, L.A. et al.: Standardization of bronchial inhalation challenge procedures. Journal of Allergy and Clinical Immunology 56: 323 (1975).

Cockcroft, D.W.; Killian, D.N.; Mellon, J.J.A. and Hargreave, F.E.: Bronchial reactivity to inhaled histamine: a method and clinical survey. Clinical Allergy 7: 235 (1977).

Dunnill, M.S.: The pathology of asthma; in Porter and Birch (Eds) Identification of Asthma, p. 35 Ciba Foundation Study Group No. 38 (Churchill Livingstone, Edinburgh 1971).

Hogg, J.C.: Bronchial asthma; in Thurlbeck and Abell (Eds) The Lung: Structure, Function and Disease, p. 000 (Williams and Wilkins, Baltimore 1978).

Lisboa, C.; Jardim, J.; Angus, E. and Macklem, P.T.: Is extrathoracic airways obstruction important in asthma? American Review of Reapiratory Disease 122: 155 (1980).

Lorber, D.B.; Kaltenborn, W. and Burrows, B.: Responses to isoproterenol in a general population sample. American Review of Respiratory Disease 118: 855 (1978).

Martin, A.J.; Landau, L.I. and Phelan, P.D.: Lung function in young adults who had asthma in childhood. American Review of Respiratory Disease 122: 609 (1980).

McFadden, E.R. and Lyons, H.A.: Arterial blood gas tensions in asthma. New England Journal of Medicine; 278: 1027 (1968).

Rebuck, A.S. and Read, J.: Patterns of ventilatory response to carbon dioxide during recovery from severe asthma. Clinical Science 41: 13 (1971).

Richardson, J. and Beland, J.: Nonadrenergic inhibitory nervous system in human airways. Journal of Applied Physiology 41: 764 (1976).

Ryan, G.; Dolovich, M.B.; Roberts, R.S. et al.: Standardization of inhalation provocation tests: two techniques of aerosol generation and inhalation compared. American Review of Respiratory Disease 123: 195 (1981).

Strauss, R.H.; McFadden, E.R.; Ingram, R.H. et al.: Influence of heat and humidity on the airway obstruction induced by exercise in asthma. Journal of Clinical Investigation 61: 433 (1978).

Szentivanyi, A.: The beta adrenergic theory of the atopic abnormality in bronchial asthma. Journal of Allergy 42: 203 (1968).

Wagner, P.D.; Dantzker, D.R.; Iacovoni, V.E. et al.: Ventilation-perfusion irregularity in asymptomatic asthma. American Review of Respiratory Disease 118: 511 (1978).

Chapter III

Measurement of the Asthmatic State

M.C.F. Pain

The Functional Defect and Its Assessment

While the complex nature of the pathophysiology of bronchial asthma is evident from Chapter II, it is useful to consider asthma and the nature of the problem under two categories. That is, the acute asthma attack and the interval status.

The Acute Attack

Airway resistance increases mainly as a result of bronchial smooth muscle constriction but also because of endobronchial oedema and intraluminal secretions. The resting lung volume increases because of expiratory prolongation and obstruction and this is recognisable as hyperinflation of the thoracic cage. The combination of increased airway resistance and lung hyperinflation increases the ventilatory work and the subject recognises this as breathlessness. The extent of breathlessness depends upon the size of the load increase, the strength of the respiratory driving forces and the perception by the subject of the interplay of these two factors. Relief of the acute episode is accompanied by lessening of airflow obstruction, reduction in resting lung volume, reduction in respiratory work and easing of breathlessness. Some coughing with expectoration of viscid bronchial secretions may continue for hours or days after relief of breathlessness, depending on the duration and severity of the attack.

Disturbing as this component of the acute episode is, it is the interference with gas exchange that imposes the threat to life. The airflow obstruction is not uniform. Not only can it involve a variable proportion of large and small airways but the degree of obstruction at any given anatomical level is unequal between regions. There are several reasons for this. Firstly, the distribution of an inhaled allergen or bronchial irritant will be non-uniform, even in normal lungs. Secondly, secretion production and non-removal will vary through the bronchial tree and thirdly, agents brought to the bronchial tree via the bloodstream, or mediators released locally producing bronchoconstriction, will be distributed unequally. The resulting non-uniform distribution of ventilation will disturb the normal relationships between alveolar ventilation and pulmonary capillary blood flow producing gas exchanging units with widely different ventilation/blood flow ratios. The consequence of this mismatching will be reduction in oxygen tension of the mixed end-capillary blood leaving the lungs and an elevation of carbon dioxide tension. Other things being equal, the usual response to the situation is an increase in minute ventilation and alveolar ventilation to return the arterial carbon dioxide tension to normal. The necessary increase in ventilation in the presence of airflow obstruction contributes an additional burden to total respiratory effort.

Improvement in gas exchange often lags behind the reduction in airflow obstruction following an asthma attack, presumably because of persisting areas of low ventilation associated with bronchial secretions.

Interval Status

Clinically, asthma is characterised by exacerbations and remissions of airflow obstruction. Indeed the most useful definition of asthma in our present state of ignorance states that asthma is 'episodic airway obstruction' without implying any specific aetiology or suggesting what degree of variation in airflow obstruction is required to be demonstrated. That return to 'normality' between attacks is the exception rather than the rule has been demonstrated by several studies which show persisting airflow obstruction, mild hyperinflation, mild to moderate or even surprisingly severe abnormalities in gas exchange in asthmatic subjects who considered they were normal or in complete remission (Cade and Pain, 1973). Thus, typically, the interval state is commonly that of 'a persisting slight amount of asthma' in the absence of symptoms and a sense of well being.

Many patients however may not return to a symptomless interval state and their clinical history is one of continuous disability with persisting significant background asthma punctuated by severe exacerbations from time to time. This latter group is particularly difficult to assess if symptoms alone are relied on as the persisting disability often leads patients to learn to live with their interval symptoms so that the actual extent of the persisting asthma may be grossly underestimated.

Despite a total lack of symptoms, and normal airway resistance and indices of gas exchange, patients with asthma between acute episodes show one characteristic which is central to the overall pathophysiology of the disease and which stamps them as being at risk. This is the property of heightened bronchial reactivity.

Bronchial Reactivity

Bronchial reactivity is the ability of the bronchial tree to alter acutely its airway resistance in response to a variety of external and internal stimuli. While there is a degree of bronchial reactivity which may be regarded as normal, in the context of asthma an acute asthma attack can be considered as an expression of that individual's bronchial hyperactivity. Heightened bronchial reactivity seems to be one of the few characteristics that all subjects with asthma have in common. Despite wide fluctuations in clinical asthma, long periods of remission and long term successful treatment with anti-asthma agents, bronchial hyper-reactivity remains fairly constantly abnormal. There are many probable explanations for the development and persistence of heightened bronchial reactivity but none, at present, totally convincing (p.14). A better understanding of the mechanisms of bronchial hyper-reactivity will necessarily assist in the understanding of the basic nature of bronchial asthma.

For practical purposes, all patients with asthma, subclinical or clinical, will have heightened bronchial reactivity. Interestingly there is a group of apparently normal subjects who can be shown to exhibit a degree of bronchial reactivity close to or overlapping that shown by patients with asthma. Whether this group is at special risk of developing asthma, given appropriate conditions, is uncertain. In the present state of knowledge, the simple equating of heightened bronchial reactivity as being exclusively diagnostic of the asthmatic state is not possible.

Assessment of the Functional Defect

Breathlessness, airflow obstruction, gas exchange impairment and bronchial reactivity can all form some basis for assessing the presence and degree of functional defect.

The assumption that an asymptomatic patient has mild asthma and that increasingly severe asthma will be associated with increasingly florid symptoms is widespread. That this is still the commonest method of assessing asthma severity reflects a disregard for well established facts, and highlights one of the common problems in the treatment of asthma today. Symptoms, of course, cannot be ignored. They have a place in the overall assessment, but total reliance on symptoms can lead to serious errors of judgement and plays a part in the incidence of 'unexpected' deaths from asthma; this is illustrated by the British Thoracic Association panel's finding (BTA Study, 1982) that in 83 of 90 patients who died of asthma, no serial peak flow measurements had been carried out.

Airflow obstruction which is potentially reversible, is the hallmark of asthma. An actual measurement of the state of airway patency with an objective test will quantitate the load to breathing and thus provide an index of severity. Gas exchange impairment can be roughly assessed by clinical examination or accurately quantitated with laboratory tests. Bronchial reactivity can be determined using one of a number of procedures and while these are briefly mentioned below it is considered that a detailed discussion is outside the scope of this chapter.

Why Bother?

Since objective assessment of the asthmatic state involves extra time and effort and demands on the time of medical practitioners are already high, this section, which should hardly be necessary, restates the benefits of the intelligent use of simple tests.

Help in Diagnosis

In many cases the diagnosis of asthma is sufficiently clear from the historical features and the findings on clinical examination. The presence of air-flow obstruction and its potentially reversible nature can be easily confirmed using measurements of peak expiratory flow rate. Reversibility can be demonstrated by repeating these measurements after the inhalation of a bronchodilator aerosol. Isoprenaline (isoproterenol) [1%] is still the quickest acting aerosol bronchodilator although the slower acting more selective β_2-adrenergic group of drugs gives less potential cardiovascular side effects.

Again, using peak expiratory flow measurements, demonstration of bronchial reactivity can be simply performed by measuring the fall in peak flow rate following a short period of exercise (Godfrey, 1975), the inhalation of nonspecific agents such as histamine or methacholine, or specific allergens. These bronchial provocation tests are not without risk and should not be performed unless measures to treat severe asthma are at hand. Bronchial provocation can be very useful in detecting heightened bronchial reactivity in subjects whose history is atypical or who have no airflow obstruction at the time of examination.

Assessment of Severity

Asthma is occasionally difficult to diagnose but it is commonly difficult to estimate its severity and experienced clinicians are constantly surprised by the degree of abnormality demonstrated by objective assessment of patients whose asthma was considered to be mild. This is partly due to the blunting of symptoms by chronic disease, variations in the perceptiveness of patients and the misleading information obtained from a cursory physical examination. Whilst some deaths from asthma apparently occur rapidly from a previously mild impairment, it remains true that most of the 'unexpected' asthma deaths are found in patients in whom objective assessment has been minimal or in whom the warning provided by that assessment has been ignored. Objective assessment can be reassuring in confirming the mildness of a particular situation or be revealing in indicating that the situation is more serious than anticipated and thus provide a basis for more appropriate treatment (Williams, 1979).

Following Progress

It is reasonable to anticipate that appropriate treatment will cause at least some improvement in control of the asthma. Lack of improvement necessitates a review of the diagnosis or adjustment of treatment. Most patients are quick to sense subjective improvement but will often tend to over-emphasise the extent of their improvement. Objective following of progress can lead to better adjustment of drug dosages or discontinuation of potentially dangerous medication in the face of objective evidence of a therapeutic failure (Epstein et al., 1969).

Patient Perception

In most chronic diseases, but particularly in asthma, the way in which the patient perceives his illness will affect his lifestyle generally and his acceptance of a suitable medication regimen. Few patients can be persuaded to take medication regularly if they feel well and some patients, however conscientious, may be undertreated over the long term if medication is taken only when the symptoms develop. Central to this is the relationship between the objectively demonstrated abnormality in lung function and the patient's perceived disability. Studies of the development of acute asthma suggest that the majority of patients with asthma are able to detect changes in airflow obstruction but to a variable degree. A small group seem quite unable to detect even considerable deviations from normal (Rubinfeld and Pain, 1976). Observations made during this study of the sensation of breathlessness during provoked asthma suggest the presence of a 'perception level'. That is, until the asthma has reached a certain degree of severity, the subject is unaware of any disability. It is easy to imagine a patient with asthma being at considerable risk if he has a high threshold of perception and thus diminished sensitivity to increasing asthma. Such a subject may have extremely severe asthma before he is aware that treatment for an acute attack is required. Perhaps more importantly, such a subject may well spend most of his life with untreated chronic impairment. Furthermore probably chronic impairment leads to upwards readjustment of threshold settings. The patient's approach to regular and sustained medication may be modified by the ability to measure and follow changes in his functional impairment.

For all these reasons, an essential part of the assessment of the patient with asthma is determination of the perception level. What is being sought is some impression about the relationship between symptoms and functional impairment (fig. 3.1). This may be obviously abnormal at the initial examination. For example, a subject may deny any breathing difficulty and at the same time demonstrate obvious and considerable airflow limitation. The relationship between objective impairment and symptoms may take several separate visits to demonstrate or alternatively, be deduced from the changes in both aspects induced by the administration of bronchoconstrictor or bronchodilator substances under controlled conditions at the initial visit.

Objectivity Without Expense: Assessment in the Acute Attack

One of the more unfortunate byproducts of the development of pulmonary function laboratories is the creation of an apparent gulf between the bedside examination of patients with asthma and their objective assessment. 'Measurement of pulmonary function' conjures up in the mind a written request form, a trip to the laboratory and the confronting of the patient with an impressive and usually expensive collection of equipment often connected to a computer. Although not wishing to disparage the value of the formal laboratory assessment, it must be said that an unfortunate reluctance to believe that anything less than this type of assessment is of value has developed. When this is coupled with a realisation that the usual 'classical' examination of the chest can be very misleading, the rapid transition from symptom assessment to laboratory assessment may seem logical.

The main message of this section is that objective assessment does not imply elaborate laboratory assessment. In the overall extraction of information about the disturbed pulmonary physiology

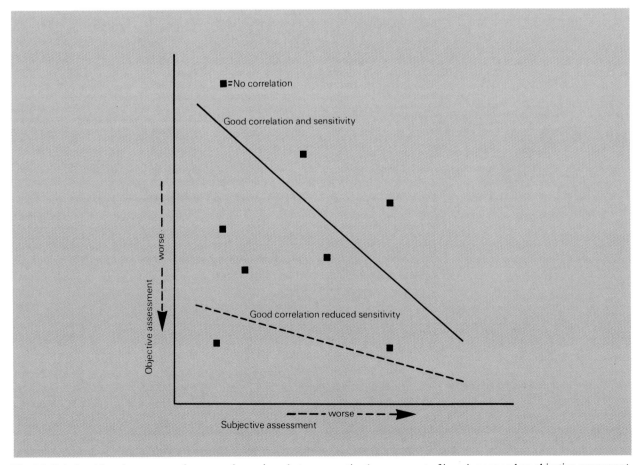

Fig. 3.1. Relationship, when measured on several occasions, between a patient's assessment of impairment and an objective assessment.

of patients with asthma, there is an asymptotic function calling for more and more effort to be expended in seeking more and more detailed information. In terms of cost effectiveness however, the bulk of information upon which clinical decisions are made can be obtained objectively using very simple equipment. This objective assessment can be made during the clinical examination and with the use of simple devices both aspects of the pathophysiology – increased load and disturbed gas exchange – investigated.

Physical Examination

For the purpose of physical examination, rather than viewing asthma as a continuous spectrum of severity, it is helpful to think of it in terms of mild, moderate and severe states, each of which may have arisen rapidly or represent a chronic, relatively stable situation. In this classification, no account is taken of symptoms or antecedent history although obviously such aspects as the immediate medication, duration of illness and precipitating events will be of importance in the overall assessment and plan of treatment.

The Forced Expiratory Time

Adequately performed, the forced expiratory time provides a surprisingly accurate indication of the severity of airflow obstruction and therefore is a most valuable bedside aid in objective assessment (Lal et al., 1964). Its performance requires some dedication on the part of the observer and the subject and the commonest fault is to underestimate the correct time because of poor patient cooperation. Usually a simple demonstration of the manoeuvre required, by the observer himself, will save many inadequate attempts by the subject thus avoiding exhaustion and frustration.

Looking directly ahead and with the mouth always kept open the subject inspires maximally and, on command, expires forcibly and maximally with observer exhortation. The time during which the expiratory phase is audible is noted. Using a stethoscope placed over the upper sternum adds somewhat to the precision and usually increases the estimation made by listening to the noise at the mouth by up to a second. The normal forced expiratory time is less than 5 seconds and in the young is usually less than 4 seconds. Inaccuracy develops from three main sources which should be guarded against: the subject may not await the expiratory command; the mouth may not be held open, or maximal effort may not continue until the residual volume is reached. Performance of the forced expiratory time manoeuvre should be taught as part of the routine examination of the chest.

Mild asthma: Patients are able to converse using quite long sentences. They are not forced to adopt any particular position and while the amount of respiratory noise generated may be alarming, actual forced expiratory manoeuvres show that the forced expiratory time is only just longer than normal. Pulse and blood pressure may be raised as a result of previous medication and there is no central cyanosis.

Moderate asthma: The patient is confined to one position and is not able to undertake even moderate physical exertion. Sentences are short but cooperation with the process of measurement of the forced expiratory time is still possible. Features of airflow obstruction are evident in the prolongation of the expiratory phase and audible continuous rhonchi.

Severe asthma: The patient is able to speak using single words only. All efforts are directed towards breathing and the position is usually one of leaning forward and obtaining some extra purchase on a table or chair. The accessory muscles of respiration (scalenes and sterno-mastoid) are obviously in use. It is often impossible to obtain sufficient cooperation for satisfactory forced expiratory time measurements. Evidence of severe airflow obstruction is reflected in the hyperinflated thorax and occasionally, paradoxical indrawing of the lower costal margin with inspiration (Hoover's sign) is seen although this is more common in severe chronic bronchitis and emphysema.

Breath sound audibility is variable. With increasing severity, the prolongation of expiration and rhonchi may diminish due to total airway closure. The large changes in intra-thoracic pressure during the respiratory cycle produce swings in jugular venous pressure and cyclical differences in systemic blood pressure. This pulsus paradoxus usually occurs only with severe airflow obstruction but its absence does not imply that airflow obstruction is not severe.

Central cyanosis while breathing air and unrelieved by oxygen enrichment is due to areas of lung with a very low ventilation/blood flow ratio and is a very significant sign of gas exchange abnormality. The situation can worsen in two directions. Either the airflow obstruction can become extreme leading to deepening cyanosis and risk of death from hypoxia, or a prolonged degree of airflow obstruction can lead to exhaustion with a failure of ventilation, carbon dioxide retention and signs of drowsiness, confusion and coma with sweating and obviously inadequate breathing.

The difficulty in assessing at the bedside the extent of gas exchange defect in asthma cannot be overstressed. The physical signs of carbon dioxide retention are of variable expression and by the time this stage has been reached, urgent intervention is required. Central cyanosis is a notoriously difficult sign to detect. Quite apart from difficulties imposed by lighting, haemoglobin level and observer competence, central cyanosis is regularly detected only when the arterial oxygen tension is about 50mm Hg. A subject with sufficient gas exchange defect to result in an arterial oxygen tension of 60mm Hg may not appear cyanosed but will be poised in terms of gas exchange, at a position in the oxygen dissociation curve for a precipitous fall in oxygen delivery with only a small further deterioration in lung function. Thus a small increase in right to left shunt from 40% to 50% will cause a marked drop in arterial oxygen tension to cyanotic levels in a patient breathing 100% oxygen by face mask.

The divisions between mild, moderate and severe asthma are artificial and difficult based on bedside physical examination alone. Patients with asthma are at risk from a general tendency to underestimate the severity of the condition either in terms of airflow obstruction or in terms of severity of gas exchange impairment in relation to a given degree of airflow obstruction since the relationship between the two is not a simple one. However, the objective assessment of these two aspects does not require great sophistication.

Simple Assessment of Airflow Obstruction

Between the measurement of forced expiratory time and the use of a spirometer, is a group of small portable instruments designed to provide some index of flow limitation. Within the group is a variation in price, complexity, accuracy and reliability but even the exclusive use of the cheapest instrument is infinitely better than no objectivity at all. The instrument should be considered as similar to the sphygmomanometer, ophthalmoscope and stethoscope, as being aids to the extension of the physical examination.

The Wright Peak Flow Meter (fig. 3.2) was the first of this group to be widely used and is still the yardstick by which the others are compared (Wright and McKerrow, 1959). It is accurate and robust, needing only infrequent calibration checks. Perhaps its main disadvantages are its relative expense and its weight and size. It is the ideal surgery instrument but is not the type of instrument normally issued to patients for home measurements. Normal values for peak expiratory flow rates (litres/minute) are now well established using this instrument (Godfrey et al., 1970; Gregg and Nunn, 1973).

A cheaper and more portable peak flow meter, also designed by Dr B.M. Wright, has recently established a respectable reputation for reliability and acceptable accuracy with a small error at very low flow rates when compared with the standard Wright peak flow meter. This Mini Wright Peak Flow Meter (Airmed, fig. 3.3) stands up well to patient use and is useful for home monitoring of air-flow obstruction. In the same category and even cheaper is the Pulmonary Monitor (Vitalograph, fig. 3.4). Its cheapness makes it more attractive for issuing to patients for home use. All these instruments provide an index in litres/minute expiratory flow indicating the maximal rate of flow achieved during maximal forced expiration.

The Airflometer works with a paddle wheel principle through a system of gears. It is cheap and quite rugged, its main disadvantage is the reading which is given in undefined 'units'. Its readout is a complex function of total volume as well as velocity of airflow, although there is a good correlation between forced expired volume (the simple spirometric standard for airflow limitation) and airflow meter units.

All these instruments are useful and none has any special advantage. In most cases the instrument is used in a longitudinal study for a particular patient so that minor inconsistencies between instruments are of no consequence. The important point is to become familiar with one instrument, be aware of its limitations and to use it frequently.

Simple Assessment of Gas Exchange Defect

This is most simply done by an analysis of the arterial blood gases. While it may seem some licence to describe arterial puncture, collection of blood and the use of a triple electrode apparatus to measure oxygen tension, carbon dioxide tension and pH as 'simple', this facility is now becoming increasingly available in even quite small hospitals and certainly in any centre accepting acute trauma cases.

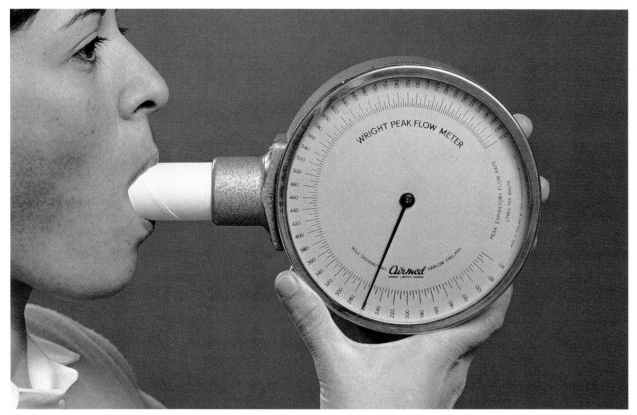

Fig. 3.2. Wright Peak Flow Meter.

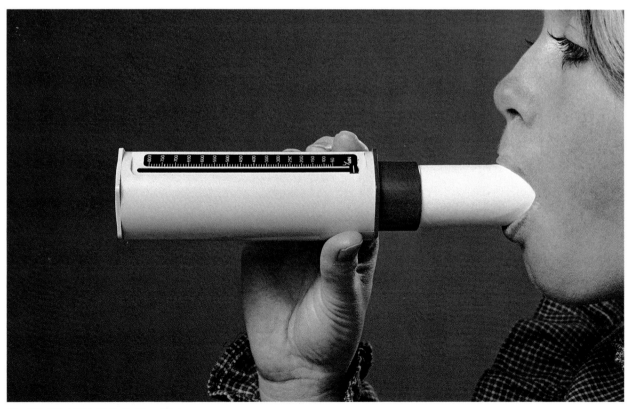

Fig. 3.3. Mini Wright Peak Flow Meter.

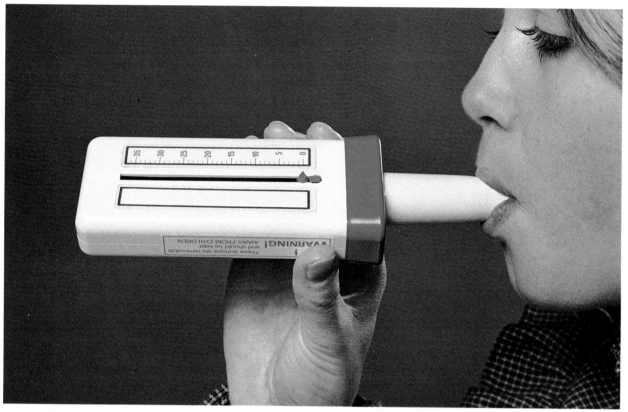

Fig. 3.4. Vitalograph Pulmonary Monitor.

A stab puncture of the brachial or radial artery using a sharp disposable 21 gauge needle and a heparinised syringe has proved to be safe and acceptable to patients without using local anaesthesia.

Arterial Oxygen Tension

The significance of the arterial oxygen tension level lies in its relationship to the inspired oxygen concentration. For example, an arterial oxygen tension of 80mm Hg is reasonably close to normal if the subject is breathing air but with the subject breathing 50% inspired oxygen, such an oxygen tension indicates a profound disturbance of gas exchange even though, with a normal cardiac output, the oxygen delivery will be potentially adequate. This is best considered as the difference between the alveolar and arterial oxygen tension. Normally this alveolar-arterial oxygen tension gradient (A-a PO_2) is very small, less than 10% of the inspired oxygen tension. Increasing disturbance of gas exchange with increased areas of low ventilation/blood flow ratio leads to increased widening of the A-a PO_2. The alveolar oxygen tension is that tension calculated for the ventilated and perfused compartment as distinct from non-perfused or non-ventilated portions of lung and is termed the 'ideal' alveolar oxygen tension. It is simply calculated from the alveolar gas equation which requires knowledge of inspired oxygen tension, carbon dioxide tension and an assumed value for R, the gas exchange ratio.

Assume alveolar oxygen tension ≃ inspired oxygen tension
                                − 1.25 × arterial carbon dioxide tension

Oxygen tension ≃ oxygen concentration % × 7

Given
1. Arterial oxygen tension, say 50mm Hg
2. Arterial CO_2 tension, say 35mm Hg
3. Inspired O_2 concentration, say 30%

What is the alveolar-arterial oxygen tension gradient?

Alveolar oxygen tension = (30 × 7) – (1.25 × 35)
                        = 210 – 44
                        = 166mm Hg
Therefore, alveolar-arterial oxygen tension gradient
                        = 166 – 50 = 116mm Hg

Discussion of arterial oxygen tension as an index of gas exchange is amplified by West (1977) but in general the greater the defect in gas exchange, the lower the arterial oxygen tension and the wider the ideal alveolar-arterial oxygen tension gradient.

Arterial Carbon Dioxide Tension

The arterial carbon dioxide tension provides information about the response of the control mechanism for respiration to the gas exchange defect. With adequate muscle power and a responsive respiratory centre, there is an increase in minute ventilation with a lowering of carbon dioxide tension. Anxiety and the respiratory stimulant action of some anti-asthma agents can also cause alveolar hyperventilation with reduction of carbon dioxide levels. A severe load, that is severe airflow obstruction, coupled with an inadequate drive or an exhausted respiratory muscle system would be associated with either a failure to lower carbon dioxide tension appropriately or an increase in carbon dioxide tension above normal. The hydrogen ion concentration and its deviation from normal is useful for deciding if the process has occurred acutely with inadequate time for compensation or represents a chronic state. Thus the hydrogen ion concentration will be below normal if acute hyperventilation has occurred and above normal with acute hypoventilation.

Although the above remarks concerning simple assessment of gas exchange apply to all lung conditions, they provide a particularly suitable basis for characterising the patient with asthma. Examples of typical values are given in table 3.1 and the pathophysiology indicated. Note the examples are with the subject breathing room air. When samples are taken from subjects breathing oxygen-enriched air, appropriate allowance must be made for the increased significance of the widened gradient. It is easy to be falsely reassured by the arterial oxygen tension in the face of a severe gas exchange defect.

Arterial pH

As well as the assessment of blood gases, pH should be measured when arterial blood is sampled. Metabolic acidosis in asthma is indicative of severe airways obstruction and is apt to be a prelude of the even more serious respiratory acidosis.

Table 3.1. Typical gas exchange values for arterial oxygen ($Pa0_2$), arterial carbon dioxide ($PaCO_2$) and alveolar-arterial oxygen (A-apO_2) for normal and asthmatic subjects.

Subject	$Pa0_2$	$PaC0_2$	A-a $p0_2$	Remarks
Normal	85-100mm Hg	36-44mm Hg	< 15mm Hg	Breathing air
Mild Asthmatic	> 80mm Hg	low normal	< 30mm Hg	Minimal disturbance in gas exchange
Moderate Asthmatic	60-80mm Hg	low normal	< 50mm Hg	Increasingly larger areas of lung which have low ventilation: blood flow ratios
Severe Asthmatic	40-60mm Hg	low or normal	< 70mm Hg	
Severe Asthmatic	40-60mm Hg	raised	< 70mm Hg	Ventilation inadequate. Life threatened from acidosis
Severe Asthmatic	< 40mm Hg	low, normal or raised	> 70mm Hg	Severe gas exchange defect. Life threatened from hypoxia

Techniques for Interval Assessment

Since asthma is usually a condition of fluctuating severity involving irregular and even infrequent reviews by the medical practitioner, it is often misleading to judge the average state of control by the history and the findings on examination at isolated visits. Memory of average control is unreliable for events which may have occurred weeks or months previously. Statements about the quality of life or severity of asthma are likely to be based on memory recall of only the previous few days. In deciding on the need for adjustment of therapy, information recorded over a period of days or weeks and brought to the next medical consultation has much to recommend it.

Information recording may be used to cover several aspects of the patient's condition since the previous visit. First, the degree of control can be assessed by recording daily activity or enforced inactivity, missed days from work, associated symptoms (cough, sputum) and/or objective measurement, usually of peak expiratory flow rate. Secondly, the action of medication can be studied by obtaining readings of peak expiratory flow rate at particular times of the day or at fixed intervals in relationship to medication, such as before and after the use of an inhaled aerosol bronchodilator. Thirdly, in a patient who is adjusting medication according to needs, an accurate record of the drugs used each day, week or month provides indirect information about the extent to which his asthma fluctuates. Finally, interval records can be used to determine the perceptive level of patients with asthma.

Diary Records

Many intelligent patients produce their own diary note of events which occur between consultations and these can form a valuable additon to our knowledge of the patients' illness. Often, very unfairly, such people are thought to be somewhat obsessional but their ability to make these observations should be used to their advantage and sometimes redirected to seeking the appropriate items of information. Recognising the need for some form of interval assessment, several commercial firms, usually those associated with the manufacture of pharmaceutical agents or laboratory instruments used in the management of asthma, have produced a printed diary card or booklet. These tend to be all-embracing and

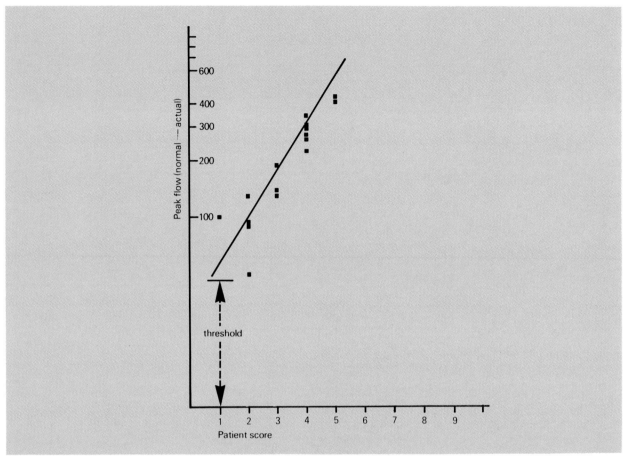

Fig. 3.5. Data obtained during interval phase assessment of an asthmatic subject to determine perceptive threshold (intercept) and discrimination (slope).

have provision for recording symptoms, drug usage, peak flow readings and graphic plotting of peak flow rate. Although a good idea in theory, there are a number of points to be considered in their use. Patients are more likely to record information successfully if the number of items to be entered is kept to a minimum. They must have adequate explanation of the reasons for the record and be convinced of its potential value. In turn, this means the practitioner must formulate in his own mind clear questions to which he is seeking answers. An example of a simplified form is shown on page 186. Diary cards do not improve patient compliance with medication nor act as a memory aid for forgetful patients.

Medication Records

Small cards with a record of medication are used mainly to remind the practitioner of changes in medication made at previous consultations and are not usually related to an objective measurement. If written with clear simple instructions, they can improve asthma therapy by ensuring that the therapy is used as intended. Many patients leave the consulting room believing they have understood instructions but simple questioning at this stage often reveals only the vaguest concept of a therapeutic plan. The confusion is directly proportional to the number of preparations prescribed.

*Perception Level
Assessment*

Valuable information can be obtained by enlisting the patient's cooperation in recording an objective measurement of airflow function – commonly the peak expiratory flow rate – and relating this to a subjective score decided by the subject. The score should be decided before the reading is taken and ideally that reading should be made and recorded by an independent observer. The recording can be made at any time and daily recording for 14 to 21 days has been adequate. For the subjective score, one can use an open-ended scale or ask the subject to decide on a number, not necessarily an integer, between 0 and 10, where 0 represents perfect well being and 10 would represent the severest asthma attack imaginable. The degree of airflow obstruction, expressed as the fall from predicted normal value, and the subjective score can be plotted as in figure 3.5. The linear relationship on semi-log plotting provides information on the threshold for recognition of asthma and on the subsequent sensitivity of the perception. These properties can be shown to differ between patients with asthma. The knowledge of these two aspects will lead to a better planning of medication and recognition of a group of 'poor perceivers' at special risk.

In Conclusion

Many of the difficulties in the management of patients with asthma are attributable to the following: lack of understanding by the patient of what medication is expected to do; incorrect inhalational techniques for aerosol administration, and a tendency to assume lack of symptoms means normality. Education of the patient is the responsibility of the practitioner providing clinical care and in this education, measurement of the asthmatic state during the interval phase is just as important as assessment at the time of an acute attack.

References

British Thoracic Associaton: Death from asthma in two regions of England. British Medical Journal 285: 1251 (1982).

Cade, J.F. and Pain, M.C.F.: Pulmonary function during remission of asthma. How reversible is asthma? Australian and New Zealand Journal of Medicine 3: 545 (1973).

Epstein, S.W.; Fletcher, C.M. and Oppenheimer, E.A.: Daily peak flow measurements in the assessment of steroid therapy for airway obstruction. British Medical Journal 1: 223 (1969).

Godfrey, S.; Kamburoff, P.L. and Nairn, J.R.: Spirometry lung volumes and airway resistance in normal children aged 5 to 18 years. British Journal of Diseases of the Chest 64: 15 (1970).

Godrey, S.: Exercise-induced asthma – clinical, physiological and therapeutic implications. Journal of Allergy and Clinical Immunology 56: 1 (1975).

Gregg, I. and Nunn, A.J.: Peak Expiratory flow in normal subjects. British Medical Journal 3: 282 (1973).

Lal, S.; Ferguson, A.D. and Campbell, E.J.A.: Forced expiratory time: a simple test for airways obstruction. British Medical Journal 1: 814 (1964).

Rubinfeld, A.R. and Pain, M.C.F.: The perception of asthma. Lancet 1: 882 (1976).

West, J.B.: Ventilation-perfusion relationships. American Review of Respiratory Disease 116: 919 (1977).

Williams, M.H.: Evaluation of asthma. Chest 76: 3 (1979).

Wright, B.M. and McKerrow, L.B.: Maximal forced expiratory flow rate as a measure of ventilatory capacity with a description of a new portable instrument for measuring it. British Medical Journal 2: 1041 (1959).

Chapter IV

The Immunological Basis of Asthma

A.B. Kay

The events which lead to airway narrowing in bronchial asthma are complex. There is little doubt that mast cell-derived pharmacological agents are involved, at least in part, in the initiation of the asthmatic response. However, it is misleading to consider bronchial asthma as being essentially an 'immunological disease'.

The IgE-mediated release of mediators from sensitised mast cells seems to play a role in pathogenesis in some individuals for some of the time, but there is now an increasing awareness that mast cells can also be triggered by a number of non-immunological stimuli. Furthermore the inflammatory response which follows mast cell activation might have more relevance to continuing asthma than the direct effects of pharmacological agents on bronchial tissue.

Asthma covers a broad clinical spectrum, ranging from mild, readily reversible, 'bronchospasm' to severe chronic intractable obstruction to airflow. There are well known difficulties in defining the disease since reversible airways obstruction may be impossible to demonstrate at the time of diagnosis. For instance, the mild episodic asthmatic may be free of symptoms for prolonged periods of time whereas individuals with acute severe asthma may take several days before airway obstruction is relieved by medication.

For these reasons an attempt will be made to discuss asthma in terms of the diverse nature of mast cell-derived chemical mediators, the various initiating factors for mast cell activation, and the relationship between the 'allergic' and inflammatory aspects of the disease.

Pathology

Because of the obvious difficulties of obtaining large quantities of bronchial tissue from asthmatics almost all our knowledge of the pathology of asthma is from autopsy studies (Dunnill, 1971). The typical features of these 'asthma deaths' have been described in Chapter II (p.12). The bronchial plugs contain inspissated mucus, cells and cell debris which includes epithelial cells shed from the basement membrane together with varying numbers of eosinophils, macrophages and lymphocytes.

Eosinophil infiltration, both in and around the walls of the bronchi, is a very characteristic feature and this is often associated with the presence of Charcot-Leyden crystals and Curshmann's spirals in the sputum plugs. The crystals are needle-like bodies consisting almost entirely of a protein, lysophospholipase, derived from the eosinophil cell membrane (Ackerman et al., 1980, 1981). The bronchial epithelium may show squamous metaplasia and there is thickening of the basement membrane and submucosal oedema. There is also an increase in the number of goblet cells in the bronchial epithelium. There is usually very marked hyperplasia of bronchial smooth muscle. Thus the principal pathological features correlate with three principal events (1) constriction of the bronchial smooth muscle, (2) oedema of the submusoca, and (3) occlusion of the lumen by mucous plugs.

Mast Cells and Basophils

Mast cells are probably of central importance in the immunological response in bronchial asthma although the role of basophils is unclear. Mast cells and basophils have high affinity receptors for immunoglobulin E. The interaction of IgE with specific allergen on the mast cell membrane leads to the release of a variety of pharmacological mediators which vary considerably both in chemical composition and modes of action (reviewed by Kay, 1981; O'Driscoll and Kay, 1982). Mediators act directly on tissues of the airway, indirectly via reflex mechanisms and also by the recruitment of inflammatory cells such as neutrophils and eosinophils.

Mast cells are associated with most mucosal surfaces (Cutz and Orange, 1977). In the human bronchi they have been observed free of the lumen, intraepithelially and beneath the basement membrane (fig. 4.1). Submucosal mast cells have been observed at all levels in the bronchial tree and are the typical connective tissue mast cells. Intraepithelial mast cells are usually located immediately above the basement membrane. Lumenal mast cells might possibly play an important role in initiating the asthmatic response since mediator release from these cells opens tight junctions between bronchial epithelial cells so allowing penetration of antigen to mast cells located deeper in the tissues (Simani et al., 1974). Recently it has been possible to prepare virtually pure suspensions of dispersed human lung mast cells from lung tissue obtained at thoracotomy (Schulman et al., 1982).

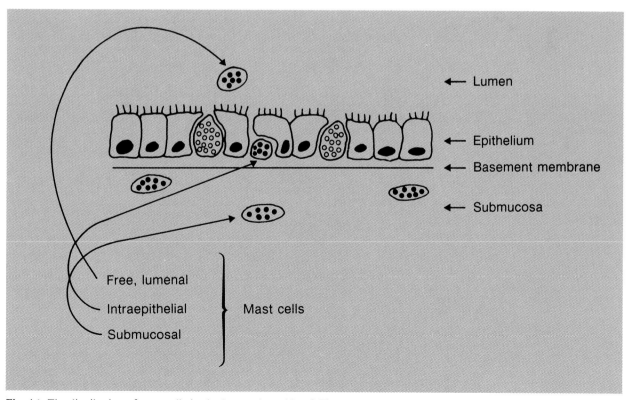

Fig. 4.1. The distribution of mast cells in the human bronchi.   © Figures 4.1 to 4.5 copyright A.B. Kay.

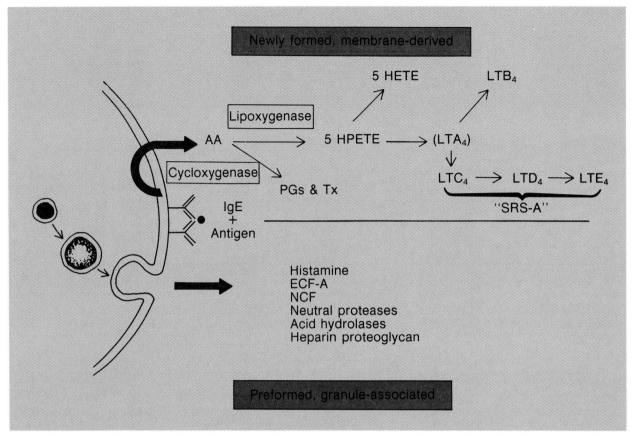

Fig. 4.2. The release of newly formed, membrane-derived and preformed, granule-associated mediators from human mast cells.

The role of blood basophils in bronchial asthma is unclear. Although basophils share many properties with mast cells and have been observed in the nasal mucosa in allergic rhinitis (Hastie et al., 1979) they do not appear to have been identified with certainty either in normal or diseased bronchial tissue.

Mast Cell-derived Mediators

Pre-formed Mediators

The pre-formed, granule-associated mediators include histamine, the peptides which comprise the eosinophil chemotactic factor of anaphylaxis (ECF-A), and a high molecular weight neutrophil chemotactic factor (HMW-NCF) in addition to various neutral proteases, acid hydrolases and heparin proteoglycan (fig. 4.2).

Histamine which in man is contained almost entirely within mast cells and basophils is derived from its precursor, histidine, by the action of histidine decarboxylase. The precise role of histamine in bronchial asthma is not understood. Under controlled laboratory conditions, such as inhalation of specific antigen or following exercise provocation, there is a rapid rise in airway resistance and in the concentration of plasma histamine which reaches a peak 10 to 15 minutes following challenge and then declines (Barnes and Brown, 1981; Lee et al., 1982a). This rapid, spasmogenic response might be due to the actions of histamine on bronchial smooth muscle acting either directly or indirectly through vagal reflexes, possibly as a result of stimulation of irritant receptors. Prior administration of sodium cromoglycate (cromolyn sodium), salbutamol or histamine H_1- and H_2-antagonists largely blocks this response (Butchers et al., 1979; Eiser et al., 1981).

Following mast cell activation a number of small acidic peptides in the molecular weight range 300 to 3000 daltons are released which preferentially attract eosinophils from a mixed leucocyte population *in vitro* (Kay, 1970; Bryant and Kay, 1977; Goetzl, 1980). This group of peptides is referred to as the eosinophil chemotactic factor of anaphylaxis (ECF-A). The peptides which have so far been chemically characterised (Val-Gly-Ser-Glu and Ala-Gly-Ser-Glu) have relatively weak chemotactic activity compared with other eosinophil-associated biological properties such as enchancement of cell membrane receptors (Anwar and Kay, 1977). ECF-A, both alone and together with other mediators (see below), might play a role in the recruitment of eosinophils to bronchial and peri-bronchial tissue.

Another mediator which is probably of mast cell origin is a high molecular weight neutrophil chemotactic factor of anaphylaxis (variously referred to as NCF, NCF-A, or high molecular weight [HMW] NCF). NCF has a molecular weight of approximately 750,000k and can be identified in the circulation of asthmatic subjects following either inhalation of specific antigen (Atkins et al., 1977) or an exercise task (Lee et al., 1982b). It has a time-course of release similar to histamine and its appearance in the circulation is blocked by prior administration of sodium cromoglycate. The *in vitro* release of NCF from lung fragments, or dispersed mast cells, is poorly documented.

A number of enzymes also are released during immediate-type reactions. These include chymase, N-acetyl-beta-glucuronidase, beta-glucuronidase and arylsulphatase A (Schwartz et al., 1979). Their precise role in disease is not yet established but they presumably have potential for local tissue damage in a manner analogous to the release of lysosomal enzyme from neutrophils. The heparin glycosaminoglycan is a macromolecule with antithrombin III activity. Mast cell heparin may play a role in local tissue homeostasis. For instance, it might combine with and dispose of platelet factor 4 released during tissue injury (McLaren et al., 1980).

Membrane-derived Mediators

The membrane-derived mediators are arachidonic acid metabolites. Arachidonic acid is derived largely, but not exclusively, from phosphatidyl choline by the action of the enzyme phospholipase A_2. Following membrane disruption, or perturbation such as the union of allergen with cell-bound IgE, there is activation of intramembranous methyltransferases which convert phosphatidyl ethanolamine to phosphatidyl choline (fig. 4.3). This event is associated with translocation or re-orientation of membrane phospholipids and the influx of extracellular calcium (Ishizaka et al., 1980). Calcium activates intramembranous permeability phospholipase A_2 and the arachidonic acid released is metabolised either by the cyclo-oxygenase pathway to form the prostaglandins, prostacyclin or thromboxanes, or by lipoxygenase enzymes to form mono-hydroxy fatty acids and the leukotrienes. The leukotrienes are of particular interest at present since they account for the activity previously referred to as 'slow reacting substance of anaphylaxis' (SRS-A) [Murphy et al., 1979]. These lipidopeptides (LTC_4, LTD_4 and LTE_4) produce smooth muscle

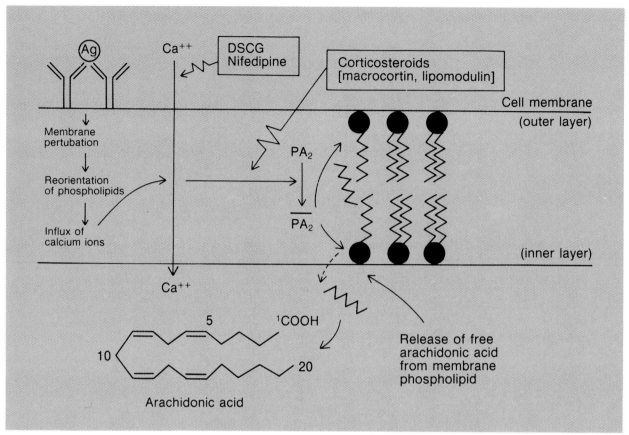

Fig. 4.3. Membrane events leading to the release of free arachidonic acid initiated as a result of membrane perturbation by antigen and IgE.

contraction at picomolar concentrations whereas the dihydroxy derivative, LTB$_4$, is a potent chemotactic agent (Ford-Hutchinson et al., 1980; Nagy et al., 1982a).

The prostaglandins also have a number of effects on bronchial smooth muscle (reviewed by Goetzl and Kay, in press). PGD$_2$, PGF$_2$ and thromboxaone A$_2$ constrict whereas PGE$_2$ has weak dilatory effects. Prostaglandins also affect the microvasculature. For instance, PGD$_2$, PGE$_2$ and PGI$_2$ augment the properties of histamine and bradykinin. Prostaglandins, especially PGD$_2$ and PGF$_2$, increase secretion of submucosal glands and are chemokinetic for neutrophils and eosinophils.

Thus the mast cell-derived mediators have a variety of biological activities as well as being diverse in their chemical structure. They also vary in their time of onset and duration of action. Histamine, for example, gives a short brisk contraction of human lung smooth muscle *in vitro* whereas the SRS-A leukotrienes cause a prolonged sustained response (Hanna et al., 1981).

Pharmacological Mediators in Relation to the Pathogenesis of Asthma

Many of the features of bronchial asthma can be explained on the basis of the known biological activities of mast cell-derived mediators. In figure 4.4 an attempt has been made to link certain clinical manifestations with pharmacological and pathological alterations. It is suggested that the events associated with obstruction of the bronchi may be divided into three main phases. These have been termed (1) a rapid, spasmogenic phase, (2) a late, sus-

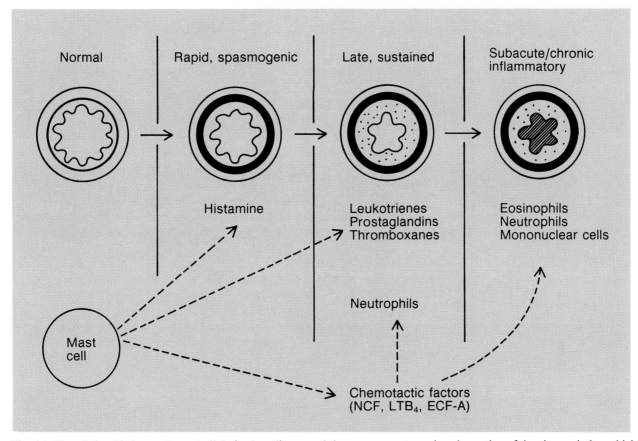

Fig. 4.4. The relationship between mast cell-derived mediators and the events accompanying obstruction of the airways in bronchial asthma.

tained phase and (3) a subacute/chronic inflammatory phase. The phases might act in sequence following the initial release of mast cell-derived agents as a result of IgE/allergen interaction or non-immunological triggers such as exercise, infection or complement activation (fig. 4.4).

Rapid, Spasmogenic Phase

When asthmatic patients are subjected to allergen challenge, an exercise task or inhalation of a nonspecific irritant such as sulphur dioxide there is an increase in airways resistance which is rapid (10-15 min) in onset. Such reactions are readily reversible, either spontaneously or by bronchodilators such as β_2-sympathomimetics. A rise in plasma histamine and NCF can also be demonstrated and the time-course parallels the changes in airways resistance (Lee et al., 1982a). As discussed above, this rapid phase is probably mediated largely through histamine acting either directly on smooth muscle or via vagal reflexes. It can be inhibited by prior administration of sodium cromoglycate, salbutamol or by histamine H_1- and H_2-receptor antagonists. This rapid increase is not affected by corticosteroids given immediately before challenge.

Late, Sustained Phase

Following bronchial challenge with specific allergen many subjects have a second, usually more severe, rise in airways resistance which is maximal 6 to 8 hours following exposure (Pepys et al., 1968). Compared with the rapid, spasmogenic phase this late reaction is slower in onset and more sustained.

The pathogenesis of late reactions is incompletely understood. There is probably some bronchial infiltration by neutrophils since, at least in human skin, IgE-dependent responses are associated with neutrophil accumulation 4 to 8 hours following antigen challenge (Dolovich et al., 1973). It was originally proposed that the late reaction was an example of a type III, or Arthus, response with neutrophil infiltration resulting from the generation of chemotactic factors following activation of complement by immune complexes. Recent evidence suggests that late reactions might be associated with re-activation of mast cells since there is also a late, sustained rise in the concentration of circulating serum NCF (Nagy et al., 1982b).

It is also possible that leukotrienes, prostaglandins and thromboxanes play a role in the late reactions as these mediators tend to have sustained biological effects and might, for instance, cause prolonged contraction of bronchial smooth muscle together with oedema of the submucosa as a result of their effects on the microvasculature. Furthermore, late reactions are inhibited by prior administration of corticosteroids (Pepys and Hutchcroft, 1975). As discussed below, one of the actions of corticosteroids is to prevent (via macrocortin) the release of free arachidonic acid which, in turn, inhibits the subsequent formation of the potent pharmacological lipid mediators.

Subacute/Chronic Inflammatory Phase

Continuing asthma in the untreated or partially controlled patient is likely to be associated, to a greater or lesser degree, with a substantial inflammatory reaction in and around the bronchi. As described above, infiltration of the bronchi with large numbers of eosinophils and mononuclear cells are characteristic findings at autopsy. Eosinophils and mononuclear cells might be recruited by mast cell-derived chemotactic factors such as ECF-A and leukotriene B_4. Eosinophils especially might contribute to tissue damage as a result of release of the basic proteins derived from their crystalloid granules. These include the eosinophil cationic protein and the major basic protein, both of which are known to be cytotoxic for a number of cell types and, in experimental animals, produce shedding of the respiratory epithelium (Gleich et al., 1979).

Continuing asthma is usually, although not invariably, responsive to corticosteroids. Corticosteroid-resistant asthma is a serious clinical problem and many of the features of these individuals have recently been described in detail (Carmichael et al., 1981). These patients have a defect in monocyte membrane markers for complement (Kay et al., 1981) indicating that cells of the monocyte/macrophage series, or other leucocytes, might have pro-inflammatory effects in bronchial asthma. Unlike cells from normal subjects and corticosteroid-responsive asthmatics, monocytes from resistant asthmatics do not respond to oral prednisolone with a diminution in complement receptor density indicating that they may have a greater potential for adherence and subsequently lysosomal enzyme release.

Plugging of the bronchial lumen with thick tenacious mucus, cells and cell debris, is a consistent finding at post mortem in asthma. Arachidonic acid products might also contribute to these events by increasing mucus secretion of already hypertrophied submucosal glands (Marom et al., 1981).

Thus mast cell mediators have the capacity to induce directly both the rapid and the late phases of bronchial obstruction. They may also play a role in perpetuating the asthmatic state by the recruitment of secondary inflammatory cells.

Trigger Factors in Asthma

It is well known that the asthma attack can be triggered by a number of mechanisms (see Chapter V) and an appreciation of the multiplicity of initiating events is central to our understanding of the asthmatic process. It is certain from clinical and experimental work that IgE-mediated mechanisms play an important role for many patients but there is now evidence that non-immunological stimuli, such as exercise, can lead to mast cell degranulation in asthmatic individuals. For instance, histamine and NCF have been detected in the circulation of asthmatic subjects following a treadmill exercise task and the release of these agents can be blocked by prior administration of sodium cromoglycate. The mechanism of exercise-induced mast cell degranulation is unknown but it is possible that these cells are unduly 'fragile' and respond more vigorously to trauma or local changes in osmolarity. Similarly, nonspecific stimuli can lead to the generation of complement fragments which trigger mast cells for the release of pre-formed and membrane-derived mediators. For example, plicatic acid, a major component of red cedar wood dust, activates the alternative pathway of complement (Chan-Yeung et al., 1980). Asthma in association with exposure to red cedar wood dust is a common problem in parts of North America. It is also known that certain external agents such as isocyanates and colophony fumes induce asthma in susceptible individuals by mechanisms which are unlikely to be dependent on IgE.

Atopy and the Role of IgE

Common environmental inhaled allergens are particularly important to the induction of asthma. In the United Kingdom the house dust mite (*Dermatophagoides pteronyssinus*) is thought to play a major role in the initiation and potentiation of asthma and rhinitis in sensitised subjects (Chapman and Platts-Mills, 1980; Tovey et al., 1981). Other common allergens include grass and tree pollens and various animal danders, particularly cats, horses and laboratory animals (these problems are dealt with in detail elsewhere – Chapter V). Allergens have certain characteristics. For instance, they usually have a molecular weight of about 20,000, are proteins or glycoproteins and are fairly large, i.e. between 12 to 25 microns. They are deposited largely in the upper airways. Allergens do not seem to have a particular chemical structure and it is probable that their accessibility to antibody forming cells is a more important factor than unique antigenic determinants. The sites of IgE formation are predominantly in the upper airways.

The contribution of specific allergen to the clinical features in an individual patient are usually suspected from the clinical history. For instance, house dust mite-induced asthma is often associated with symptoms of rhinitis and is precipitated by activities such as bedmaking and in relation to old, dusty or damp premises, where there is high prevalence of *D. pteronyssinus*. Asthma features which are seasonal and correspond with the grass pollen season, or less commonly to high tree pollen counts, are usually obvious, as are contacts with animals such as cats and horses. The diagnosis of allergen-induced, IgE-mediated asthma has to be substantiated by a positive skin prick test, and if this is not possible, a radio-allergosorbent-test (RAST) test using the appropriate allergen. Other allergens such as moulds and foods are sometimes important factors in individual patients. It is important to stress that allergy may be the trigger for asthma attacks for a relatively short part of the natural history of the disease. Allergen-induced asthma is more common in childhood but subjects may either 'grow out' of their wheeziness or proceed to a more chronic form of the disease in which allergy seems to become less and less important.

The contribution of atopy and the atopic state to asthma has given rise to some confusion. An atopic individual is one who gives a positive immediate skin prick test to common inhalant allergens regardless of whether symptoms are present. In the UK an atopic individual usually reacts to one or more of the following allergens: mixed grass pollens, the house dust mite, cat fur and *Aspergillus fumigatus*. Atopic persons tend to have raised serum IgE concentrations, but not invariably so. Although it is recognised that atopics have a tendency to develop various clinical syndromes such as asthma, hay fever and eczema, the demonstration of immediate skin responses in a single individual is not, by itself, particularly helpful in the identification of triggering factors. For instance, it is known that 10 to 20% of the population react in this way but only 1 to 5% have asthma symptoms. Although there is a clear link between asthma and the atopic state, genetic studies suggest that atopy and asthma are inherited independently but that the inheritance of atopy, in many subjects, increases the expression of clinical asthma (Sibbald et al., 1980a, b). Thus the presence of atopy does not necessarily imply that this is directly or causally associated with all of the asthmatic symptoms developing in a single individual. Generally speaking, allergy often plays an important role in young, atopic episodic asthmatics and this will usually be obvious from the clear clinical history supported by positive skin tests. On the other hand, the role of allergens and atopy in chronic asthma is far less clear since these patients rarely give a clear history of allergen-induced wheeze, may or may not have positive skin tests and the positive skin tests themselves, if present, often bear little relation to triggering factors as judged by the clinical history.

Measurements of total serum IgE concentrations are of little use in the day to day management of asthma. On the other hand, a low total IgE, i.e. less than 50 IU/ml, may be helpful evidence against an allergic basis for the disease. The range of IgE levels found in normal healthy non-atopic individuals is <0.1 to 150 IU/ml. The range of IgE levels found in clinical practice is very wide and is sometimes greater than 30,000 IU/ml. These high values are rarely seen in bronchial asthma unless they are accompanied by other conditions such as atopic dermatitis or helminthic disease.

There has been considerable interest over the past few years in antibodies other than IgE which might sensitise mast cells for the release of chemical mediators. Some investigators have reported that sera from certain allergic individuals contain a heat stable, short term sensitising IgG (STS-IgG) and it has been suggested that this immunoglobulin belongs to the IgG_4 subclass (Gwynn et al., 1982). There is other evidence, however, which indicates that IgG_4 antibodies are part of the normal immune response to various antigens (van Toorenebergen and Aalberse, 1981) and efforts to isolate and characterise STS-IgG have so far been unsuccessful.

At present, other immunological tests such as RAST, *in vitro* histamine release from leucocytes and complement profiles appear to be of little, if any, value in the management and diagnosis of bronchial asthma.

The Role of Challenge Tests in Asthma Management

Although the many forms of challenge test have increased considerably our understanding of the pathogenesis of asthma and the mode of action of various drugs used in its treatment, these procedures have a limited place in its routine diagnosis and management. As stated, the contribution of common inhalants such as the house dust mite, grass pollens and animal danders to the aetiology of the disease in an individual patient is obvious from a clear clinical history and positive skin prick tests. Very occasionally, the true nature of a common environmental allergen has to be established by the use of bronchial provocation tests but this is rarely indicated.

In contrast, bronchial challenge tests are often very useful in identifying a causative agent in various forms of occupational asthma. This is because in many instances a number of agents could be incriminated in a given environment and skin prick tests to the suspected allergen are often negative. Occupational and other environmental factors implicated in bronchial asthma are discussed in Chapter V.

Challenge tests can also be useful in the field of food-induced wheeze especially where skin tests and RAST are negative. In many individuals a diagnosis of food-induced wheeze, which is very suggestive from the clinical history, can be confirmed by skin prick tests and RAST tests and the patient often improves with the appropriate elimination diet. On the other hand, a number of patients appear to have IgE independent food-induced bronchospasm which can only be satisfactorily documented by an appropriate 'blind' study under hospital conditions (Papageorgiou et al., in press). Furthermore, these patients can be protected by oral sodium cromoglycate or oral beclomethasone dipropionate if elimination diets prove difficult or unsatisfactory.

Therapeutic Implications

It has already been stated that although mast cells may play a central role in the initiation of the asthmatic response, the triggering of mast cells by IgE and specific allergen probably plays a limited part in the disease overall. Nevertheless, in the few cases where an allergen is a clear, major precipitating factor the general principles for the treatment of allergic diseases should be observed. These include allergen avoidance (which to a large extent is self-explanatory but in practice often very difficult), desensitisation (which should only be considered in very special circumstances and when one, or at the most, two allergens are incriminated) and anti-allergic drugs. The term 'anti-allergic drugs' is misleading since it implies that if a particular compound is beneficial then the disease necessarily has an allergic basis. For instance, sodium cromoglycate prevents exercise- as well as antigen-induced airways obstruction and whilst part of its mode of action is associated with mast cells and the inhibition of mast cell-derived mediators, it probably has other equally important actions, such as inhibition of vagal reflexes and reversal of bronchial hyper-reactivity.

The mode of action of many compounds used in the treatment of bronchial asthma is incompletely understood. Nevertheless, an attempt has been made to relate the various biochemical pathways discussed above to the mode of action of drugs which either have an established place in the treatment of asthma (such as sodium cromoglycate and corticosteroids) or which have potential because of their known mode of action (fig. 4.5).

Calcium Antagonists and Cromoglycate

Drugs such as verapamil or nifedipine which are calcium antagonists, partially inhibit exercise-induced bronchospasm (Patel, 1981). They may act by reducing smooth muscle responsiveness but in high concentrations verapamil also inhibits SRS-A release (Butchers et al., 1981). Sodium cromoglycate also inhibits calcium flux in certain *in vitro* systems (Foreman and Garland, 1976) and part of its mode of action might be explained by its ability to prevent indirectly the activation of phospholipase A_2 and subsequent arachidonic acid metabolism. This view is supported by *in vitro*

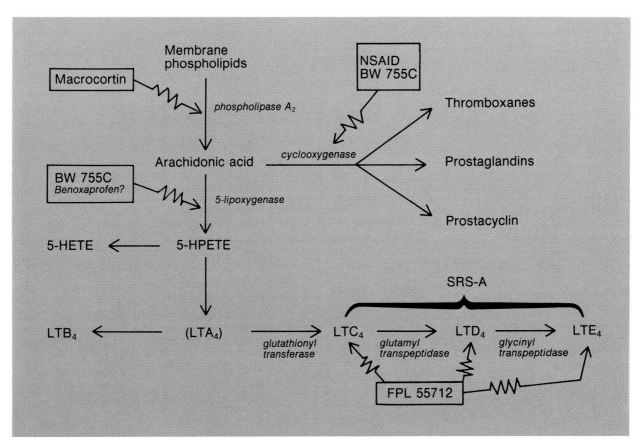

Fig. 4.5. Pathways of arachidonic acid metabolism and the sites of action of various inhibitors and antagonists. See text for description of experimental compounds.

experiments in which cromoglycate was shown to reduce the amount of SRS-A released by sensitised human lung fragments after exposure to specific antigen (Dawson and Tomlinson, 1974).

Corticosteroids

Despite the usefulness of cromoglycate-like drugs and bronchodilators in the relief and prevention of asthma, corticosteroids are the mainstay of therapy in moderate to severe disease. Although the precise modes of action of corticosteroids remain incompletely understood, it is now realised that many of their actions might be explained by their ability to generate certain newly synthesised proteins which inhibit the action of phospholipase A_2. One of these, macrocortin, has been shown to be a 15,000 molecular weight, acid resistant, protease sensitive, heat resistant, protein (Blackwell et al., 1980). Another, termed lipomodulin, has a molecular weight of 40,000 (Hirata et al., 1981). Thus macrocortin and lipomodulin, by inhibiting phospholipase A_2 prevent the formation of leukotrienes, prostaglandins, thromboxanes, and other metabolites of arachidonic acid. Other actions of corticosteroids which are relevant to bronchial asthma include eosinophilopoeisis, inhibition of eosinophil chemotaxis, inhibition of neutrophil chemotaxis and the release of lysosomal enzymes. Whether these actions are dependent on the generation of new proteins such as macrocortin is yet to be established. Therefore, corticosteroids might dampen, or abolish, the generation of membrane-derived mediators as well as preventing the influx of neutrophils, eosinophils and possibly other leucocytes.

Benoxaprofen and Experimental Compounds

Drugs which inhibit the metabolism of arachidonic acid, either by the lipoxygenase or cyclo-oxygenase pathways or compounds which are specific antagonists of the SRS-A leukotrienes are of considerable theoretical interest but at the present time have no place in therapy. Benoxaprofen is a non-steroidal anti-inflammatory drug which has been used as an anti-arthritic agent although, in the UK, its product licence has recently been suspended. In certain animal models it is a potent inhibitor of lipoxygenase enzymes, but has relatively weak effects on cyclo-oxygenase pathways (Walker et al., 1980). BW755C is an experimental drug which inhibits both the lipoxygenase and cyclo-oxygenase pathways, thus preventing the synthesis of both prostaglandins and leukotrienes (Walker et al., 1980). FPL 55712 is a specific antagonist of the leukotrienes LTC_4 and LTD_4, probably acting by competitive antagonism (Sheard et al., 1982). It is not absorbed orally and has a very short half-life. A small open trial showed a minimum degree of improvement when FPL 55712 was administered by aerosol to patients with severe asthma (Lee et al., 1981). A new product, FPL 59257, is orally active and has a longer pharmacological half-life (Sheard et al., 1982).

In Summary

Mast cells probably play a central role in the pathogenesis of asthma. The mechanism of release of potent mast cell-derived mediators may be specific (i.e. immunological) or nonspecific. Chemical mediators are either preformed within granules or generated from membrane-bound phospholipids. The immediate spasmogenic effect is largely the result of histamine release acting directly on bronchial tissue or indirectly through reflexes. Mediators also recruit secondary inflammatory cells and this is probably particularly important in late reactions and continuing asthma. Although the inheritance of atopy increases the expression of clinical asthma, atopy and asthma are inherited independently. Challenge tests play a limited role in the diagnosis of bronchial asthma but they have contributed considerably to our understanding of the pathogenesis of the disease. A number of chemical compounds with therapeutic potential are now available which either prevent the formation of mast cell-derived agents or inhibit their action.

References

Ackerman, S.J.; Gleich, G.J.; Weller, P.F. and Ottesen, E.A.: Eosinophilia and elevated serum levels of eosinophil major basic protein and Charcot-Leyden crystal protein (lysophospholipase) after treatment of patients with Bancroft's filariasis. Journal of Immunology 127: 1093 (1981).

Ackerman, S.J.; Leogering, D.A. and Gleich, G.J.: The human eosinophil Charcot-Leyden crystal protein: biochemical characteristics and measurement by radioimmunoassay. Journal of Immunology 125: 2118 (1980).

Anwar, A.R.E. and Kay, A.B.: The ECF-A tetrapeptides and histamine selectively enhance human eosinophil complement receptors. Nature 269: 522 (1977).

Atkins, P.C.; Norman, M.; Weiner, H. and Zweiman, B.: Release of neutrophil chemotactic activity during immediate hypersensitivity reactions in humans. Annals of Internal Medicine 86: 415 (1977).

Barnes, P.J. and Brown, M.J.: Venous plasma histamine in exercise and hyperventilation-induced asthma in man. Clinical Science 61: 159 (1981).

Blackwell, G.J.; Carnuccio, R.; Di Rosa, M.; Flower, R.J.; Parente, L. and Persico, P.: Macrocortin: a polypeptide causing the anti-phospholipase effect of glucocorticoids. Nature 287: 147 (1980).

Bryant, D.H. and Kay, A.B.: Cutaneous eosinophil accumulation in atopic and non-atopic individuals: the effect of an ECF-A tetrapeptide and histamine. Clinical Allergy 7: 211 (1977).

Butchers, P.R.; Fullarton, J.R.; Skidmore, L.E.; Thompson, L.E.; Vardey, C.J. and Wheeldon, A.: A comparison of the anti-anaphylactic activities of salbutamol, disodium cromoglycate in the rat, the rat mast cell and in human lung tissue. British Journal of Pharmacology 67: 23 (1979).

Butchers, P.R.; Skidmore, I.F.; Vardey, C.J. and Wheeldon, A.: Calcium antagonists in exercise-induced asthma. British Medical Journal 282: 1792 (1981).

Carmichael, J.; Paterson, I.C.; Diaz, P.; Crompton, G.K.; Kay, A.B. and Grant, I.W.B.: Corticosteroid-resistance in chronic asthma. British Medical Journal 282: 1419 (1981).

Chan-Yeung, M.; Giclas, P.C. and Henson, P.M.: Activation of complement by plicatic acid, the chemical compound responsible for asthma due to western red cedar (*Thuja plicata*). Journal of Allergy and Clinical Immunology 65: 333 (1980).

Chapman, M.D. and Platts-Mills, T.A.E.: Purification and characterisation of the major allergen from *Dermatophagoides pteronyssinus* antigen. Journal of Immunology 125: 587 (1980).

Cutz, E. and Orange, R.P.: Mast cells and endocrine (APUD) cells of the lung; in Lichtenstein and Austen (Eds) Asthma: Physiology, Immunopharmacology, and Treatment, p. 51 (Academic Press, New York 1977).

Dawson, W. and Tomlinson, R.: Effects of cromoglycate and ETYA on release of prostaglandins and SRS-A from immune challenged guinea pig lung. British Journal of Pharmacology 52: 107P (1974).

Dolovich, J.; Hargreave, F.E.; Chalmers, R.; Shier, K.J.; Gauldis, J. and Bienenstock, J.: Late cutaneous allergic reactions in isolated IgE-dependent reactions. Journal of Allergy and Clinical Immunology 52: 38 (1973).

Dunnill, M.S.: The pathology of asthma; in Porter and Birch (Eds) Identification of Asthma. CIBA Foundation Study Group 38, p. 35 (Livingstone, Edinburgh 1971).

Eiser, N.M.; Mills, J.; Snashall, P.D. and Guz, A.: The role of histamine receptors in asthma. Clinical Science 60: 363 (1981).

Ford-Hutchinson, A.W.; Bray, M.A.; Doig, M.V.; Shipley, M.E. and Smith, M.J.H.: Leukotriene B_4, a potent chemotactic and aggregating substance released from polymorphonuclear leukocytes. Nature 286: 264 (1980).

Foreman, J.C. and Garland, L.G.: Cromoglycate and other antiallergic drugs: a possible mechanism of action. British Medical Journal 1: 820 (1976).

Gleich, G.J.; Frigas, E.; Loegering, D.A.; Wassom, D.L. and Steinmuller, D.: Cytotoxic properties of the eosinophil major basic protein. Journal of Immunology 123: 2925 (1979).

Goetzl, E.J.: Mediators of immediate hypersensitivity derived from arachidonic acid. New England Journal of Medicine 303: 822 (1980).

Goetzl, E.J. and Kay, A.B.: Humoral and cellular components of human allergic reactions; in Goetzl and Kay (Eds) Current Perspectives in Allergy, p.1 (Churchill Livingstone, Edinburgh, 1982).

Gwynn, C.M.; Ingram, J.; Almousawi, T. and Stanworth, D.R.: Bronchial provocation tests in atopic patients with allergen-specific IgG$_4$ antibodies. Lancet 1: 254 (1982).

Hanna, C.J.; Bach, M.K.; Pare, P.D. and Schellenberg, R.R.: Slow reacting substances (leukotrienes) contract human airway and pulmonary vascular smooth muscle *in vitro*. Nature 290: 343 (1981).

Hastie, R.; Heroy, J.H. and Levy, D.: Basophil leucocytes and mast cells in human nasal secretions and scrapings studied by light microscopy. Laboratory Investigation 40: 554 (1979).

Hirata, F.; Del Carmine, R.; Nelson, C.A.; Axelrod, J.; Schiffman, E.; Warabi, A.; De Blas, A.L.; Nirenberg, M.; Manganiello, V.; Vaughan, M.; Kumagi, S.; Green, I.; Decker, J.L. and Steinberg, A.D.: Presence of autoantibody for phospholipase inhibitory protein, lipomodulin, in patients with rheumatic diseases. Proceedings of the National Academy of Sciences USA 78: 3190 (1981).

Ishizaka, T.; Hirata, F.; Ishizaka, K. and Axelrod, J.: Stimulation of phospholipid methylation, Ca^{2+} influx and histamine release by binding of IgE receptors on rat mast cells. Proceedings of the National Academy of Sciences, USA 77: 1903 (1980).

Kay, A.B.: Studies on eosinophil leucocyte migration. II. Factors specifically chemotactic for eosinophils and neutrophils generated from guinea-pig serum by antigen-antibody complexes. Clinical and Experimental Immunology 7: 723 (1970).

Kay, A.B.: Basophils and mast cells: function and role in inflammation; in Venge and Lindbom (Eds) The Inflammatory Process, p. 293 (Almquist and Wiksell International, Stockholm 1981).

Kay, A.B.; Diaz, P.; Carmichael, J. and Grant, I.W.B.: Corticosteroid-resistant chronic asthma and monocyte complement receptors. Clinical and Experimental Immunology 44: 576 (1981).

Lee, T.H.; Walport, M.J.; Wilkinson, A.H.; Turner-Warwick, M. and Kay, A.B.: The SRS-A antagonist (FPL 55712) in chronic asthma. Lancet 2: 304 (1981).

Lee, T.H.; Brown, M.J.; Nagy, L.; Causon, R.; Walport, M.J. and Kay, A.B.: Exercise-induced release of histamine and neutrophil chemotactic factors in atopic asthmatics. Journal of Allergy and Clinical Immunology 70: 73 (1982a).

Lee, T.H.; Nagy, L.; Nagakura, T.; Walport, M.J. and Kay, A.B.: The identification and partial characterisation of an exercise-induced neutrophil chemotactic factor in bronchial asthma. Journal of Clinical Investigation 69: 889 (1982b).

McLaren, K.; Holloway, L. and Pepper, D.S.: Human platelet factor 4 and tissue mast cells. Thrombosis Research 19: 293 (1980).

Marom, Z.; Shelhamer, J.H. and Kaliner, M.: Effects of arachidonic acid, monohydroxyeicosatetraenoic acid and prostaglandins on the release of mucous glycoproteins from human airways *in vitro*. Journal of Clinical Investigation 67: 1695 (1981).

Murphy, R.C.; Hammarstrom, S. and Samuelsson, B.: Leukotriene C: a slow reacting substance from murine mastocytoma cells. Proceedings of the National Academy of Sciences USA 76: 4275 (1979).

Nagy, L.; Lee, T.H.; Goetzl, E.J.; Pickett, W.C. and Kay, A.B.: Complement receptor enhancement and chemotaxis of human neutrophils and eosinophils by leukotrienes and other lipoxygenase products. Clinical and Experimental Immunology 47: 541 (1982a).

Nagy, L.; Lee, T.H. and Kay, A.B.: Neutrophil chemotactic activity in antigen-induced late asthmatic reactions. New England Journal of Medicine 306: 497 (1982b).

O'Driscoll, B.R.C. and Kay, A.B.: Leukotrienes and lung disease. Thorax 37: 241 (1982).

Papageorgiou, N.; Lee, T.H.; Nagakura, T.; Wraith, D.G. and Kay, A.B.: Inhibition of food-induced asthma by oral disodium cromoglycate. Submitted for publication.

Patel, K.R.: Calcium antagonists in exercise-induced asthma. British Medical Journal 282: 932 (1981).

Pepys, J. and Hutchcroft, B.J.: Bronchial provocation tests in etiologic diagnosis and analysis of asthma. American Review of Respiratory Diseases 112: 829 (1975).

Pepys, J.; Hargreave, F.E.; Chan, M. and McCarthy, D.S.: Inhibitory effects of disodium cromoglycate on allergen inhalation tests. Lancet 2: 134 (1968).

Schulman, E.S.; MacGlashan, D.W.; Peters, S.P.; Schleimer, R.P.; Lichtenstein, L.M. and Newball, H.H.: Purification and characterization of human lung mast cells. Federation Proceedings 41: Abstr. 628. 377 (1982).

Schwartz, L.B.; Austen, K.F. and Wasserman, S.I.: Immunologic release of beta-glucuronidase from purified rat serosal mast cells. Journal of Immunology 123: 1445 (1979).

Sheard, P.; Bantick, J.R.; Holroyde, M.C. and Lee, T.B.: Antagonists of SRS-A and leukotrienes; in Samuelsson and Paoletti (Eds) Proceedings of the Symposium on Leukotrienes and Other Lipoxygenase Products (Raven Press, New York 1982).

Sibbald, B.; Horn, M.E.C.; Brain, E.A. and Gregg, I.: Genetic factors in childhood asthma. Thorax 35: 671 (1980a).

Sibbald, B.; Horn, M.E.C. and Gregg, I.: A family study of the genetic basis of asthma and wheezy bronchitis. Archives of Disease in Childhood 55: 354 (1980b).

Simani, A.S.; Inoue, S. and Hogg, J.C.: Intracellular junctions of the tracheal epithelium in guinea pigs. Laboratory Investigation 31: 68 (1974).

Tovey, E.R.; Chapman, M.D.; Wells, C.W. and Platts-Mills, T.A.E.: The distribution of dust mite allergen in the houses of patients with asthma. American Review of Respiratory Diseases 124: 630 (1981).

Van Toorenenbergen, A.E. and Aalberse, R.C.: IgG$_4$ and passive sensitization of basophil leukocytes. International Archives of Allergy and Applied Immunology 65: 432 (1981).

Walker, J.R.; Booth, J.R.; Cox, B. and Dawson, W.: Inhibition of the release of slow reacting substance of anaphylaxis by inhibitors of lipoxygenase activity. Journal of Pharmacy and Pharmacology 32: 866 (1980).

Chapter V

Trigger Factors in Asthma

P. Sherwood Burge

The current concept of asthma is of hyper-reactive bronchi with, in many patients, specific triggers mediated by IgE antibodies. Some nonspecific triggers of asthma are present in virtually all asthmatics, the most common being respiratory infections and exercise. Specific triggers are present in the great majority of younger asthmatics but are less common in asthma developing in middle age. Specific IgE (or short term sensitising IgG) antibodies are, in general, not enough to cause asthma without co-existing bronchial hyper-reactivity. This chapter deals with nonspecific triggers of asthma, and then the more important specific triggers with the aim of providing a basis for the taking of a useful medical history from asthmatic patients.

Exercise

Most asthmatics have a deterioration in their asthma triggered by exercise, provided that the exercise is hard enough (p.18). The exercise required varies from walking slowly for some patients, to sustained hard running for others. Sustained exercise for about 6 minutes is more likely to provoke asthma than exercise broken up into short 1 to 2 minute episodes. The asthma may come on during exercise but more commonly starts immediately afterwards, and lasts for 15 to 60 minutes. The occasional patient develops a late asthmatic reaction, starting more than one hour after the exercise, but such reactions are uncommon. Sometimes exercise induced asthma is only a problem during cold, damp weather. Both cold, dry air (McFadden, 1981) and the inhalation of ultrasonically nebulised water (Schoeffel et al., 1981) can induce asthma independently of exercise, and both are likely to be important contributors to exercise induced asthma.

Swimming causes less asthma than running, perhaps because the air in swimming pools is warm and fully saturated with water vapour. There are, however, a few swimmers who have asthma for the first time after swimming in pools which have been overtreated with chlorine, which can induce nonspecific bronchial hyper-reactivity (Pickering and Mustchin, 1979).

Respiratory Infections

Respiratory infections are one of the most common factors provoking severe asthmatic attacks, accounting for about two-thirds of severe attacks in children and about one-third in adults (Lambert and Stern, 1972). Viruses account for the great majority of these infections; there is little evidence that bacterial infection is relevant. In a prospective study of children with asthma, Minor et al. (1974) found that 42/61 episodes of asthma were precipitated by symptoms of respiratory tract infection and in 35 of these infection was confirmed by laboratory tests. The more severe the virus infection the more likely asthma was to result from it. Most of the attacks were related to rhinovirus infection. Other identified viruses have included influenza, parainfluenza, adenovirus, respiratory syncitial virus and mycoplasma infections. The situation with adults is less well documented. Gregg (1975) found that less than 10% of previously healthy adults developed wheeze during rhinovirus infection whereas in an asthmatic group over 80% wheezed with a similar infection. In a recent study of adults admitted to hospital with acute asthma without other obvious precipitating factors (such as reduction in treatment), 37% said that they had had a recent upper respiratory infection and a further 23% possible upper respiratory infection (Jones, D.; personal communication). Positive virus isolation was only achieved in about one-third of those with a history of respiratory infection; however, it is more difficult to isolate viruses from adults than children. All those with a proven viral infection had a short history of deterioration before admission (usually less than 5 days). During the study there was an outbreak of influenza A2/Texas infection in the ward which affected 7 of the previously admitted asthmatics. The

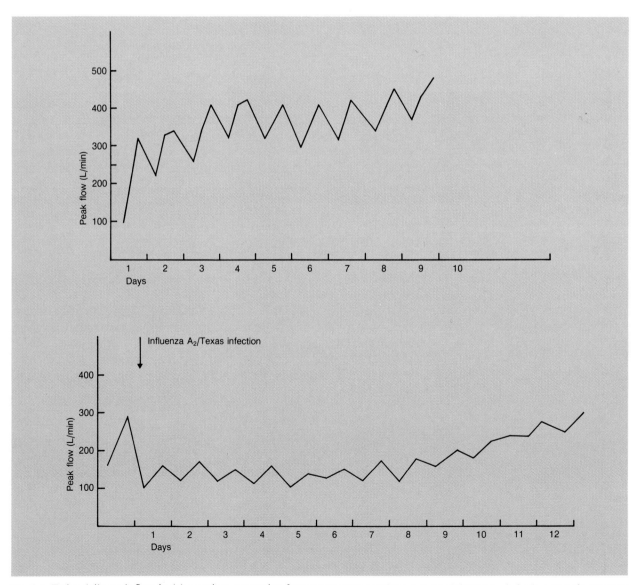

Fig. 5.1. Twice daily peak flow in (*a*) a patient recovering from acute severe asthma not precipitated by infection and (*b*) recovery in a patient developing influenza A2/Texas infection in hospital. (The figure was kindly supplied by Dr Dai Jones.)

pattern of recovery appeared to be different in these 7 from that in those without virus infection (fig. 5.1). Those with proven virus infection showed a slower recovery (mean 10.7 days) compared with the others in whom the mean period was 4.9 days. Also, during the recovery phase, the diurnal swings in peak flow were much reduced in the infected group.

Psychological Triggers

The role of psychological factors in asthma has been reviewed recently by Matus (1981). There used to be a widely held view that asthma was a disease of the mind, and that controlling an asthmatic's emotional behaviour could abolish the asthma. This view led to the patient being blamed for his disease and called a failure if the asthma remained. It was also associated with considerable under-treatment with drugs. Although this psychosomatic theory of asthma is no longer believed by most doctors, it is still widely held by patients. It is now clear that psychological abnormalities and stress are not enough on their own to cause asthma; in a patient with pre-existing asthma, however, psychological factors may make the asthma worse. Asthmatic attacks can be very frightening, causing considerable difficulty in separating stressful stimuli which provoke attacks from stress induced by an asthmatic attack precipitated by other factors.

There is an excess of psychopathic and inadequate patients amongst severe asthmatics. These patients are often the most difficult to treat because they are unable or unwilling to take prescribed treatment, they frequently miss clinic appointments and run out of medication. There is no evidence that their psychopathology is a cause of their asthma, although it certainly adds to the difficulties of treating it. Some patients have voluntary control of their airway calibre and can induce asthmatic attacks at will.

The role of suggestion has been investigated in interesting double-blind studies using deception (Luparello et al., 1970). Isoprenaline and carbachol were given by inhalation to 20 asthmatics; each drug was given twice, on one occasion the patient being told it was a bronchodilator, and on the other occasion a bronchoconstrictor. Suggestion of bronchodilatation caused greater improvement with isoprenaline and less deterioration with carbachol than when bronchoconstriction was suggested. Other studies have shown that the effects of suggestion can be blocked by intravenous atropine, indicating that suggestion is working via the vagal pathways (McFadden et al., 1969).

In childhood the psychopathology of the parents may be more important than that of the child. Some parents need to keep their children ill. There are a number of studies showing improvement in childhood asthma when the child is taken to a residential school. Many will receive better medication in the schools, which could account for the improvement. The most interesting study was carried out in Denver where asthmatic children were left at home with a foster parent while the parents were removed to a motel for 2 weeks (Purcell et al., 1969). Pets and other sources of allergen at home remained largely unchanged. The children were divided (by an unspecified assessment) into those in whom emotional factors appeared clinically highly relevant to their asthma, and those in whom emotional problems were thought to be less relevant. There was improvement in the first group but not in the second. Unfortunately the design of this experiment is open to criticism. It is unclear on what grounds allocation to the groups was decided and whether the assigning was done before or after the parents were removed. The results could be interpreted as half the children randomly improving.

In summary, there are a number of asthmatics who spontaneously suggest stressful periods as times when their asthma is worse. The balance of evidence points to stress as an aggravating factor, but not as the cause of the asthma. When the asthma is controlled medically the psychological problems usually improve.

Menstruation and Pregnancy

About one-third of women have deterioration of their asthma with, or just before their periods (Hanley, 1981). Menstrual deterioration is not affected by taking oral contraceptives. Affected women are of the same age and degree of atopy as those not affected, but have shorter cycle lengths, although the duration of menstruation appears not to differ between the two groups.

Pregnancy may be associated with deterioration or improvement in asthma (Turner et al., 1980). In one prospective study 43% deteriorated during pregnancy (Gluck and Gluck, 1976), a similar proportion to those showing menstrual deterioration. If deterioration occurs it is most likely to start around the fourth month of pregnancy. In general a patient who deteriorates during one pregnancy is likely to deteriorate during the next, while one who improves is also likely to improve during subsequent pregnancies.

Gastro-oesophageal Reflux

There is an established relationship between gastro-oesophageal reflux and asthma but it is not yet clearly documented whether individual episodes of acid reflux are associated with airways obstruction or whether the relationship is less direct. Both medical and surgical treatment of reflux can improve asthma

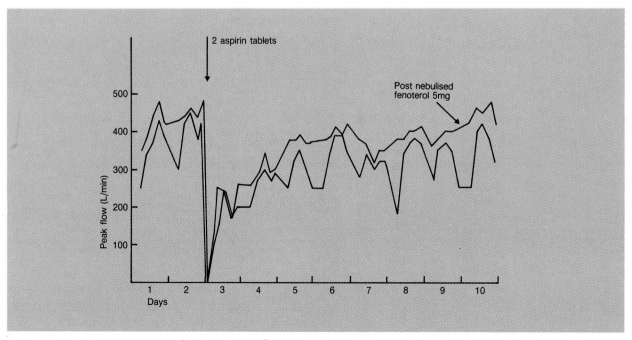

Fig. 5.2. Four-hourly measurements of peak expiratory flow rate before and after bronchodilation. On day 3 of the record the patient took two aspirin tablets to which she was known to be sensitive. She was admitted within 20 minutes, moribund and has not reached her baseline values 8 days later.

(Kjellen et al., 1981). Reflux may be made worse by medical treatment for asthma, particularly by taking oral theophyllines which dilate the lower oesophageal sphincter. These drugs can cause acid reflux even in normal people. A similar situation is at least theoretically possible with oral β_2-adrenergic agonists.

Drug-induced Asthma

Drugs are an important cause of asthma, and enquiry about this possibility should be made in all patients. Salicylates and other non-steroidal anti-inflammatory agents are the most common drugs precipitating asthma. A history of aspirin-induced asthma is obtained in about 2% of adult asthmatics, but challenge testing results in bronchoconstriction in as many as 13% of children and 19% of adults with asthma (Vedanthan et al., 1977; Spector et al., 1979). Some patients show small changes with normal doses of aspirin, while others may develop life threatening asthma after small doses (fig. 5.2). The capacity of analgesic drugs to cause asthma seems to depend on their ability to block the cyclo-oxygenase pathway of arachidonic acid metabolism.

β-Adrenergic blocking drugs are also common precipitators of asthma. Asthma is probably less common following the use of selective β_2-blockers such as atenolol and metoprolol, but nevertheless can be severe even with these drugs. All β-adrenergic blockers may provoke wheeze, even used topically as eye drops, and should be avoided in asthmatics. Important reactions to other drugs are much less common. Some drugs precipitating asthma are shown

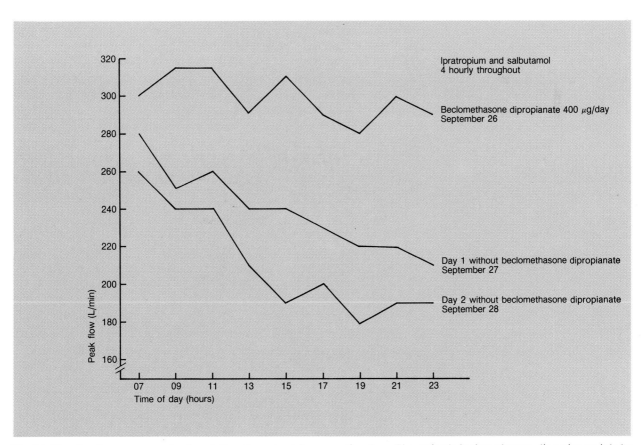

Fig. 5.3. Two-hourly measurements of peak flow throughout 3 consecutive days. The patient's beclomethasone dipropionate inhaler failed to function on the second day resulting in rapid deterioration in his asthma.

Table 5.1. Drugs, diagnostic agents etc. which may cause asthma

Category	Examples
Common causes of asthma	Aspirin and other non-steroidal anti-inflammatory drugs, β-adrenergic blockers
Causes of anaphylactic reactions and associated asthma	Dextrans, iodinated contrast media, penicillin, gamma globulin, desensitising allergen extracts
Rare causes of asthma	Pituitary snuff, quinine and quinidine, pancreozymin and other enzymes, ispaghula, dyes, gums and preservatives in many drugs
Asthma drugs which have themselves caused asthma	Hydrocortisone, methyl prednisolone, ACTH, aminophylline, β_2-agonists, cromoglycate, inhaled corticosteroids, ipratropium bromide

in table 5.1. Drugs liable to cause anaphylactic reactions should be given with care in asthmatics. Acquired hypersensitivity to drugs given orally is uncommon, but may be due to dyes, gums and preservatives which they contain. Allergy initially induced by inhalation of a drug (such as in penicillin manufacturers) may subsequently be provoked by ingesting that drug.

Drugs given in the treatment of asthma can sometimes cause asthma. Although reactions are rare they are important and warrant space here. Inhaled bronchodilators and corticosteroids may induce asthmatic attacks, probably due to the propellants (Bryant and Pepys, 1976) or to material leached from the valve mechanism (Godin and Malo, 1979) rather than the active drugs. Sodium cromoglycate (cromolyn sodium) fairly often causes transitory cough or wheeze, which is prevented by using the compound preparation containing isoprenaline. However, occasionally a severe asthmatic attack can follow its use (Paterson et al., 1976). The reaction is caused by the drug itself and not the lactose filler. Aminophylline may occasionally precipitate asthma and other allergic reactions, due either to the theophylline component or to the ethylenediamine with which it is conjugated (ethylenediamine is not present in anhydrous theophyllines).

ACTH preparations have caused both anaphylactic reactions, with some deaths, and exacerbations of asthma, when used in the treatment of asthma and for other diseases (Forssman et al., 1963). Anaphylactic reactions with accompanying asthma may also occur with hydrocortisone and methyl prednisolone (Mendelson et al., 1974).

Failure to take maintenance treatment for asthma is also an important cause of acute severe asthma, accounting for 10 to 20% of hospital admissions. This may be provoked by the malfunctioning of a pressurised inhaler. An example is shown in figure 5.3.

Air Pollution

The quality of outdoor and indoor air can have major effects on asthmatics. The most important nonspecific pollutants are sulphur dioxide and oxidants. Asthma can be provoked by relatively low concentrations of sulphur dioxide in susceptible individuals. Such levels of sulphur dioxide are found downwind of some smelters, making it very difficult for asthmatics to live there. There is probably also a relationship between asthmatic attacks and levels of photochemical oxidants in the air. This has been studied in the Los Angeles area (Whittemore and Korn, 1980), where air pollution levels were related to symptoms in a group of asthmatics. The best correlation was with days with high oxidant and high particulates; symptoms were also worse on cool days. The sulphur dioxide content of the air was not measured frequently enough to provide figures for this correlation.

The indoor air can be greatly affected by humidifiers either in individual rooms or from central air conditioning units in buildings. Humidifiers classically produce alveolitis or humidifier fever but asthmatic reactions are probably at least as common (fig. 5.7 on p.75). Many humidifiers are grossly contaminated with bacteria, fungi, algae and other organisms. The exact cause of the resulting respiratory disease is unclear but may be related either to endotoxins or to an allergic response to the micro-organisms in the humidifiers.

Many asthmatics are unable to tolerate either smoking themselves or cigarette smoke passively inhaled from others. Cigarette smoke induces transient bronchoconstriction in normal people (Rees et al., 1982); asthmatics sometimes show a much greater and more prolonged bronchoconstriction than normal individuals.

Specific Triggers

Inhaled allergens are the most important specific triggers of asthma. They can be divided into seasonal allergens, mostly derived from plant pollens, and perennial allergens from such sources as the house dust mite, animals and foods. The important inhaled allergens vary greatly in different parts of the world. For instance, in Britain and much of continental Europe house dust mites are the most common cause of inhalant allergy and the most common allergen identified on skin prick testing. In dry, desert areas such as Arizona, they are relatively unimportant, being only the sixth most common cause of positive skin tests, the first 5 all being pollens (Barbee et al., 1976).

Allergen exposure in the first 6 months of life, when immune mechanisms may be poorly functioning, may determine the future pattern of sensitivity. It has been shown that with grass pollens, house dust mites and birch pollens, those who are born shortly before the main season of these allergens are more likely to become sensitised to them subsequently (Björkstén et al., 1980).

As well as the allergens differing, their seasons also vary from place to place. Each physician needs to know his local allergens and their seasons. This chapter will concentrate on allergens important in Britain, mentioning other allergens which are of overriding importance in other parts of the world. For a general guide to aeroallergens (Roth, 1978) and a description of US allergens and their seasons (Solomon and Mathews, 1978) see the Further Reading list at the end of this chapter.

Pollens

Plants are either pollinated by insects or by airborne pollination. Not surprisingly the plants pollinated by insects produce relatively little pollen whereas the plants pollinated by the wind produce vast amounts of pollen and are more relevant to the production of asthma.

Grass Pollens

Most grass pollens have cross-reacting group 1 allergens making a mixed grass pollen extract suitable for skin testing and diagnosis. In dry areas Bermuda grass is prevalent. This does not contain group 1 allergens and requires a specific skin testing extract. Bermuda grass is the most common cause of a positive skin test in Tucson, Arizona. Grass pollens are the traditional causes of hay fever and in Britain are far the most important pollen causing asthma and rhinitis. Their main season is in the spring between May and July. Grass pollen grains are large (15-60 μm) and therefore do not reach the lungs. They may be deposited in the nose, eyes, or oropharynx and it is probable that most of the asthma is triggered by soluble material which leaves the pollen grain rapidly on contact with moisture in the upper respiratory tract.

Tree Pollens

In Britain trees pollinate before grasses and have their main season between February and May, depending on the species. Tree pollen is a less frequent cause of asthma than grass pollen in England but in other parts of the world the situation is the reverse. Birch pollinosis is of major importance in Scandinavia; a major allergen has been identified from birch pollen with a molecular weight of about 20,000 (Belin, 1972). In the Mediterranean littoral olive tree pollen is thought to be the most common cause of pollinosis while in Kuwait there are good studies of the mesquite tree (*Prosopus*), widely planted for their shade when water became more freely available. An extract from the pollen of these trees is the most common cause of positive skin tests and symptoms in those living in Kuwait, accounting for 73% of all positive skin tests (the next most common being Bermuda grass). Mesquite tree pollen affects both indigenous Kuwaitis and immigrants; the mean period of residence before symptoms develop is 6 years. The mesquite tree does not cause widespread pollen contamination, the symptoms occur with fairly close contact with the trees. These findings show how a manmade change of the environment can cause radical alterations in allergens (Al-Awadi, 1973).

Weed Pollens

Weed pollens are an important cause of allergy; the most important weed allergens are from the family of rag weeds (*Ambrosia*) which are present throughout the warmer portions of the western hemisphere but in particular East and central North America where the season is from the end of July to October. At least 5 major antigens have been extracted from short rag weed pollen, the most important of which is antigen E which accounts for 8.5% of the total proteins extracted from this pollen. Antigen E is present in many rag weeds and some other Compositae but is not found in melons and bananas which can cause rhinitis or oral reactions in patients sensitive to rag weed. Short rag weed has now spread outside North America to the upper Rhone Valley near Lyons in France and to several Balkan countries. However, most of the rest of Europe, Africa and Great Britain is free of rag weed. Western rag weed is becoming established in Southern and Eastern Australia. Other weeds such as the careless weed and Russian thistle are important allergens in arid regions.

Moulds

Moulds are undoubtedly important aeroallergens but there are more problems with standardisation of allergen extracts than there are with pollens. Cladosporium spores are some of the most widespread. *Cladosporium* grows on moulding vegetation and its main sporing season is in later summer and autumn. It is closely associated with *Alternaria* which is a particular problem on growing grain. These two spores have a common season and are the most common cause of rhinitis and asthma in late summer in areas which do not have rag weed. *Aspergillus* species, in particular *Aspergillus fumigatus*, can be found all the year round but in greater concentrations in the winter months. They are of particular significance since they are able to grow at body temperature, in the lungs, and can not only cause rhinitis and asthma but also can adhere to the bronchial lumen and elicit a tissue damaging reaction (broncho-pulmonary aspergillosis). Other Aspergilli can also cause alveolitis when very large quantities of the spores are inhaled, as in malt workers alveolitis.

The role of *Candida albicans* as a fungal allergen is uncertain. IgE antibody is quite frequently found to extracts of *Candida albicans*; in Britain the significance of this is unclear. In Japan *Candida albicans* is regarded as the most important allergen provoking asthma (Akiyama et al., 1981).

House Dust Mites

The major allergen in house dust and feathers is derived from a number of house dust mites. In northern countries *Dermatophagoides pteronyssinus* is the most common. *Dermatophagoides farinae* becomes more important as the altitude increases and is the major allergen in many Far Eastern countries. *Euroglyphus maynei* is able to withstand dry atmospheres more than the other two and is the major mite found at higher altitudes in Europe. The house dust mites live off human skin scales and require a relatively warm, humid environment. They are rare in cold, dry climates and in desert environments. In Europe there appears an altitude above which mites become uncommon, about 1500 metres in Central Europe (Vervoet et al., 1982). The mites are mainly found in bedding, soft furnishings, pillows and soft toys. They are the most common cause of positive skin tests in England. The main allergens are found in the faecal pellets which are covered in peritrophic membrane, a situation analgous to the locust allergens. Mites are also a major source of allergens in farmers who store grain which has become moulded. There are a number of mites which feed on moulds, in particular *Glycyphagus domesticus* and to a lesser degree *Tyrophagus putrescentiae* and *Acarus siro*. It is likely that these cross-react at least to some extent with *Dermatophagoides pteronyssinus* (Cuthbert et al., 1979).

Animal Danders

Domestic pets are a major source of preventable and removable allergen (Dewdney, 1981). Some individuals are exquisitely sensitive to these allergens so that dander left on furnishings or horse hair left on riding clothes is enough to provoke severe reactions. Horse hair was formerly used widely in furnishing and mattresses and still finds its way into felting. Cat allergens are particularly potent; they are found in the saliva and urine of the cat. Although the washed hair is probably an unimportant source of allergens they may be derived from the pelt of the cat. It is possible that Siamese cats have distinct allergens from other sorts of cat. The situation with dogs is a more complicated one since there seems to be more species difference in the allergens, although they perhaps cause slightly fewer reactions than horses and cats. Many other animals are kept as pets, in particular hamsters, gerbils, rabbits, rats and mice. All of these have important allergens in the dander, saliva and urine and are a particular problem in those who breed the animals. Birds are frequently forgotten when enquiring about domestic pets. Asthma is probably at least as common as the more severe allergic alveolitis in people who keep birds indoors or pigeons out of doors. The major allergen is probably avian IgA which appears in the droppings of the birds and also as a bloom on their feathers. It is likely, at least with pigeons, that the bloom is a more relevant source of allergen than the droppings which rarely become dry and capable of being inhaled in any large amount.

Arthropods

Arthropods are important causes of allergy. Asthma results mainly from inhalation of insect particles but allergic reactions can also occur to stinging insects, particularly to wasps, bees and mosquitoes. The reactions to stinging insects commonly involve large local and systemic reactions with hypotension and angio-oedema, but asthma can also be provoked. There is a considerable problem in identifying non-stinging insects that cause disease in the general population because the insects are rarely recognised by the patient, most of the evidence coming from occupationally exposed groups. However, there are two situations where insects cause an epidemic type of allergy in the general population. The most recently investigated is the green nimitti, a non-biting midge found in the Nile. This insect has become much more prevalent since the Nile has been dammed, resulting in its flow becoming sluggish at the end of the autumn rains. The insect appears in huge quantities at this time and provokes rhinitis or asthma in about one-quarter of the population living close to the Nile. The insects are only able to fly a few kilometres and so the problem is fairly localised. A similar situation happens with the caddis fly around the Great Lakes and rivers of Northern America.

Locusts are now the most common insect studied in schools, universities and research establishments because they are large and breed all the year round. Occupational asthma develops in about one-quarter of those who handle locusts and rhinitis occurs in about one-third (Burge et al., 1980). There appear to be cross-reacting antibodies with the house dust mite which make skin test reagents relatively nonspecific for making the diagnosis.

Asthma may also result from contact with larvae and caterpillars. Many caterpillars cause urticarial reactions due to toxins in their hairs but some also cause allergic reactions including asthma. Asthma is most common with the larvae of blue bottles, green bottles and the common house fly which are used as fish bait. Contact urticaria is usually associated with the asthma and occurs on the hands, face, neck and genitalia. Asthma is a particular problem in those who breed the larvae.

Food Hypersensitivity

Foods are a less common cause of asthma than they are of eczema and bowel disturbances; asthma induced by foods is more common in children than in adults. The identification of offending foods is made difficult by generally poor skin testing reagents which are not properly standardised or evaluated. Food induced asthma may be due to the food itself, its breakdown products or the colouring and preservatives in it. The types of reaction differ slightly from those provoked by inhaled agents in that the most common immediate reaction starts 20 to 30 minutes after ingesting the food and lasts for 1 to 2 hours. A few patients have reactions within seconds of putting food into their mouth, when the allergen is presumably absorbed from the buccal cavity. Both of these varieties of immediate asthma can usually be attributed with reasonable certainty to the foods that cause them. Nuts, fish and pip containing fruits are the most common causes of immediate reactions in adults. Tartrazine, a yellow dye present in many foods, is the most common additive giving similar reactions. The skin testing reagents for nuts and cod are particularly good. Late asthmatic reactions due to foods are much more difficult to evaluate but nevertheless occur. They are most commonly due to eggs and milk but may also be due to basic cereals, e.g., flour, rice etc. There are many false positive and false negative skin tests with foods causing late asthmatic reactions.

Reactions induced by foods seem to be less reproducible than those due to inhaled allergens. In particular, patients seem to become tolerant of food ingested regularly and only react severely when the particular food is re-introduced after a period without it. Patients who have been sensitised by inhalation may sometimes react to the same material when taken orally. This particularly occurs in patients with occupational asthma due to antibiotics who may subsequently develop asthma when that antibiotic is taken orally or even when present in small quantities in meat.

Alcoholic drinks are a frequent cause of asthma, usually resulting in immediate reactions (Gong et al., 1981). They have been described for a wide range of alcoholic drinks including beer, red wines, white wines, champagnes, whisky, gin, sherry, campari etc. The reactions are usually caused by the congeners in the drink and not the alcohol itself (Breslin et al., 1973). An example is shown

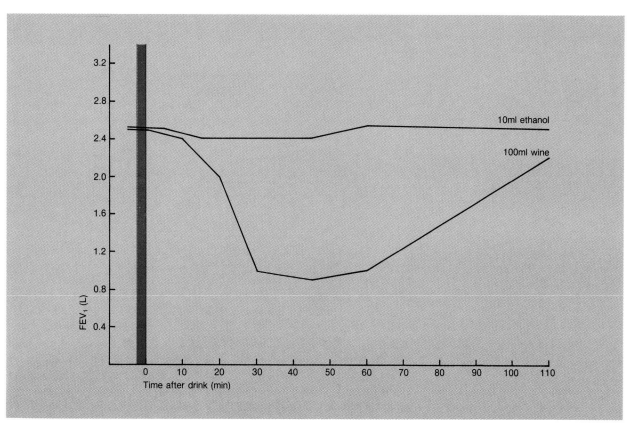

Fig. 5.4. Bronchial provocation testing with 100ml of wine and 10ml of ethanol, both producing similar blood alcohol levels. There is an immediate asthmatic reaction, the onset delayed for about 20 minutes, following ingestion of the wine, but no reaction to the ethanol.

in figure 5.4. Ethanol itself is generally a bronchodilator (Ayres and Clark, 1982).

Occupational Asthma

Occupational asthma is said to account for about 5% of adult-onset asthma. This figure will vary widely depending on the local industry. In some factories more than 50% of workers have developed occupational asthma (such as in platinum refineries with workers exposed to the complex salts of platinum and in workers making biological detergents in the early years of this process). At the other extreme only individual cases may occur amongst large workforces. Occupational asthma is important both because of the severe consequences to the livelihood of those affected and because of the insights it gives us to the relationships between exposure and symptoms. With most of the trigger factors of asthma so far discussed, the degree and duration of exposure are unlikely to be known; it is even difficult to know whether a particular allergen is in the air or not. The situation with occupational allergens from this point of view is much clearer as it is nearly always possible to date the onset of exposure and to define the periods of daily exposure. It is also often possible to measure the levels of allergen in the air. This section will be used to illustrate some of these general principles as well as to delineate some of the most important causes of occupational asthma.

The Latent Interval Between First Exposure and the Onset of Symptoms

If the occupational agent is working by allergic mechanisms then a period of symptomless exposure is experienced during which a specific antibody is formed. Following sensitisation the worker will react to concentrations of the occupational agent far below those to which he was exposed beforehand without symptoms. This latent interval varies with the potency of the allergen, the degree of exposure and the atopic status of the worker. With the most potent occupational allergen, such as complex salts of platinum, this latent interval may be as short as a few weeks and has an average time of about 3 months. The median period for sensitisation in workers exposed to isocyanates is about 2 years, whereas for colophony (rosin) the median period is over 4 years with some workers first developing symptoms after more than 10 years of exposure.

Atopy may be defined either in terms of having an atopic disease such as asthma, allergic rhinitis or flexural eczema, or in immunological terms as having the capacity to produce specific IgE antibody to common allergens met with in an ordinary way. If this second definition of atopy is used, and interpreted as having positive skin prick tests to common environmental inhalant allergens, then somewhere between 30% and 50% of the population will be atopic (clearly most of these having no disease related to these specific antibodies). Workers with positive skin tests to ordinary inhaled allergens may have shorter latent intervals and a greater tendency to become sensitised to some occupational allergens. This has been well demonstrated for workers exposed to biological detergents (Juniper et al., 1977; fig. 5.5), platinum salts, laboratory animals and insects and perhaps colophony. There are other situations where no relationship between atopy and disease has been found, particularly in workers exposed to isocyanates. For many occupational agents the role of atopy has not been examined.

Many small molecular weight occupational agents capable of

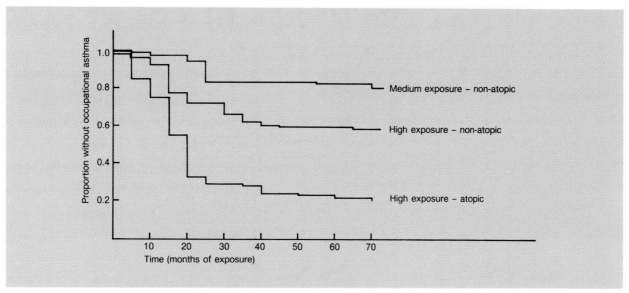

Fig. 5.5. The proportion of workers exposed to the biological detergent enzyme alcalase without occupational asthma, according to the degree of exposure and atopic status. (Re-drawn from Juniper et al., 1977.)

causing asthma are also irritant, particularly formaldehyde, iso-cyanates, phthalic anhydride and colophony. The concentration at which they are irritant is usually considerably higher than the concentration at which they are capable of causing asthma in sensitised individuals. However, a single large accidental exposure may be sufficient to sensitise some individuals so that they subsequently react to very small concentrations. This has been reported particularly with toluene di-isocyanate. If concentrations at work are very high then irritant reactions may occur without a latent interval.

Relationship Between Exposure and Symptoms in a Sensitised Individual

A normal person has a diurnal variation in airway calibre, related to sleep. Airways obstruction is maximal during the latter part of sleep or on waking and minimal 6 to 8 hours later. This normal diurnal variation is exaggerated in asthmatics where it exceeds 20% as measured by peak flow or FEV_1. This means that a worker will tend to improve in the first few hours after waking and will deteriorate in the evening, irrespective of any occupational exposure. The patterns of reaction related to work exposure will be superimposed upon this normal diurnal variation. Exposure at work is usually for many hours and is repeated from day to day and so is in many ways unlike the single exposures given in laboratory bronchial provocation studies. It is likely to resemble much more closely the types of exposure to ordinary environmental allergens such as grass pollen etc. As exposures are continued day by day, the effect of repeated exposures must also be examined. The patterns of reaction can be divided into those that occur within an individual day's exposure and those that occur with repeated day to day or week to week exposure.

Daily Patterns of Reaction

There are 3 main patterns – the immediate reaction, the late asthmatic reaction and the 'flat' record. The immediate reaction resembles the immediate reaction seen on bronchial provocation testing except that deterioration usually continues throughout the exposure with some improvement after leaving work (fig. 5.6). Recovery from an immediate reaction is usually quicker than from a late asthmatic reaction. The late asthmatic reactions start more than an hour after exposure. If the worker is on a morning shift, then the first part of work exposure will be superimposed on the improving airways obstruction from the normal diurnal variation and late reactions may not occur at work at all; they may only occur in the evening at home or may be first noted during the night after work. The same worker on an afternoon shift may well experience symptoms sooner after arriving at work because the work deterioration will be superimposed on the downward phase of the normal diurnal variation. Late asthmatic reactions at work are more common than immediate reactions. The relationship between the work and symptoms is frequently overlooked by the patient particularly when the reactions occur only at night (fig. 5.7).

The most difficult pattern is the 'flat' reaction which is somewhat of a 'non-event'. In this situation the airways obstruction appears relatively fixed throughout the 24 hours and is usually unresponsive to bronchodilators. In this way the worker resembles a patient with chronic obstructive bronchitis without an asthmatic element. It is only when the worker is taken away from exposure to the causative agent for a considerable period of time that the true reversibility of the airways obstruction becomes apparent. On re-exposure such a worker may show obvious reactions to the occupational allergen but with repeat exposures this may again be lost. An example is shown in figure 5.8.

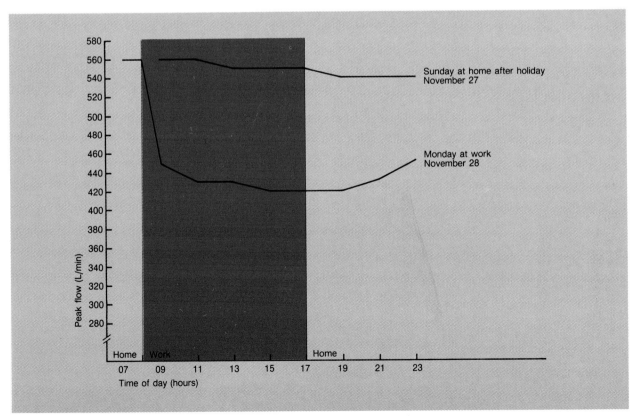

Fig. 5.6. Immediate asthmatic reactions at work in a worker exposed to diphenyl methane di-isocyanate.

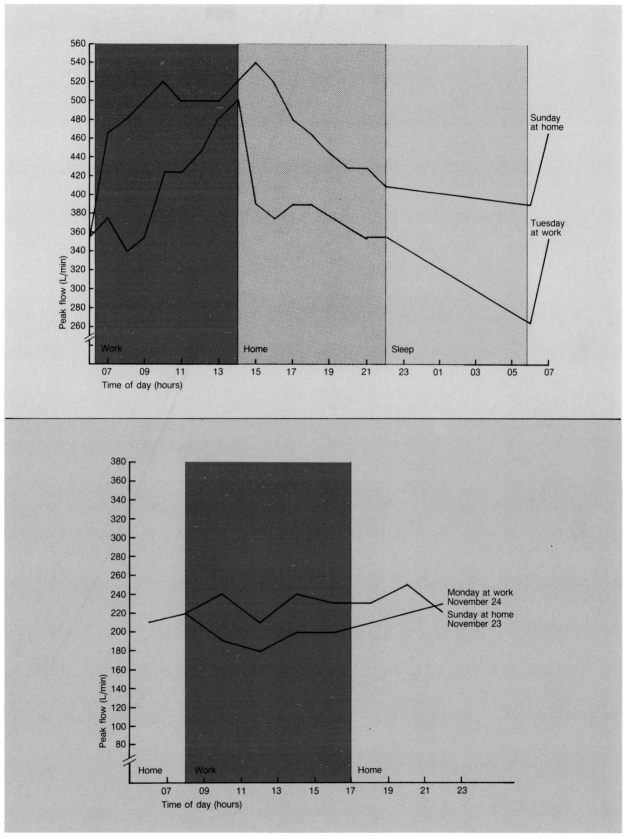

Fig. 5.7. A late asthmatic reaction, predominantly during the night, in a worker exposed to a contaminated humidifier.

Fig. 5.8. A 'flat' asthmatic reaction at work in a tool setter exposed to oil mists. A further record of his peak flow is shown in figure 5.10.

Weekly Patterns

The patterns resulting from exposure day by day depend on the rate of recovery. If recovery is rapid and effectively complete by the following morning then each workday results in equivalent deterioration (fig. 5.9). If recovery is incomplete by the following morning, but is substantial within 2 to 3 days rest period at the weekend, then symptoms become more severe day by day at work (fig. 5.10). Symptoms may be present only at the end of each working week. Symptoms which progress with daily exposure are the most common pattern. A special situation occurs in cotton workers and in some workers exposed to contaminated humidifiers, where the reaction is maximal on the first day after a rest period. It may even be confined to the first day at work after a holiday. An example is shown in figure 5.11. These diseases fit the physiological definition of asthma, but are likely to be produced by different mechanisms.

The patterns of reaction from day to day not only depend on the rate of recovery but also on the level of exposure, which is likely to vary from day to day. Perhaps because of this the records are not always consistent from week to week. In general, workers become more sensitive day by day with repeated exposures to their occupational allergens. This is likely to be similar to common environmental allergens.

Long Term Interval Patterns

Workers with the most severe occupational asthma may deteriorate to such a stage that the airways obstruction appears fixed and does not vary greatly during days at work and does not improve over a short period of time away from work. The start of recovery may be delayed for up to 10 days after leaving work and

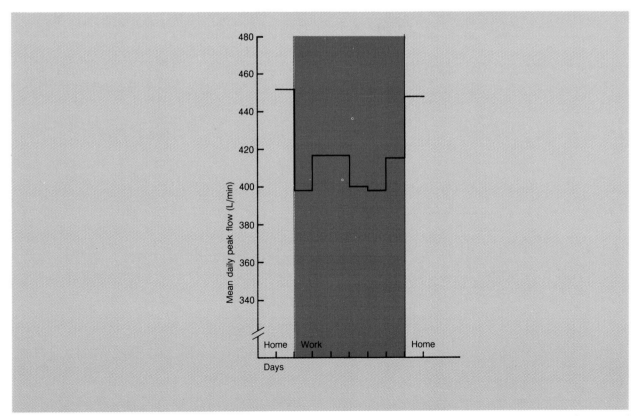

Fig. 5.9. Equivalent daily deterioration in mean daily peak flow in a foreman in a printing works exposed to a contaminated humidifier.

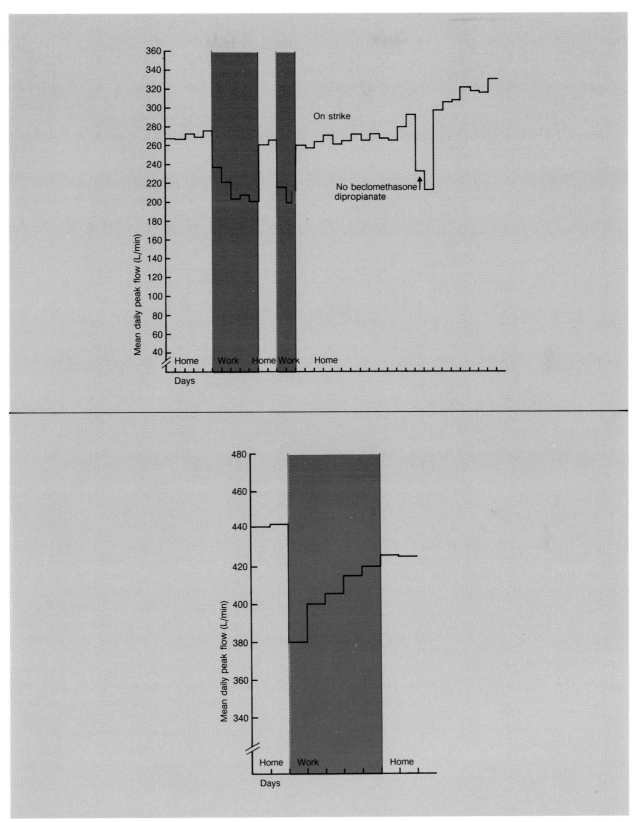

Fig. 5.10. Progressive daily deterioration in mean daily peak flow in the tool setter treated with salbutamol, ipratropium and beclomethasone dipropionate shown in figure 5.8. After the second work period the factory went on strike. This was followed by continuing improvement for 20 days with a 2 day deterioration when his steroid inhaler failed to work.

Fig. 5.11. Asthma, worse on the first day of work, in a clerk in a printing works exposed to a contaminated humidifier. There is improvement with successive days at work despite the continuing exposure.

Table 5.2. Causes of occupational asthma usually associated with specific IgE antibodies

Agents	At-risk groups
Grains and flour	Farmers, millers, dockers, bakers
Enzymes	Biological detergent makers, food tenderisers, drug and chemical workers
Proteins from animals, birds, insects and other invertebrates	Particularly laboratory animal workers; insect (and larvae) breeders for science, fish bait, etc.; bird breeders, feather merchants, hat makers, prawn shuckers
Pollens	Farmers and market gardeners handling sugar beet, strawberries, rape, etc.
Green coffee beans and castor beans	Millers, farmers, etc.
Tobacco and tea	Farmers, pickers, processors
Micro-organisms	Where there are humidifiers, mushroom factories, timber processing works and single cell protein manufacture, soup manufacturers
Silk	Farmers, hairdressers (sericin) and processors
Platinum salts	Refiners and scrap recoverers
Chloramine T	Sterilisers, particularly in breweries
Synthetic and natural dyes	Those involved in making and handling materials, including users of pen recorders
Gum acacia	Drug manufacturers, printers and food processors

may continue for several months. Such patterns are particularly common in isocyanate workers who often seem to have a severe form of occupational asthma. Figure 5.10 shows continuing improvement 21 days after the last work exposure.

The degree of exposure necessary to cause symptoms with occupational allergens varies widely. In some situations such as with workers exposed to colophony the exposure at work is relatively high, and may be several milligrams of particulate fume per mm³ of air. In other situations the levels of exposure may be truly minute with reactions produced by allergen carried home on the clothes and hair. Workers sensitised to laboratory animals may continue to have occupational asthma after removal from exposure because of contact in the canteen or elsewhere with workers with animal allergens on their clothes. Occasionally contact with workers outside the workplace is enough to produce such reactions. Such extreme sensitivity has been found in platinum refinery workers and workers manufacturing antibiotics.

Causes of Occupational Asthma

Some of the more important causes of occupational asthma are shown in tables 5.2 and 5.3. The list is rapidly increasing. It is often surprisingly difficult to find out what a worker is exposed to, particularly where small molecular weight chemicals are the cause. The allergens listed in table 5.2 are mainly biological agents which resemble common inhalant allergens in many ways. The antigens are often medium molecular weight proteins and IgE antibodies can usually be found, although the relationship between antibodies and disease is rarely very close. Those in table 5.3 are mainly small molecular weight chemicals which may be working as haptens. They are unlikely to be working as antigens in their own right because of their small molecular weight. Little is known about the immunology of these agents although antibodies to protein conjugates of some of them have been found, particularly to trimellitic anhydride.

Table 5.3. Causes of occupational asthma for which tests for IgE antibodies are not available or not established

Agents	At-risk groups
Isocyanates:	
Toluene di-isocyanate (TDI)	Polyurethane foam manufacture, chemical workers,
diphenylmethane di-isocyanate (MDI)	wire coating, paints, adhesives, printing
hexamethylene di-isocyanate (HDI)	Paint makers and handlers
napthylene di-isocyanate (NDI)	Synthetic rubber production workers
Cotton	Ginners, millers and weavers
Wood dusts	Workers handling particularly western red cedar and hard woods
Colophony (rosin)	Workers using electronic solder and hot melt glues, chemists, feather pluckers
Metals:	
chromates	Workers involved in chromium plating, cement manufacture, stainless steel welding, painting
cobalt	Workers involved in hard metal manufacture and grinding, refining
nickel sulphate	Nickel platers
vanadium	Boiler cleaners (oil fired)
Epoxy resin curing agents	Workers handling phthalic and trimellitic anhydrides, triethylene tetramine etc., e.g. in adhesives, paints, surface coatings, plastics
PVC (and plasticisers)	Hot cutters of PVC wrapping, meat wrappers
Formaldehyde	Workers involved with a range of products including urea formaldehyde, phenol formaldehyde, melamine formaldehyde in plastic moulding, glueing, cavity wall insulation, etc.; also medical users
Ethylenediamine	Colour photograph processors
Henna, persulphates, sericin, etc.	Hairdressers
Penicillin, cephalosporins, sulphonamides, cimetidine, etc.	Drug manufacturers

Grain and Flour Dust

Occupational asthma is widespread at many stages in the process from harvesting through to grain storage, milling and baking. This is one of the earliest recognised causes of occupational asthma described by Ramazzini in 1714. The causes of occupational asthma and other respiratory diseases due to grain dusts are largely unresolved but are likely to vary considerably in the various stages of its processing. Farmers harvesting grain are thought to be affected largely by the moulds which grow on the grain. During storage they initially proliferate and then are eaten by a number of storage mites, most related to the house dust mite, which seem responsible for much of the asthma in the later half of the winter in farmers using stored grain to feed cattle. Millers are exposed to the grain, its fungi, mites and other additives put in at this stage. Baker's asthma is perhaps mostly due to the actual flour as by the time they handle it the concentrations of fungi, mites and other materials are relatively low.

Laboratory Animal Allergy

It is perhaps surprising that an area in which so many doctors are directly involved at work has been so long in being investigated. Occupational asthma is common in workers handling laboratory mammals, particularly rats and mice but also rabbits, guinea pigs and other animals. Various studies have estimated the prevalence of occupational asthma to be between 3% and 14% of exposed workers with up to about one-third having some sort of allergic reaction. There is a clear relationship between atopy and the development of occupational asthma but not between atopy and the development of occupational rhinitis or urticaria, which are also common. A major advance has been in studies of the antigens. Clean rodent hair seems to be an unimportant cause of asthma in exposed workers. Some of the most potent allergens are urinary proteins, particularly those excreted by rats and mice. These urinary proteins may contaminate the animals' hair, so extracts that are produced from uncleaned hair may well show positive reactions. Saliva may also contain important allergens, which may also be present on unwashed rodent hair.

Isocyanates

Isocyanates are used in the production of polyurethanes in which a polyol cross links with an isocyanate to form a foam or rigid structure. Toluene di-isocyanate (TDI) was the most widely used but has now largely been replaced by diphenyl methane di-isocyanate (MDI), which is less volatile at room temperature. Hexamethylene di-isocyanate (HDI) is the most volatile of all the isocyanates and is being increasingly used as a paint spray, particularly for aircraft and cars. As well as being used to make flexible and rigid foams isocyanates are also widely used as adhesives, surface coatings and as a lacquer on the outside of electrical wires. Exposure may result from the manufacture of the basic isocyanate, from their use as a resin, either in foaming or surface coating, or from the breakdown of fully reacted polyurethanes when heated at relatively low temperatures. High concentrations of TDI vapour may cause an irritant rhinitis and chest tightness on first exposure. More commonly, low concentrations well below the threshold limit value of 0.02 ppm, may induce asthma in sensitised workers. Occupational asthma may develop in about 5% of workers regularly exposed to TDI; this figure will clearly depend on the degree of exposure encountered. Much of the occupational asthma resulting from isocyanate exposure is particularly severe with prolonged recovery periods.

Enzymes

A variety of enzymes have caused occupational asthma. The most widespread have been enzymes from *Bacillus subtilis* used in biological detergents. Enzymes (e.g. trypsin) are also widely used in food processing, drug manufacture and in scientific research establishments. Alcalase, one of the enzymes from *Bacillus subtilis*, is probably the main agent responsible for the occupational asthma in biological detergent manufacturers. More than half of highly exposed workers were sensitised to alcalase in one factory manufacturing biological detergents (Juniper et al., 1977). The problem was controlled by enclosing the areas where the enzyme was present as a dry dust, by encapsulating the enzyme into large particles and by providing efficient exhaust extraction. Atopic workers were also removed from exposure and the problem largely disappeared.

Colophony

Colophony is the resin produced from pine resin after the turpentine has been distilled off. Its main uses are now as an adhesive and as a soldering flux although it is present in many other substances including paper size, deodorants, emulsifiers and semi-synthetic plastics. It is the adhesive on standard Elastoplast and the material that violinists use on their bows. As an adhesive in the cold it is unlikely to be inhaled in sufficient quantities to cause asthma but as a hot adhesive or electronic soldering flux, large

amounts of resin acids and their decomposition products are inhaled by those close by. Occupational asthma has occurred in about
20% of workers heavily exposed in one electronics factory (Burge,
1982).

In Conclusion

Individual patients usually have multiple triggers of their
asthma, which vary in importance during their lifetime. This chapter has tried to detail the more important trigger factors.

References

Akiyama, K.; Yui, Y.; Shida, T. and Miyamoto, T.: Relationship between the results
of skin, conjunctival and bronchial tests and RAST with *Candida albicans* in
patients with asthma. Clinical Allergy 11: 343 (1981).

Al-Awadi, A.R.A.: The study of allergy in Kuwait. Ministry of Public Health, Kuwait
(local publication) (1973).

Ayres, J. and Clark, T.J.H.: Alcohol in asthma and the bronchoconstrictor effect of
chlorpropamide. British Journal of Diseases of the Chest 76: 79 (1982).

Barbee, R.A.; Lebowitz, M.D.; Thompson, H.C. and Burrows, B.: Immediate skin test
reactivity in a general population sample. Annals of Internal Medicine 84: 129
(1976).

Belin, L.: Separation and characteristics of birch pollen antigens with special reference
to the allergenic components. International Archives of Allergy and Applied Immunology 42: 329 (1972).

Björkstén, F.; Suoniemi, I. and Koski, V.: Neonatal birch-pollen contact and subsequent
allergy to birch-pollen. Clinical Allergy 10: 587 (1980).

Breslin, A.B.X.; Hendrick, D.J. and Pepys, J.: Effect of disodium cromoglycate on asthmatic reactions to alcoholic beverages. Clinical Allergy 3: 71 (1973).

Bryant, D.H. and Pepys, J.: Bronchial reactions to aerosol inhalant vehicle. British
Medical Journal 1: 1319 (1976).

Burge, P.S.: Occupational asthma due to soft soldering fluxes containing colophony.
European Journal of Respiratory Diseases 63 (Suppl.) (in press).

Burge, P.S.; Edge, G.; O'Brien, I.M.; Harries, M.G.; Hawkins, R. and Pepys, J.: Occupational asthma in a research centre breeding locusts. Clinical Allergy 10: 355
(1980).

Cuthbert, O.D.; Brostoff, J.; Wraith, D.G. and Brighton, W.D.: Barn allergy – asthma
and rhinitis due to storage mites. Clinical Allergy 9: 229 (1979).

Dewdney, J.M.: Allergy induced by exposure to animals. Journal of the Royal Society
of Medicine 74: 928 (1981).

Forssman, O.; Korsgren, M.; Nordh, B. and Paulsen, F.: Allergy to ACTH of animal
and human origin. Acta Allergologica 18: 462 (1963).

Gluck, J.C. and Gluck, P.A.: The effects of pregnancy upon asthma – a prospective
study. Annals of Allergy 37: 164 (1976).

Godin, J. and Malo, J-L.: Acute bronchoconstriction caused by Beclovent and not Van-
ceril. Clinical Allergy 9: 585 (1979).

Gong, H.; Tashkin, D.P.; Calvaresse, B.M.: Alcohol-induced bronchospasm in an asthmatic patient. Chest 80: 167 (1981).

Gregg, I.: The role of virus infection in asthma and bronchitis; in Symposium on Virus
Infection. Publication No. 46, p.82 (Royal College of Physicians, Edinburgh 1975).

Hanley, S.P.: Asthma variation with menstruation. British Journal of Diseases of the
Chest 75: 306 (1981).

Juniper, C.P.; How, M.J.; Goodwin, B.F.J. and Kinshott, A.K.: *Bacillus subtilis* enzymes: A 7 year clinical, epidemiological and immunological study of an industrial allergen. Journal of the Society of Occupational Medicine 27: 3 (1977).

Kjellen, G.; Tibbling, L. and Wranne, B.: Effect of conservative treatment of oesophageal dysfunction on bronchial asthma. European Journal of Respiratory Diseases
62: 190 (1981).

Lambert, H.P. and Stern, H.: Infective factors in exacerbations of bronchitis and asthma.
British Medical Journal 3: 323 (1972).

Luparello, T.; Leist, N.; Lourie, C.H. and Sweet, P.: The interaction of psychologic
stimuli and pharmacologic agents on airway reactivity in asthmatic subjects. Psychosomatic Medicine 32: 509 (1970).

Matus, I.: Assessing the nature and clinical significance of psychological contributions
to childhood asthma. American Journal of Orthopsychiatry 51: 327 (1981).

McFadden, E.R.: An analysis of exercise as a stimulus for the production of airways obstruction. Lung 159: 3 (1981).

McFadden, E.R.; Luparello, T.; Lyons, H.A. and Bleeker, E.: The mechanism of action of suggestion in the induction of acute asthma attacks. Psychosomatic Medicine 31: 134 (1969).

Mendelson, L.M.; Meltzer, E.O. and Hamburger, R.N.: Anaphylaxis-like reactions to corticosteroid therapy. Journal of Allergy and Clinical Immunology 54: 125 (1974).

Minor, T.E.; Dick, E.C.; De Meo, A.N.; Ouellette, J.J.; Cohen, M. and Reed, C.E.: Viruses as precipitants of asthmatic attacks in children. Journal of the American Medical Association 227: 292 (1974).

Paterson, I.C.; Grant, I.W.B. and Crompton, G.K.: Severe bronchoconstriction provoked by sodium cromoglycate. British Medical Journal 2: 916 (1976).

Pickering, C.A.C. and Mustchin, C.P.: 'Coughing water' – bronchial hyper-reactivity induced by swimming in a chlorinated pool. Thorax 34: 682 (1979).

Purcell, K.; Brady, K.; Chai, H.; Muser, J.; Mock, L.; Gordon, N. and Means, J.: The effect on asthma in children of experimental separation from the family. Psychosomatic Medicine 31: 144 (1969).

Rees, P.J.; Chowienczyk, P.J. and Clark, T.J.H.: Immediate response to cigarette smoke. Thorax 37: 417 (1982).

Schoeffel, R.E.; Anderson, S.D. and Altounyan, R.E.: Bronchial hyper-reactivity in response to inhalation of ultrasonically nebulised solutions of distilled water and saline. British Medical Journal 283: 1285 (1981).

Spector, S.L.; Wangaard, C.H. and Farr, R.S.: Aspirin and concomitant idiosyncrasies in adult asthmatic patients. Journal of Allergy and Clinical Immunology 64: 500 (1979).

Turner, E.S.; Greenberger, P.A. and Patterson, R.: Management of the pregnant asthmatic patient. Annals of Internal Medicine 93: 905 (1980).

Vedanthan, P.K.; Menon, M.M.; Bell, T.D. and Bergin, D.: Aspirin and tartrazine oral challenge – incidence of adverse response in chronic childhood asthma. Journal of Allergy and Clinical Immunology 60: 8 (1977).

Vervoet, D.; Penaud, A.; Razzouk, H.; Senft, M.; Arnaud, A.; Boutin, C. and Charpin, J.: Altitude and house dust mites. Journal of Allergy and Clinical Immunology 69: 290 (1982).

Whittemore, A.S. and Korn, E.L.: Asthma and air pollution in the Los Angeles area. American Journal of Public Health 70: 687 (1980).

Further Reading

Roth (Ed) Allergy in the World (University Press, Hawaii 1978).

Solomon, W.R. and Mathews, K.P.: Aerobiology and inhalant allergens; in Middleton et al. (Eds) Allergy: Principles and Practice, p.899 (Mosby, St Louis 1978).

Chapter VI

Therapeutic Choices in Asthma

Trevor Gebbie

The treatment of asthma has been a controversial topic for many years and it remains today one of the problem areas in medicine. Treatments as diverse as hypnotherapy, acupuncture, and alteration of the ion content of the air have had their supporters, and perhaps the diversity of these treatments and their apparent lack of a logical basis reflect our inability to define asthma precisely. While allergic mechanisms are widely accepted in the aetiology of asthma, in clinical practice – certainly in adult medicine – the number of patients in whom an allergic basis can be clearly identified is a relatively small fraction of the total, and so measures such as immunotherapy have very limited indications. Even in those cases where an allergic basis is clear cut with an offending allergen identified, immunotherapy seems at best only 'useful' and often only of marginal benefit (Lichtenstein, 1978). The present pharmacological approach to treatment, however, while originating with empirical observations, has a solid basis in extensive controlled clinical and experimental studies and is the only satisfactory way of managing the great majority of asthmatic patients.

In the treatment of asthma, once reversible airways obstruction has been clearly identified, certain important principles of management should be recognised:

1) Treatment should be aimed at restoring airways function to normal, and maintaining normal function.

2) Monitoring ventilatory function with tests such as the FEV_1 or peak expiratory flow rate provides vital information on the patient's functional state, and this monitoring can often be made the patient's responsibility.

3) It is important to determine the best functional level for any individual patient as a guide to management.

4) There is a logical progression with treatment from the occasional use of a bronchodilator aerosol to regular treatment with oral and inhaled agents.

5) Treatment may need to be continuous to maintain normal function. It is unsatisfactory to treat exacerbations of symptoms as they occur unless they are infrequent and minor and there is good function during remission.

It is clear that most asthmatics have continuing functional abnormalities even during remission (McFadden et al., 1973) and Rubinfeld and Pain (1976) have shown that many patients are unreliable perceivers of disability and cannot sense the presence of quite severe airways obstruction (p.35). Persisting functional abnormality in patients who do not recognise its presence is almost certainly the explanation for many sudden 'acute' episodes of asthma and possibly an explanation for unexpected sudden death. Bellamy and Collins (1979) in a study of hospital admissions due to acute severe asthma, showed that inadequate control of symptoms had occurred over a period of 5 weeks with a more rapid deterioration 24 hours immediately prior to admission. Sudden deterioration from a background of good control is uncommon in adults with asthma, and the use by the patient of home monitoring of pulmonary function can alert both patient and medical practitioner to the need for intensified treatment.

Since asthma can be produced by a wide range of stimuli such as exercise, inhaled irritants, allergens, drugs, and infection, an understanding of the mechanisms common to these provoking factors makes for a more rational basis for therapeutic decisions (see Chapter V).

Bronchial hyper-reactivity is the characteristic feature of asthma with the airways abnormally responsive to many different influences which normally produce little or no reaction. This hyper-reactivity may be the result of either a disorder of the immune system (Chapter IV) or an abnormality of autonomic nervous system function or a combination of both. The concept of release of chemical mediators as the result of antigen/antibody reaction is based on studies of more than 70 years ago on the actions of histamine. Many other mediator substances have since been identified, but the exact role of many of these in asthma is not clear (p.48). Abnormal function of the autonomic nervous system due to defective β-receptor function was suggested by Szentivanyi (1968) and there is a great deal of experimental and clinical evidence in support. As a corollary, there is evidence that the parasympathetic nervous system may be hyperactive in some asthmatics with cholinergic induced bronchoconstriction as a result. These concepts concerning the basis of bronchial hyper-reactivity are not mutually exclusive, but there is at present no clear-cut unified relationship established between immune and non-immune mechanisms. In a review of the biochemical and immunological basis of bronchial asthma, Aas (1978) has pointed out that it is possible the primary defect of bronchial asthma is to be found in mediator systems or regulatory functions not yet defined. The various hypotheses concerning the cause of the bronchial hyper-reactivity of asthmatics are discussed in more detail in Chapter II (p.14).

The direction of pharmacological research in asthma in recent years has been towards drugs with an effect on immune processes or with actions mediated through the sympathetic or parasympathetic nervous system. A simplified representation of the pharmacological mechanisms in asthma is shown in figure 6.1. In general, anti-asthma drugs can be classified as either:

1) Bronchodilators, drugs with a direct action on the bronchial wall, relieving airways obstruction. These drugs can be given for immediate symptomatic relief or for continuous control if indicated.

2) Drugs which may prevent the development of airways obstruction, if used appropriately, by suppressing the basic pathological processes producing the obstruction.

Bronchodilators

The factors producing airways obstruction in asthma include (1) bronchial smooth muscle constriction, (2) mucous plugging of the airway lumen, (3) oedema of the bronchial mucous membranes, (4) thickening of the basement membrane, (5) cellular infiltration, (6) vascular congestion. With these multiple possible factors involved it is obvious that there is much more to the relief of airways obstruction than simply the relaxation of constricted

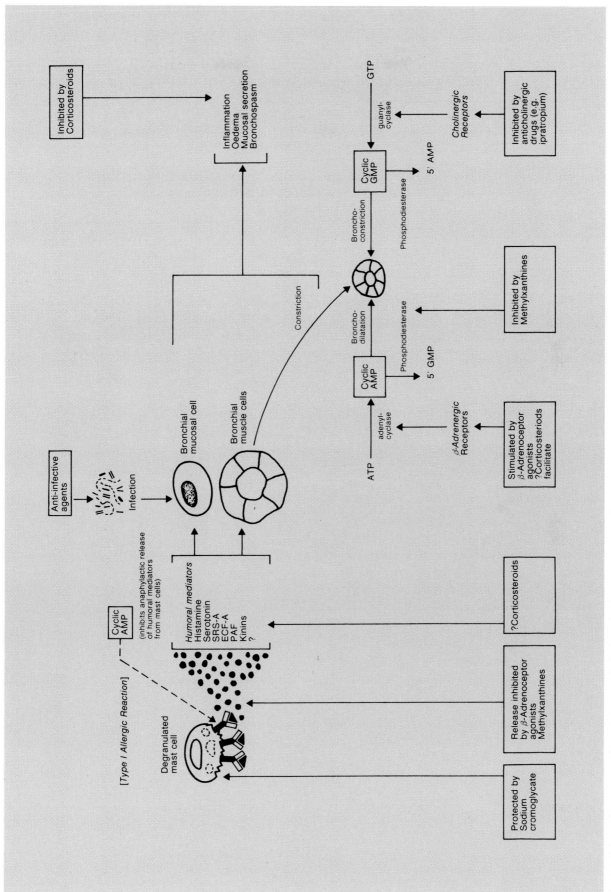

Fig. 6.1. Schematic representation of pharmacological mechanisms and modes of action of antiasthmatic drugs (adapted from Palmer and Petrie, 1980).

smooth muscle. In addition, the factors may be present in varying degrees on any one occasion, and each may resolve with differing time courses. This is one explanation for the observation that bronchodilator drugs may vary in their effectiveness from time to time – if 'spasm' is a major contributing factor, then this may respond more rapidly to bronchodilator therapy than mucous plugging of the airway for instance.

Bronchodilator drugs are classified as:

1) Sympathomimetics – which act on the β-adrenergic component of the sympathetic nervous system.

2) Anticholinergic agents – which block the effect of the parapathetic system on bronchomotor tone.

3) Methylxanthines – which affect the respiratory system in a number of ways in addition to relaxing bronchial smooth muscle.

Sympathomimetics

These drugs have been the mainstay of treatment for asthma since adrenaline (epinephrine) was shown to be effective subcutaneously in 1903 and by inhalation 7 years later (Barger and Dale, 1910). As constituents of various asthma remedies, their use goes back even further. Ephedrine had been in use in China for several thousand years before its introduction into Western medicine in 1924 by Chen and Schmidt. The sympathomimetics (fig. 6.2) have a wide range of pharmacological actions and are among the most extensively studied therapeutic agents. Modern receptor theory

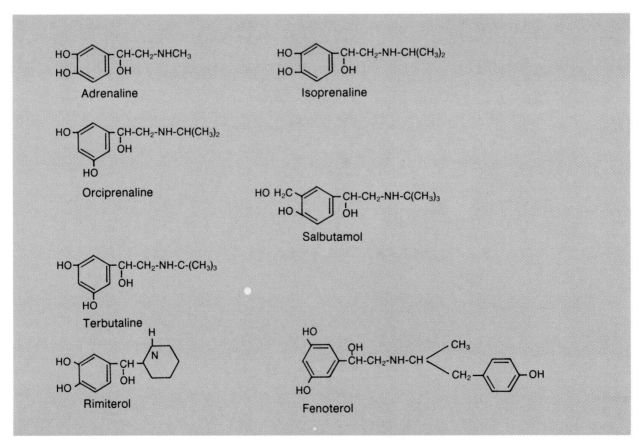

Fig. 6.2. Structural formulae of some sympathomimetic bronchodilators. Through modification of the constituents and their location on the basic catecholamine ring, breakdown by catechol-O-methyl transferase is prevented and prolonged action results. By substituting at the N-alkyl position on the catechol ring and enlarging the moiety attached here greater β_2 specificity results. The smaller this group the more nonspecific $\alpha\beta$ stimulation results.

offers an explanation for their differing effects on various organ systems and has given an important impetus to the development of drugs with greater specificity as bronchodilators.

The concept of a 'receptor' as the molecular component of the cell which combined with a drug to produce a biological response dates from the late 19th century, but in 1948 Ahlquist suggested the presence of two kinds of adrenergic receptor, α and β, to account for the differing effects of sympathomimetic agents on a variety of physiological processes. It was subsequently shown by Lands et al. (1967) that β-receptors could not be regarded as a single population, and could be subdivided into two groups, β_1 and β_2. Recent work indicates that α-receptors are of two sub-types also. Thus it is now held that adrenergic receptors are of 4 types, α_1, α_2, β_1 and β_2 (Motulsky and Insel, 1982).

α-Receptors are predominantly located in blood vessels, the alimentary tract and the uterus, and their activation generally results in smooth muscle contraction. There is no clear evidence for the presence of α-receptors in the bronchial muscle of normal man, but they have been identified in some animal species. However, α-adrenergic blocking drugs have significantly reduced histamine-induced bronchoconstriction in asthmatics. This suggests that α-adrenergic receptors may be present in the bronchi of asthmatic patients and that histamine sensitivity may be mediated through these receptors (Gaddie et al., 1972). There is, however, little clinical evidence of the value of α-blocking drugs in the treatment of asthma.

β_1-Receptors are present in cardiac muscle and intestinal smooth muscle, and β_2-receptors mainly in bronchial smooth muscle, skeletal and uterine muscle and blood vessels.

The β-adrenergic receptor has been identified with the cell membrane enzyme adenyl cyclase, and this enzyme itself may well be the receptor. When stimulated by either neural or hormonal impulses, adenyl cyclase catalyses the formation within the cell of increased amounts of cyclic-AMP from ATP. The effect of increased cyclic AMP upon the smooth muscle cell is to decrease cell tension and produce smooth muscle relaxation. Cyclic-AMP appears to produce muscle relaxation by binding Ca^{++} ions to the cell membrane and the cytoplasmic reticulum, stabilising the cell membrane, lowering the myoplasmic concentration of calcium, resulting in cell relaxation.

Cyclic-AMP is broken down by a cytoplasmic enzyme phosphodiesterase. Apparently opposing the action of cyclic-AMP in the smooth muscle cell is cyclic guanosine monophosphate, cyclic-GMP, which is induced by parasympathetic activity. Vagal stimulation or cholinergic drugs increase cyclic-GMP levels causing smooth muscle contraction and bronchoconstriction. Thus the particular level of bronchomotor tone at any time appears to be a delicate balance between cyclic-AMP and cyclic-GMP levels – or between β-adrenergic and parasympathetic influences.

The subdivision of adrenergic receptors into α and β groups suggested that these were functionally and morphologically separate structures in the cell membrane. Increasingly, evidence suggests that a more dynamic concept of adrenergic receptors is necessary. It may well be that α and β receptors simply represent different molecular conformations of a single receptor and that interconversion between α and β adrenoceptors can occur. Considerable experimental evidence supports the likelihood of inter-conversion and this has been considered to be a mechanism which would allow an organ or tissue to adapt its response according to its metabolic state (Nickerson and Kunos, 1977).

Nonspecific β-Agonists

With the recognition that stimulation of β_2-adrenergic receptors relaxes bronchial smooth muscle while β_1 stimulation produces unwanted cardiac effects such as tachycardia, the emphasis in pharmacological research has been on producing drugs with specific β_2-agonist properties. To a large extent this has been achieved with a number of recently developed sympathomimetic bronchodilators, but the apparent specificity of these drugs in clinical practice is probably only dose-related, side effects being common if big enough doses are used. With the development of these more specific compounds, there is now little justification for the continued use of the nonspecific β-agonists such as ephedrine and isoprenaline (isoproterenol). Ephedrine has been frequently used in combinations with other drugs but is an inferior bronchodilator to the specific β_2-agonists and it commonly produces side effects which are often enhanced when it is combined with theophylline. Also, in such combination products the amount of theophylline present is usually inadequate to produce therapeutic blood levels.

Isoprenaline is a rapidly effective bronchodilator when inhaled, but is relatively ineffective orally as it is metabolised in the gut wall and during first-pass through the liver. Because it acts on both β_1- and β_2-receptors, there is a significant incidence of side effects such as palpitation and tremor. Rightly or wrongly, isoprenaline was blamed for the reported rise in deaths of young asthmatics in the United Kingdom from 1960 to 1966. Although many doubt that isoprenaline per se was to blame, the development of newer β_2-agonists of at least equal efficacy has made isoprenaline obsolete in clinical practice. It remains, however, a standard bronchodilator for the laboratory assessment of the comparative efficacy of bronchodilator drugs.

Orciprenaline, while lacking the specificity of the newer agents, produces virtually no side effects when administered as an aerosol and has a considerably more prolonged effect than isoprenaline. It has been in use now for 20 years with no evidence of significant drug tolerance or other ill effects from prolonged use.

Specific β_2-Receptor Agonists

There are now a number of drugs with clinical effects almost entirely resulting from β_2-receptor stimulation. This selectivity of action is largely based on laboratory studies of drug action on isolated tissues but is borne out in clinical practice. The drugs most widely used are: salbutamol, terbutaline, fenoterol and rimiterol. When inhaled these drugs have a rapid action, the major part of their bronchodilating effect being produced in 10 to 15 minutes. Rimiterol has a relatively short half-life and its bronchodilator effect begins to wane after 1 hour. The others maintain their effect for approximately 4 to 6 hours.

The preferred route of administration obviously depends on whether inhaled or oral medication produces the most effective bronchodilatation and fewer side effects. The side effects of muscle tremor and tachycardia are much more common after oral administration than after inhalation. This is a dose-related phenomenon – the effective oral dose with all the agents being significantly greater

Table 6.1. A comparison of some β-agonist bronchodilators

Compound	Peak effect after inhalation (min)	Duration of effect (h)	Dose per puff (mg)	Dose per tablet (mg) (max daily)	Nebuliser solution
Orciprenaline	30	2-4	0.75	20 (80)	–
Salbutamol	10-15	4-6	0.1	8, 4, 2 (16)	5 mg/ml
Terbutaline	10-15	4-6	0.25	5:2.5 (15)	10 mg/ml
Fenoterol	10-15	4-6	0.2	–	5 mg/ml
Rimiterol	10-15	1-2	0.25	–	–

than that by the inhaled route of administration (table 6.1). It is quite clear from a number of studies that better and more prolonged bronchodilatation results from inhalation rather than oral administration.

Inhalation: Aerosol or Nebuliser?

Since it is always desirable to achieve maximal therapeutic effect with the least risk of side effects and at the smallest dose level, inhalation is the preferred route of administration whether for intermittent or regular maintenance therapy. In addition to these considerations, recent studies demonstrating the presence of mast cells actually within the airway lumen and in the epithelium of the airways (p.47), gives further emphasis to the value of inhalation as a method of treatment. If the initial antigen/antibody reaction in allergic asthma occurs on the mast cell within the airway lumen or on the epithelial surface as has been suggested, inhalation therapy aimed at modifying this reaction seems most logical.

Having established that inhalation therapy has significant advantages over oral, how best should an aerosol be administered? Alternative methods of inhalation are:

1) A metered dose from pressurised aerosol using volatile hydrocarbons (Freons) as propellant. This requires coordination and activation of the aerosol by the patient during inspiration so that medication enters the airways with the inspired airstream.

2) A metered dose from a breath actuated dry-powder device is now available for salbutamol and fenoterol. This is an advantage for the very young, the elderly and others who may find coordinating inspiration with firing difficult using the standard aerosol.

3) Nebulisation of an aqueous solution either in a hand inhaler (now largely superseded) or from a nebulising unit attached to a compressed air supply. In this way a wet aerosol is produced which enters the airway during tidal breathing.

4) Using an intermittent positive pressure breathing (IPPB) machine, such as a Bird respirator, with the machine triggered by the patient's inspiratory effort. The inspiratory pressure and flow rate can be adjusted (usually 15mm Hg and 15 L/min respectively).

For an aerosol to be inhaled effectively and distributed widely through the airways, particle size is important, the optimum range being 1 to 7μm. Smaller particles penetrate furthest and larger particles are deposited proximally. The particle size in the commonly used metered dose pressurised aerosols is 3 to 5μm and a similar appropriate particle size is achieved by various nebulisers. Other factors which affect aerosol deposition are rate of airflow and airway calibre. It has been clearly shown that with high inspired flow rates there is increased deposition of particles in the pharynx and larynx and reduced overall delivery of aerosol to the lung compared to inhalation during quiet breathing. Dolovich et al. (1977) have shown that IPPB delivered 32% less aerosol to the lungs than quiet breathing from a compressed air nebuliser. Thus the assumption that IPPB will produce better penetration of the airways or more peripheral deposition of aerosol is unwarranted, and this method has nothing to recommend it in the delivery of therapeutic aerosols.

For a full discussion of inhalation techniques likely to give the best therapeutic response, see Appendix I.

There has been an increased use recently of compressed air nebulisers. Originally used in paediatric departments and emergency rooms, inhalation by this method has the advantage of not requiring the cooperation of the patient. The drug is nebulised over a period of minutes, depending on the flow rate through the nebuliser, it is carried in the tidal airstream and requires no coordinated effort by the patient. This technique will produce bronchodilatation and consequent relief of symptoms when use of the metered aerosol appears to have failed, but its success is almost certainly due to the much larger dose of drug delivered via the nebuliser. Weber et al. (1979), using a Maxi-myst compressor, showed that 6 to 8 times the dose of terbutaline had to be given by nebulisation to achieve the same degree of bronchodilatation as when administered by metered dose aerosol, and they could see no advantages in the use of compressor powered nebulisation in routine management.

Tachyphylaxis

While there is no doubt that the β_2-agonists continue to produce bronchodilatation during prolonged administration, the development of a decreased response to these agents, or subsensitivity, has been a matter of importance and some controversy. Jenne et al. (1977) showed the development of a mild degree of bronchial receptor tolerance after prolonged administration of terbutaline. Svedmyr et al. (1976) in both *in vitro* studies on bronchial muscle preparations, and *in vivo* studies involving patients under treatment for 1 year, did not show any resistance to bronchial β-adrenergic stimulation and suggested that the development of 'resistance' may be due to other factors causing airways obstruction.

Nelson et al. (1977) showed that the mean response of patients to the first dose of salbutamol was consistently greater than the response after a period of regular administration. Maximal decrease in response occurred after 2 weeks' treatment and there was no further decrease in response after regular treatment for as long as 1 year. Recently Harvey and Tattersfield (1982) have shown normal and asthmatic subjects differ in response to regularly inhaled large doses of a β-agonist. After 4 weeks inhalation of salbutamol, in a dose increasing from 100μg 4 times a day to 500μg 4 times a day, normal subjects developed a progressive fall in airway response to the drug where as asthmatic subjects maintained their response. There seems no doubt that the side effects of β-agonist administration diminish with prolonged use.

Anticholinergic Bronchodilators

The parasympathetic system via the vagus nerve exerts a major influence on airway calibre with bronchoconstriction resulting from stimulation of cholinergic receptors. It is logical therefore to expect that parasympathetic blockade would produce bronchodilatation, and atropine in various forms has been used for this purpose for many years in the treatment of asthma. Atropine methonitrate as an aerosol has similar bronchodilating effects to salbutamol and when combined with it significantly prolongs its action.

The systemic effects of anticholinergic drugs – interference with ocular accommodation, depression of salivary and bronchial secretion, increased mucus viscosity with decreased mucociliary clearance from the lung – have prejudiced the clinical use of these agents. Until recently the anticholinergics had been largely superseded by β_2-agonists. However, the isomer of one of the isopropyl derivatives of atropine, ipratropium, has been shown to have excellent bronchodilator properties with virtually none of the central anticholinergic effects of atropine. No impairment of lung mucociliary clearance occurs and there are no ill effects on mucus viscosity. Ipratropium has a prolonged action producing bronchodilatation for 6 to 8 hours, but the response is generally a little less marked than with the β_2-agonists. The onset of effect is a little slower than for the β_2-agonists, being 15 to 30 minutes. There are varying reports of the effectiveness of a combination of β_2-agonists and ipratropium, a combination which in theory ought to be additive as a bronchodilator.

Ward et al. (1981) in treating hospital patients with acute asthma showed that ipratropium and salbutamol inhalation given in sequence produced greater bronchodilatation than either used alone, and concluded that ipratropium enhanced the bronchodilator effect of salbutamol. In a double blind trial, however, Pierce and colleagues (1982) could show no significant increase in effect with a combination of terbutaline and ipratropium compared to either drug used alone in short or long term use.

The exact role of ipratropium in relation to the β-agonists in the treatment of asthma has yet to be determined.

Methylxanthines as Bronchodilators

Mode of Action

Theophylline is clinically the most important of the 3 naturally occurring methylxanthines and, as with theobromine and caffeine, is found in dietary constituents. Apart from its action as a bronchodilator, it is a central nervous system stimulant and will abolish periodic respiration. It produces a mild diuresis due to a self-limiting effect on the renal tubules, and has an unpredictable effect on the pulmonary circulation, generally producing vasodilatation in poorly ventilated regions of the lung. It produces a decrease in central venous pressure possibly due to an inotropic effect on the heart. Convulsions, due to its central stimulant effects, may result from an overdose and CNS manifestations of toxicity are more common than cardiotoxic effects.

The effectiveness of theophylline as a bronchodilator is attributed to its ability to relax bronchial smooth muscle, but the exact mechanism of this has not been clearly established. It is widely described as an inhibitor of the enzyme cyclic nucleotide phosphodiesterase – an enzyme which catalyses the conversion of $3'$ $5'$ cyclic-AMP to the inactive $5'$-AMP. In this way it produces increased levels of cyclic-AMP within the cell and thus enhances bronchial smooth muscle relaxation. It also inhibits the release of histamine from sensitised mast cells. On these grounds it should act synergistically with the β_2-agonists which stimulate increased formation of cyclic-AMP through the adenyl cyclase system (fig. 6.1). Although its action as a phosphodiesterase inhibitor is said to be the basis of its therapeutic effectiveness, it has been shown to be only a mild inhibitor of bronchial phosphodiesterase and yet potent inhibitors of bronchial phosphodiesterase such as papavarine do not show any bronchodilator action. It has recently been pointed out by Estenne et al. (1980) that intravenous aminophylline (theophylline ethylene diamine) in therapeutic doses does not influence resting bronchomotor tone in the normal lung, whereas other bronchodilators such as the β_2-agonists have a significant and measurable effect. They suggest that their findings are consistent with the theory that theophylline effects are not due to a direct action on bronchial smooth muscle.

It may well be that the recently described ability of theophylline to inhibit the release of histamine from mast cells may account, at least in part, for its action in asthma. In addition the work of Aubier et al. (1981) showing that in usual therapeutic doses aminophylline enhances the contractile force of the normal human diaphragm and reverses diaphragmatic muscle fatigue, indicates that the value of theophylline in asthma may well relate to factors other than its bronchodilating capabilities.

While theophylline is an effective bronchodilator of considerable value in certain clinical situations – it has been shown to reverse pharmacologically induced airways obstruction unresponsive to salbutamol – there are problems with its use which must be appreciated if the drug is to be employed to its best effect. The plasma half-life of theophylline varies considerably between patients, from 3 to 10 hours with a mean of 5 hours. This tends to vary with age, and in children, because of a high metabolic clearance of theophylline, the half-life is only 3 to 4 hours; thus children require a higher maintenance dose per 24 hours.

Metabolism

Theophylline is primarily metabolised by the liver with a small proportion (10%) of the drug excreted unchanged by the kidney. Many factors influence the hepatic handling of theophylline: cigarette smoking increases liver metabolism and thus may alter dose requirements; liver disease impairs metabolism meaning lower doses must be used, and impaired hepatic function in congestive heart failure may result in reduced theophylline clearance. A number of drugs may influence the hepatic metabolism such as allopurinol and the macrolide antibiotics triacetyl oleandomycin and erythromycin. These drugs may decrease hepatic metabolism with consequent rise in serum levels and the possibility of toxic effects. Since both the therapeutic effect of theophylline and the incidence of toxicity correlate directly with the plasma concentration, it is necessary to monitor serum levels to allow for the wide variation of the individual patient's ability to metabolise the drug. Failure to do this means the likelihood of sub-optimal therapeutic blood levels or alternatively the risk of toxic effects.

Plasma theophylline levels can now be measured in most laboratories, and a plasma level of 10 to 20mg/L (50-100μmols/L) is accepted as a therapeutic range which is a compromise between ineffectiveness and toxicity. Some patients show a therapeutic response at blood levels below the accepted therapeutic range, and others tolerate high levels without clinical evidence of side effects, although the incidence of these increases markedly above the range.

Side Effects and Toxicity

Side effects with theophylline are commonly gastrointestinal with anorexia, nausea, vomiting and abdominal discomfort, but headache, malaise, nervousness and tachycardia also occur. Rapid intravenous administration may produce tachyarrhythmias and even cardiac arrest (Camarath et al., 1971). Most serious side effects, however, result from plasma levels well above the therapeutic range.

Because of its poor solubility the ethylene diamine salt of theophylline (aminophylline) is used for intravenous administration. When a 'loading' dose of aminophylline is given intravenously, it is strongly recommended that it be given over at least 15 minutes and be well diluted in, say, a 50ml IV infusion, rather than given as a series of small boluses from a syringe. Intramuscular injection should be avoided – the high pH of the solution makes this an extremely painful injection and absorption from this route is unpredictable.

Absorption

Theophylline given orally is generally about 90 to 100% absorbed; the recently developed microcrystalline formulations ensure almost complete bioavailability and the rapid attainment of peak plasma levels. Because of the low water solubility of theophylline a number of theophylline compounds have been developed and the actual theophylline content of these varies considerably, between 50 and 80%. As theophylline is the active pharmacological agent, these compounds are not necessarily therapeutically equivalent and varying plasma levels may result if treatment is changed from one to another without appreciating their theophylline equivalence. With the microcrystalline forms of theophylline now available, there is little justification for the continued use of these derivatives. There is certainly no longer any place for the mixed combinations of theophylline, ephedrine and a barbiturate; the dangers of administering a respiratory depressant, coupled with the inadequacies of ephedrine as a bronchodilator compared to the newer β_2-agonists, and the fact that the theophylline dose in these combinations is usually too small to achieve a therapeutic blood level, has made them obsolete.

Similarly, while aminophylline suppositories have been used in the treatment of asthma – particularly for nocturnal symptoms – for many years, absorption from suppositories is unpredictable and erratic and thus potentially hazardous, and there is no justification for this form of therapy in modern management.

Sustained release forms of theophylline are now available and are reportedly useful in the treatment of patients with high rates of theophylline clearance. These sustained release forms have been shown to produce a therapeutic plasma level 10 hours after ingestion and to lead to significant improvement in nocturnal wheezing when they are taken before going to bed. Subjects with a slow plasma clearance may maintain satisfactory therapeutic levels with standard formulations.

Dosage

Bearing in mind that the final decision on dosage for continuous theophylline therapy calls for measurement of serum theophylline concentration, the recommendations of Wyatt et al. (1978) provide a useful guide:

- children less than 9 years, 24 mg/kg/day
- between 9 and 12 years, 20 mg/kg/day
- 12 to 16 years, 18 mg/kg/day
- over 16 years, 13 mg/kg/day.

These dosages may be used to start therapy and adjusted, if necessary, after serum theophylline measurement.

The intravenous dosage of theophylline in an emergency is 5 to 6 mg/kg bodyweight given over 15 to 30 minutes, preferably diluted in 50ml infusion. If the patient is already on theophylline the IV dose should be reduced to at least half the above. In an emergency, an infusion of the above dose over 5 to 10 minutes is justifiable, but a more rapid IV injection should not be given. This IV dose can be repeated at 6-hourly intervals or alternatively continuous infusion of aminophylline at a dose of 0.9mg/kg bodyweight per hour is recommended for maintenance by some authorities, with a higher dose recommended in children: 1 to 1.5 mg/kg/hour. The dosage of intravenous aminophylline should not exceed 1g/24 hours unless serum theophylline levels are available.

Because of problems with toxicity in patients already on oral theophylline, and the difficulty in obtaining information on serum levels in an emergency, it is now our practice to avoid continuous infusion altogether and simply to give the drug intravenously, *ad hoc*, as a slow bolus, or avoid its use whenever possible.

Comparative Efficacy

There is no doubt about the effectiveness of theophylline as a bronchodilator, but in practice it is generally only of medium potency compared to the specific β_2-agonists. Its relatively slow onset of action when given orally compared to inhaled β_2-agonists, the incidence of side effects and the problems inherent in the monitoring of drug plasma levels make it very much a 'second line' drug in the management of asthma in the writer's opinion. It is extensively used in North America, where most of the research into its pharmacokinetics has been carried out, but this is probably a consequence of the delayed availability of the new β_2-agonists. Rossing et al. (1980) in a study comparing the effectiveness of intravenous aminophylline, inhalation of isoprenaline, and subcutaneous adrenaline in the emergency treatment of asthma, showed IV aminophylline to be considerably inferior as a bronchodilator to inhaled isoprenaline and subcutaneous adrenaline. In addition to illustrating that the β-agonist drugs were superior as bronchodilators, they noted that the mean duration of treatment required before discharge from the emergency room was significantly longer for patients receiving aminophylline (5.4 hours) than for patients who were treated with either adrenaline subcutaneously (3.5 hours) or isoprenaline by inhalation (3.0 hours). Their results quite clearly demonstrated that sympathomimetic agents are more effective bronchodilators in acutely ill asthmatics, and that inhaled β-agonists are highly effective in this situation.

Sodium Cromoglycate

Mode of Action

When sodium cromoglycate (cromolyn sodium) became available in 1968 it introduced an important new approach to the management of asthma. Here was a drug which was not a bronchodilator, had no apparent anti-inflammatory action, and did not antagonise the action of histamine, SRSA, or the other known mediators of anaphylaxis. Some explanation for its therapeutic action was found to lie in its stabilising effect on mast cells. Mast cells are recognised as having a major role to play in the basic mechanisms of allergic disease (see Chapter IV p.47) and cromoglycate appears to stabilise the mast cell membrane, preventing degranulation of the cell and the release of mediators. The drug does not prevent antigen/antibody combination, nor does it affect the fixation of antibody to the mast cell wall, but this inhibition of cell degranulation and mediator release prevents the manifestations of the allergic reaction. For cromoglycate to be effective it must be given before exposure to the antigen so that the drug is present in the airway before antigen-antibody combination takes place.

While at first it was thought that cromoglycate exercised its inhibitory effect only on those immunological reactions which involved reaginic antibody and mast cells, it has been suggested that it has several types of blocking activity including inhibitory effects on some non-antigenic stimuli (Altounyan, 1980).

Clinical Efficacy

Sodium cromoglycate can be regarded as the first prophylactic agent for use in asthma. The drug has no place in the management of the acute attack, but it can prevent asthma developing if used appropriately and in the right clinical circumstances.

In addition to its undoubted action on mast cells, another important therapeutic effect of cromoglycate is reduction in bronchial hyper-reactivity. According to Altounyan (1980) this is an indirect effect of the drug which occurs after several weeks' use and is only observed in allergic patients when exposed to antigen challenge.

Although cromoglycate's major benefit is in preventing allergen-induced bronchoconstriction, reports have shown significant benefit in non-atopic asthma although the clinical effectiveness of the drug in these circumstances varies considerably. Initial reports in the late 1960s were enthusiastic and favourable, and there are now several hundred reported trials of sodium cromoglycate in asthma with results varying from favourable to equivocal. The fact that even allergic asthma may be the result of non-immune or non-allergic mechanisms at times, may account for the response to the drug varying considerably.

Apart from the effectiveness of sodium cromoglycate in preventing asthma due to inhaled allergens, it has been shown to prevent exercise-induced asthma. The drug must be inhaled before exercise; there is no benefit if it is taken immediately afterwards.

Dosage and Indications

Sodium cromoglycate is inhaled as a dry powder from a special inhaler. Gelatine capsules containing 20mg of the powder are inserted into a 'spinhaler', the capsule sides are pierced, and the inspired breath spins the capsule so that the powder is released and inhaled. About 10% of the inhaled dose reaches the lung, the rest being swallowed, and about 10% of the inhaled drug is absorbed and excreted unchanged in the urine and bile. There is no breakdown of the drug in man or evidence of accumulation in the lung or tissues. The maximum duration of effectiveness of a single inhaled dose is 4 to 6 hours, and so regularly spaced inhalations throughout the day are necessary. An alternative dosage form available in some parts of the world delivers a metered dose of 1mg per actuation and a nebuliser solution is also made containing 10mg sodium cromoglycate per ml.

Clinical benefit from cromoglycate may not be apparent for a varying time, depending on the nature of the asthma being treated. It may be as long as 4 weeks before a definite therapeutic effect is seen although predictable seasonal asthma may respond quickly, within 2 or 3 days. In patients with chronic asthma, it may be possible to reduce oral steroids, and bronchodilator use, but it is sometimes necessary to use cromoglycate for several weeks before this can be done.

A reasonable practice is to use the drug for a month and if there is no therapeutic response to stop treatment. Sodium cromoglycate has no place in the treatment of non-compliant patients and patients should be taught fully to understand the role the drug plays in the management of their condition or treatment failure will be likely. Sodium cromoglycate should not be used in the management of acute severe asthma, and it may in fact aggravate asthmatic attacks through an irritant effect of the dry inhaled powder.

Its effectiveness in controlling chronic asthma seems about comparable with oral theophylline (Hambleton et al., 1977) but with the advantage of being largely free from side effects. This freedom from side effects makes it a particularly attractive drug for use in children where the success rate is considerably higher than adults. Cromoglycate is a relatively non-toxic drug, the most common side effect being due to irritation by the inhaled powder. Rare hypersensitivity reactions have been reported with skin eruptions, pulmonary infiltrates and angioneurotic oedema.

Corticosteroids in the Treatment of Asthma

It is more than 30 years since the first report of the value of corticosteroids in the treatment of asthma and in spite of the general acceptance of their value as the most potent therapeutic agents in the suppression of asthmatic symptoms, the exact mechanism of their action remains to be established (Chapter IV, p. 57; fig. 6.1). The major therapeutic benefits probably result from (1) the suppression of inflammation, and (2) the facilitation of sympathetic nervous system function, particularly relating to β-adrenergic receptor stimulation.

Anti-inflammatory Mechanisms

The anti-inflammatory action of steroids is nonspecific in that they will inhibit the inflammatory response from both immunological and non-immunological stimuli. Thus experimentally, pretreatment with steroids will suppress the inflammatory reaction from almost any kind of injury. Steroids reduce inflammation by:

1) Blocking increased capillary permeability induced by acute inflammation and maintaining the integrity of the microcirculation. As a result there is reduced leakage of fluid and protein into an area of injury and swelling is minimised.

2) Tending to stabilise lysosomes, preventing damage to lysosome walls and the release of enzymes.

3) Decreasing neutrophil chemotaxis and inhibition of the migration of neutrophils and monocytes to areas of inflammation. Following steroid administration there is a brisk neutrophil leucocytosis associated with a distinct fall in the number of circulating eosinophils, lymphocytes and monocytes. This fall is probably the result of redistribution of cells to other body compartments.

Antigen/antibody union is not influenced by steroids, nor is the formation of antibodies affected, but there is suppression of the inflammatory response following antigen/antibody union. The inhibition of neutrophil chemotaxis and the depression of monocyte-macrophage function results in decreased mobilisation and accumulation of these cells in inflammatory regions. The action of steroids in correcting increased capillary permeability associated with inflammation reduces the leaking of protein and fluid into the bronchial lumen and has a decongestant effect on bronchial mucous membranes.

Although corticosteroids have no specific receptor organs, they are taken up by the target cell and bound to a specific receptor protein within the cell. The resulting complex is then transported to the cell nucleus where it is bound to specific acceptor sites on the nuclear chromatin. The transcription apparatus of the cell is activated and new specific messenger RNA is formed. The new mRNA molecules are then transported to the ribosomes in the cytoplasm. Here new protein molecules are synthesised which are considered responsible for the steroid mediated functional response of the particular target cell or tissue. This mechanism is consistent with the observation that steroid effects are not manifest for some hours after administration.

Permissive Mechanisms

The 'permissive' effects on β-adrenergic receptors were pointed out by Brodie et al. (1966) who showed in experimental animals that in the absence of corticosteroids many of the metabolic responses to adrenaline were severely impaired but with cortisone replacement were restored. Townley et al. (1970) also demonstrated the facilitation of sympathetic nervous system function by corticosteroids when they reported an apparently synergistic effect of hydrocortisone and catecholamines on bronchial smooth muscle preparations. At a clinical level it was observed by Rebuck and Read (1971) that there was apparent potentiation of the response to inhaled sympathomimetics during steroid treatment of acute severe asthma.

There is thus both clinical and experimental evidence to indicate that corticosteroids have a permissive effect on β-adrenergic receptor response to catecholamines.

Other Mechanisms

The administration of corticosteroids is associated with an increased accumulation of 3' 5' cyclic-AMP in bronchial smooth muscle cells. This appears to enhance the effect of β-adrenergic stimulation and as a consequence there will be (1) direct relaxation of bronchial smooth muscle, and (2) inhibition of mediator release. Improved mucociliary clearance and decreased mucus viscosity have also been suggested, perhaps by the same enhancement of adrenergic activity.

Table 6.2. Relative anti-inflammatory potency and plasma half-life for some systemic steroids

Compound	Anti-inflammatory potency	Plasma half-life (min)
Cortisone	1	90
Prednisone, prednisolone	5	200-240
Cloprednol	10	90-100
Methylprednisolone	5	200
Betamethasone	25	300
Dexamethasone	25	300

To summarise, corticosteroids do not affect antibody formation or interfere with antigen/antibody union; they do not antagonise histamine or SRSA; they restore cell membrane permeability towards normal, reducing the accumulation of fluid and protein in tissues, and possibly reducing the penetration of antigen into the respiratory mucous membrane. Steroids inhibit both the movement of phagocytes to inflamed tissues and the release of lysosomal enzymes. While they are not bronchodilators, steroids enhance the bronchodilating effects of β-adrenergic drugs.

Corticosteroid Side Effects

The potent anti-inflammatory actions of corticosteroids are associated with major metabolic side effects. This has led to modification of the original steroid molecule in an attempt to produce derivatives with minimal side effects. Derivatives which are mineralocorticoid have no anti-inflammatory activity, while those with a potent glucocorticoid action (i.e. predominantly affect carbohydrate metabolism) have high anti-inflammatory activity.

There are now a number of synthetic steroid preparations in clinical use with minimal metabolic side effects, but retaining the characteristics necessary for therapeutic benefit. A serious complication of continued systemic therapy is suppression of the hypothalamic-putuitary-adrenal axis. Suppression of the HPA axis can be minimised by using steroids with a short half-life (a major reason for the general use of prednisone and prednisolone in asthma) and avoided by not administering them continuously or for prolonged periods. In a minority of patients, however, it is necessary to continue systemic corticosteroid therapy indefinitely, but wherever possible – consistent with satisfactory maintenance of ventilatory function – oral steroids should be used only intermittently to control severe exacerbations.

Alternate-day therapy with corticosteroids may allow satisfactory control with minimal HPA suppression and few side effects. Fauci (1978) provides a logical argument for alternate-day therapy with a single early morning dose of prednisone on alternate days as a form of maintenance therapy once control has been established. A recent study (Change et al., 1982) indicated that children treated for 2 years or more with daily or alternate-day steroids had a similar degree of growth retardation.

A report from Shapiro et al. (1979) suggests that the new oral corticosteroid cloprednol which has a plasma half-life of only 100 minutes, produces significantly less suppression of the HPA axis than prednisone while maintaining at least comparable relative control of chronic steroid-dependent asthma. The relative potency and half-life of a number of commonly used corticosteroids is shown in table 6.2.

Apart from the suppression of the HPA axis, the most common and important side effects of steroid therapy which have been reported are as follows:

1) Musculoskeletal – osteoporosis, aseptic necrosis of bone, myopathy

2) Endocrine – failure of growth in children, adrenal suppression

3) Circulation – sodium and water retention, hypertension, hypokalaemia

4) Metabolic – buffalo hump obesity and facial mooning, precipitation of diabetes mellitus

5) Gastrointestinal – peptic ulceration

6) Ocular – development of posterior subcapsular cataracts

7) Nervous system – psychiatric disturbances

8) General – atrophy of subcutaneous tissues, impairment of wound healing, development of opportunistic infections.

The importance of recognising the small group of patients who are corticosteroid-resistant has been pointed out by Carmichael et al. (1981). They describe a group of patients with demonstrable, reversible airways obstruction, resistant to oral and inhaled steroids in high doses. These patients are at risk from needless exposure to steroid side effects for little therapeutic benefit.

Prolonged corticosteroid therapy in children has an inhibitory effect on growth, although it should be appreciated that asthma itself results in growth retardation in children (Chang et al., 1982). This emphasises the need to balance the risk of continued steroid treatment with the benefits. It has been shown that less than half of the daily dose necessary to control severe asthma will produce growth retardation (Kerrebijn and De Kroon, 1968).

The use of daily corticotrophin injections is reported to correct growth retardation in children and provide satisfactory control of asthma, but does not prevent the development of Cushingoid side effects. Hydrocortisone powder inhalations 7.5 to 15mg daily were first reported in 1955 as being effective in the treatment of asthma, but it was soon shown that absorption occurred and there was no advantage over oral steroids. With the development of potent topically acting corticosteroids with poor absorption characteristics, such as beclomethasone dipropionate and betamethasone valerate, it became possible to reconsider the aerosol delivery of steroids and reduce steroid side effects. Numerous trials have confirmed the effectiveness of steroid aerosols and in a dose of 300 to 400μg per day, beclomethasone dipropionate provides effective control for a large number of asthmatics without the effect on growth in children and HPA axis suppression seen with oral steroids. In doses greater than 500μg/day sufficient absorption occurs to result in some HPA suppression (Wyatt et al., 1978). The side effects of inhaled steroids are discussed fully in Chapter X.

Dosage and Indications

The dosage and indications for systemic corticosteroid treatment of asthma are discussed in Chapter VII. These aspects of inhaled steroids are discussed in Chapters XI and XII.

Table 6.3. A suggested approach to drug selection for asthma

Mild symptoms		
	Little functional disturbance	Occasional β_2-agonist aerosol
	Symptoms more frequent	Regular β_2-agonist aerosol
	in children	Regular sodium cromoglycate
Moderate symptoms		
	Significant functional impairment	β_2-agonist aerosol
		+ inhaled steroids (standard dosage)
		+ ? theophylline
	Symptoms occasionally severe	Intermittent oral steroids
Chronic severe asthma		
		β_2-agonist aerosol regularly
		+ inhaled steroids (standard to high dosage)
		+ daily theophylline
		+ prednisone ? alternate day

A Management Plan

Having reviewed the available pharmacological choices in asthma therapy, certain important points should be emphasised concerning the management of individual patients.

Simplicity

It is important to keep treatment as simple as possible, using the least number of agents which will control symptoms and maintain satisfactory respiratory function.

Education

It is essential that patients understand their treatment and that they know the nature of the drugs prescribed and the reasons for their use. The likelihood of non-compliance with medication is high if patients are ill informed. Poor understanding of the correct use of aerosols is widespread and largely reflects a failure on the profession's part to discharge satisfactorily its responsibility to educate. Apparent treatment failure, particularly with prophylactic agents such as cromoglycate and inhaled steroids, is frequently due to non-compliance.

24-Hour Treatment

In patients with chronic asthma, treatment must be tailored so that there is medication cover continuously, throughout each 24 hours.

Self-reliance

Particularly in those subject to severe asthma, patients should be given a large degree of responsibility for controlling their own treatment following guidelines given to them by their medical practitioner. This is obvious in the case of agents such as bronchodilators, but applies equally to the use of oral steroids if these are necessary to control severe asthma. Patients should be given clear advice on the dose increment recommended, told to initiate such increments themselves and then to seek further advice subsequently. Such responsibility on the part of the patient is best coupled with home monitoring of ventilatory function with, for example, a peak expiratory flow meter (p. 39). If the patient is taught to monitor function at home and keep a record of changes in function (p.186), modifications to treatment can be made much more satisfactorily than by relying on symptoms alone.

Prescribing Guidelines

A suggested prescribing scheme for asthma is set out in table 6.3. The mainstay of the management of asthma is the appropriate use of a β_2-agonist aerosol for virtually all cases, supplemented where appropriate with prophylactic measures such as daily sodium cromoglycate or inhaled steroids. Where the response is less than ideal oral theophylline or ipratropium aerosol is added and, if necessary, oral steroids in severe cases.

References

Aas, K.: Biochemical and immunological basis of bronchial asthma. Triangle. Sandoz Journal of Medical Science 17: 103 (1978).

Ahlquist, R.P.: A study of the adrenotropic receptors. American Journal of Physiology 153: 586 (1948).

Altounyan, R.E.C.: Review of clinical activity and mode of action of sodium cromoglycate. Clinical Allergy 10(Suppl.): 481 (1980).

Aubier, M.; De Troyer, A.; Sampson, M.; Macklem, P.T. and Roussos, C.: Aminophylline improves diaphragmatic contractility. New England Journal of Medicine 305: 249 (1981).

Barger, G. and Dale, H.H.: Chemical structure and sympathomimetic action of amines. Journal of Physiology 41: 19 (1910).

Bellamy, D. and Collins, J.V.: Acute asthma in adults. Thorax 34: 36 (1979).

Brodie, B.B.; Davies, J.I.; Hynie, S.; Krishna, G. and Weiss, B.: Interrelationships of catecholamines with other endocrine systems. Pharmacological Reviews 18: 273 (1966).

Camarath, S.J.; Weil, M.H.; Hanashiro, P.K. and Shubin, H.: Cardiac arrest in the critically ill – a study of predisposing causes in 132 patients. Circulation 44: 688 (1971).

Carmichael, J.; Paterson, I.C.; Diaz, P.; Crompton, G.K.; Kay, A.B. and Grant, I.W.B.: Corticosteroid resistance in chronic asthma. British Medical Journal 282: 1419 (1981).

Chang, K.C.; Milich, D.R.; Barwise, G.; Chai, H. and Miles-Lawrence, R.: Linear growth in chronic asthmatic children: the effects of the disease and various forms of steroid therapy. Clinical Allergy 12: 369 (1982).

Dolovich, M.B.; Killian, D.; Wolff, R.K.; Obminski, G. and Newhouse, M.T.: Pulmonary aerosol deposition in chronic bronchitis: intermittent positive pressure breathing versus quiet breathing. American Review of Respiratory Disease 115: 397 (1977).

Estenne, M.; Yernault, J.-C. and De Troyer, A.: Effects of parenteral aminophylline on lung mechanics in normal human. American Review of Respiratory Disease 121: 967 (1980).

Fauci, A.S.: Alternate day corticosteroid therapy. American Journal of Medicine 64: 729 (1978).

Gaddie, J.; Legge, J.S.; Petrie, G. and Palmer, K.N.V.: The effect of an alpha-adrenergic receptor blocking drug on histamine sensitivity in bronchial asthma. British Journal of Diseases of the Chest 66: 141 (1972).

Hambleton, G.; Weinberger, M.; Taylor, J.; Cavanaugh, M.; Ginchasky, E.; Godfrey, S.; Tooley, M.; Bell, T. and Greenberg, S.: Comparison of cromoglycate and theophylline in controlling symptoms of chronic asthma. Lancet 1: 381 (1977).

Harvey, J.E. and Tattersfield, A.E.: Airway response to salbutamol: effect of regular inhalations in normal, atopic and asthmatic subjects. Thorax 37: 280 (1982).

Jenne, J.W.; Chick, T.W.; Strickland, R.D. and Wall, F.J.: Subsensitivity of beta responses during therapy with a long acting beta$_2$ preparation. Journal of Allergy and Clinical Immunology 59: 383 (1977).

Kerrebijn, K.F. and De Kroon, J.P.M.: Effect on height of corticosteroid therapy in asthmatic children. Archives of Disease in Childhood 43: 556 (1968).

Lands, A.M.; Arnold, A.; McAuliff, J.P.; Luduena, F.P. and Brown Jr., T.G.: Differentiation of receptor systems activated by sympathomimetic amines. Nature 214: 597 (1967).

Lichtenstein, L.M.: An evaluation of the role of immunotherapy in asthma. American Review of Respiratory Disease 117: 191 (1978).

McFadden Jr., E.R.; Kaiser, R. and DeGroot, W.J.: Acute bronchial asthma. New England Journal of Medicine 288: 221 (1973).

Motulsky, H.J. and Insel, P.A.: Adrenergic receptors in man. New England Journal of Medicine 307: 18 (1982).

Nelson, H.S.; Raine, D.; Donor, H.C. and Posey, W.C.: Subsensitivity to the bronchodilator action of albuterol produced by chronic administration. American Review of Respiratory Disease 116: 871 (1977).

Nickerson, M. and Kunos, G.: Discussion of evidence regarding induced changes in adrenoceptors. Federation Proceedings 36: 2580 (1977).

Palmer, K.N.V. and Petrie, J.C.: Respiratory diseases; in Avery (Ed) Drug Treatment, 2nd Edn. p.767 (Adis Press, Auckland 1980).

Pierce, R.J.; Holmes, P.W. and Campbell, A.H.: Use of ipratropium bromide in patients with severe airways obstruction. Australian and New Zealand Journal of Medicine 12: 38 (1982).

Rebuck, A.S. and Read, J.: Assessment of management of severe asthma. American Journal of Medicine 51: 788 (1971).

Rossing, T.H.; Fanta, C.H.; Goldstein, D.H.; Snapper, J.R. and McFadden Jr., E.R.: Emergency therapy of asthma: comparison of the acute effects of parenteral and inhaled sympathomimetics and infused aminophylline. American Review of Respiratory Disease 122: 365 (1980).

Rubinfeld, A.R. and Pain, M.C.F.: Perception of asthma. Lancet 1: 882 (1976).

Shapiro, G.G.; Tattoni, D.S.; Kelley, V.C.; Pierson, W.E.; Dorsett, C.S. and Bierman, C.W.: Cloprednol therapy in steroid dependent asthma. Pediatrics 63: 747 (1979).

Svedmyr, N.; Larsson, S. and Thiringer, G.: Development of 'resistance' in beta adrenergic receptors of asthmatic patients. Chest 69: 479 (1976).

Szentivanyi, A.: The beta adrenergic theory of the atopic abnormality in bronchial asthma. Journal of Allergy 42: 203 (1968).

Townley, R.G.; Reeb, R.; Fitzgibbons, T. and Adolphson, R.L.: The effect of corticosteroids on the beta adrenergic receptors in bronchial smooth muscle. Journal of Allergy 45: 118 (1970).

Ward, M.J.; Fentem, P.H.; Roderick-Smith, W.H. and Davies, D.: Ipratropium bromide in acute asthma. British Medical Journal 282: 598 (1981).

Weber, R.W.; Petty, W.E. and Nelson, H.S.: Aerosolised terbutaline in asthmatics. Journal of Allergy and Clinical Immunology 63: 116 (1979).

Wyatt, R.; Weinberger, M. and Hendeles, L.: Oral theophylline dosage for the management of chronic asthma. Journal of Pediatrics 92: 125 (1978).

Chapter VII

Systemic Steroids in Asthma

G.M. Cochrane

Since the introduction of inhaled corticosteroids the place of systemic steroids in asthma has become obscured. Although corticosteroids given systemically are generally accepted as effective in the treatment of asthma, especially in the severely ill, there are in fact few conclusive studies. However, systemic corticosteroids are considered to be of benefit in the management of asthma in the following circumstances: in the severely ill patient; in patients whose asthma is getting progressively worse; for long term prophylaxis, and to determine whether or not there is any reversibility of obstruction in patients with chronic airflow impairment (table 7.1). These categories are inevitably rather artificial, but provide a framework for examining the role of systemic steroids in the treatment of asthma. The possible mechanisms of action of corticosteroids have been discussed in the previous chapters (p.57, 96). Table 7.2 lists commonly available corticosteroids, their sodium retaining characteristics, glucocorticoid activity and biological half-lives. Their characteristics will not be discussed further here but referred to later in the appropriate section.

Acute Severe Asthma

Do Corticosteroids Work in Acute Severe Asthma?

Clark (1977) defined acute severe asthma as an episode of increased severity failing to respond to more than average treatment. When patients suffer from such an increase in symptoms it has become generally accepted that they require corticosteroids to treat the attack effectively. While steroid therapy has been shown to be effective in the treatment of continuous symptomatic asthma, there are few studies investigating their use in acute severe asthma (MRC, 1956). In fact, two studies suggest that steroids either as a single injection of hydrocortisone or as a full course of intravenous and oral therapy, do not significantly improve the treatment of acute asthma (McFadden et al., 1976; Luksza, 1982). Grant (1982) suggests that this is not the case and a study has shown a more rapid recovery in patients treated with corticosteroids compared with a control group who received bronchodilator therapy only (Fanta et al., 1982a). Although conclusive evidence is not available, most physicians feel that corticosteroids should be given to patients with severe asthma.

The assessment of the patient who is at most risk of dying from an attack of asthma is difficult. It is, however, important to determine such at-risk patients as it is they who may well be helped by parenteral corticosteroids, the risks being outweighed by the possible benefit.

Assessment of Severity of Asthma

Clinical Assessment

Jones (1980) suggested clinical grading of the severity of asthma on an exercise tolerance system (table 7.3). Patients whose asthma has reduced their exercise potential to Grade IIb (i.e. confined to a chair or bed but able to get up with great difficulty) or worse are more likely to die. The increasing frequency of use of β_2-stimulant aerosols is an excellent guide to the severity of the attack. Observing the patient undressing for a physical examina-

Table 7.1. Indications for systemic corticosteroids

1) Acute severe asthma

2) Worsening chronic asthma

3) Long term maintenance therapy

4) Diagnostic trial of reversibility in a patient with chronic airflow obstruction

tion often helps one appreciate how severely their exercise tolerance is impaired. The signs indicative of acute severe asthma are listed in table 7.4 and the measurement of these indices is discussed fully in Chapter III.

Respiratory Rate

Cyanosis occurs very late in severe asthma and suggests impending death. A respiratory rate greater than 30 per minute in a child or 25 per minute in an adult is associated with severe asthma and it is surprising how frequently respiratory rate is not measured. Recently, clinical physiologists have been reminded that even during a severe attack of asthma, the work of breathing is greatest during inspiration (Morris, 1981) and most patients complain of difficulty in breathing in. Tracheal tug and intercostal muscle indrawing are maximum at the onset of inspiration, when the respiratory muscles generate the greatest pleural pressures and the inspiratory airflow obstruction does not allow air to enter the alveoli fast enough. During the recovery phase from an attack of acute asthma, the peak expiratory flow at first does not change, but tracheal tug and intercostal recession decreases.

Abnormalities of Pulse

Pulse rate remains an important sign of severity with a pulse rate of above 110 per minute in an adult and 120 per minute in a child suggesting severe asthma. Frequently the rapid pulse is taken to be a sign of 'excessive' use of β-stimulants or theophyllines but this is not the case. Treating the attack of asthma and decreasing airflow obstruction, albeit with additional bronchodilators, leads to a fall in pulse rate. In patients with asthma who are over 55 years of age, a low pulse rate can lead to a false sense of security as, with age, a sinus tachycardia in response to asthma does not always occur. Bradycardia precedes hypoxaemic cardiac arrest and hence is an ominous sign in severely ill patients of any age. In acute asthma, there is a respiratory cycled systolic pressure difference (or pulsus paradoxus). A difference of 18mm Hg between inspiration and expiration suggests severe asthma. The mechanism for pulsus paradoxus is still obscure, but explanations vary between diminished venous return associated with high intrathoracic pressures or cardiac tamponade secondary to pulmonary hyperinflation, and diaphragmatic flattening.

Wheeze

Obvious wheezing clearly suggests airflow obstruction but frequently 'silent' chests are more worrying as the patients' asthma is so severe that they are unable to generate adequate airflow to produce a wheeze. Signs of pneumothorax or mediastinal emphysema are associated with a poor prognosis. Peak expiratory flow rate should be measured; values below 100 litres/minute only occur in the presence of severe airflow obstruction. If possible the

Table 7.2. Some more commonly used corticosteroids

Compound	Anti-inflammatory effect	Approximate potency (mg)	Sodium-retaining potency	Biological half-life (hours)[1]	Regular daily dose (mg) above which HPA axis[2] suppression likely	
					male	female
Hydrocortisone	1	20	1	8-12	20-30	15-25
Prednisolone	4	5	0.25	18-36	7.5-10	7.5
Methyl prednisolone	5	4	±	18-36	7.5-10	7.5
Triamcinolone	5	4	±	18-36	7.5-10	7.5
Betamethasone	25-30	0.6	±	36-54	1- 1.5	1- 1.5
Dexamethasone	25	0.8	±	36-54	1- 1.5	1- 1.5

1 Biological half-lives are based on the duration of pituitary adrenal suppression.
2 These values are given only as a guideline and are dependent on total body surface area.

forced expired volume in one second (FEV_1) is measured; a value of less than a litre or below 30% of predicted normal is considered by some to be the best indication of the need for hospital care.

Gas Exchange

Although arterial blood gas estimation facilities are seldom available to the primary physician, patients are often referred directly to emergency departments where they should exist. Patients with acute asthma frequently have apparent hyperventilation because the $PaCO_2$ is less than the usually accepted normal of 40mm Hg. However, this alveolar hyperventilation is frequently a 'normal' response in asthma. Cochrane et al. (1980) have suggested that a $PaCO_2$ of 35mm Hg in the presence of a PaO_2 of 50mm Hg suggests significant alveolar underventilation if the arterial pH is normal, as the 'normal' response to such arterial hypoxaemia would predict a $PaCO_2$ of 27mm Hg. Any $PaCO_2$ value above 35mm Hg in the presence of a PaO_2 below 60mm Hg is a sign of severe asthma. See also p.39.

Severely ill patients should where possible be transferred to hospital. However, as many studies have shown that a considerable number of patients die in the actual course of transfer, therapy should be given beforehand.

Treatment of Acute Severe Asthma Before Hospital Transfer

β_2-stimulants

Patients should be given adequate doses of β_2-stimulant therapy even though they may well have already taken many more 'puffs' than usual from their metered dose aerosol. It has been suggested that 0.5mg salbutamol intramuscularly or 0.25mg terbutaline subcutaneously should be given and where available, β_2-stimulant via a nebuliser system in the dose equivalent of 5mg salbutamol (only about 10% of which will actually reach the lungs). Aminophylline injections have for many years been considered first line therapy in this situation but there is now data suggesting that theophylline is a less potent bronchodilator than inhaled β-stimulants (Rossing et al., 1980; Fanta et al., 1982b). Also, because of the increase in the number of patients receiving maintenance treatment with slow-release methylxanthines, the safe dose required in an emergency is often difficult to estimate (see p.174). Fast injections of methylxanthines are dangerous, but even when given slowly, in the presence of hypoxia and hypokalaemia, the risks of serious cardiac arrhythmias are significant. It has been suggested that using a standard selective β_2-aerosol, 2 puffs every 5 minutes during transfer may be safer than intravenous aminophylline, especially when used in conjunction with intravenous hydrocortisone.

Corticosteroids

In acute severe asthma, corticosteroids should be given parenterally. Hydrocortisone should be given in a dose which will produce a plasma cortisol level which is at least that which can be obtained by maximal stimulation of the adrenal cortex. The usually recommended intravenous emergency dose is 100mg for a child or 200mg for an adult, and does not take account of body surface area. This dose is likely to maintain cortisol levels, similar to those achieved by maximum stimulation, for 2 to 4 hours (Collins et al., 1975).

Oxygen

During the transfer of patients to hospital controlled oxygen therapy (inspired oxygen 35-40%) should be given as this may well diminish the risks of cardiac arrhythmias, and is unlikely to induce life-threatening carbon dioxide retention in patients with severe asthma.

Treatment of Acute Severe Asthma in Hospital

Intravenous Hydrocortisone

Argument persists about the optimal dose of steroids for acute asthma. The dose suggested above stems from the earlier cited work and it would appear desirable to achieve a plasma cortisol level in excess of 100 $\mu g/100ml$. Patients with asthma do not (as once suggested) appear to have an impaired adrenal response to stress, although acute severe asthma does not always produce a maximal

Table 7.3. A classification of asthma severity (after Jones, 1980)

Grade I	Able to carry out housework or job with difficulty
Grade II	Confined to a chair or bed but able to get up with moderate difficulty (IIA) or with great difficulty (IIB)
Grade III	Totally confined to a chair or bed
Grade IV	Moribund

Table 7.4. Indices of asthma severity

Cyanosis

Respiratory rate/minute > 25 (adult) > 30 (child)

Pulse rate/minute > 110 (adult) > 120 (child)

Pulsus paradoxus > 18mm Hg

Tracheal tug with intercostal recession

Severe wheezing or 'silent' chest

PEFR < 100 litres/minute

PaO_2 < 60mm Hg

$PaCO_2$ > 35mm Hg in the presence of a PaO_2 < 60mm Hg

$PaCO_2$ > 40mm Hg in the presence of a PaO_2 < 70mm Hg

adreno-cortical response. One trial has suggested that in the majority of patients there is no advantage in using massive doses of corticosteroids, rather than those that produce a cortisol level equivalent to the maximum (100-150 μg/100ml) that can be achieved by stress or ACTH or tetracosactrin stimulation (Britton et al., 1976).

Without doubt the intravenous route has the advantages of certain and rapid access to the circulation, whereas oral absorption may be reduced in the acute attack, and the use of adrenal cortex stimulating hormones (ACTH) is highly unreliable. The *speed of response* to hydrocortisone intravenously is normally considered to be within 6 to 8 hours in the severely ill asthmatic (less in the less severely ill). Oral prednisolone appears not to have any effect in less than 9 hours; even when given intravenously prednisolone appears to take 8 hours to work. However, many patients feel that the combination of inhaled and intravenous bronchodilators and intravenous corticosteroids can diminish their symptoms appreciably in 2 to 3 hours, although changes in PEFR and FEV_1 take longer. Perhaps we are not yet aware of what to measure when determining the response to treatment in asthma.

Dosage and Concomitant Drugs

To achieve a blood level of hydrocortisone between 100 and 150 μg/100ml requires a dosage regimen of approximately 3 to 4 mg/kg bodyweight given every 6 hours. The author's practice is to give (if not already given before admission) 200mg hydrocortisone as a bolus; this is normally the equivalent of 3 to 4 mg/kg bodyweight. The cortisol levels are then maintained by 6-hourly infusions of 4 mg/kg bodyweight for the next 24 hours (usually between 200-300mg hydrocortisone 6-hourly). The total dose of hydrocortisone for the first 24 hours is thus 1 to 1.5g. Frequently patients respond dramatically to this regimen over the course of the first 24 hours, especially when it is allied to maximum doses of inhaled β_2-stimulant (5mg of nebulised salbutamol or equivalent 4-hourly), intravenous methylxanthines if indicated (the dose being related to blood levels) and the atropine derivative ipratropium bromide given by nebulised inhalation (1mg 4-6 hourly). The dose of hydrocortisone is usually decreased by 3 mg/kg bodyweight 6-hourly over the next 24 hours if there is improvement in the indices outlined in table 7.4; the patient is started on 40 to 60mg prednisolone orally during the second 24 hours. If there is no significant response in pulse rate, pulsus paradoxus or PEFR then the initial high dose of intravenous hydrocortisone is continued. In patients who are responding to therapy, intravenous hydrocortisone is stopped after 48 hours and oral prednisolone maintained at a level of 60 to 40 mg/day depending on bodyweight (over 80kg, 60mg; 70-80kg, 50mg; below 70kg, 40mg). In the poorly responsive, intravenous hydrocortisone is usually continued until adequate signs of clinical improvement justify transfer to oral prednisolone. Theoretically methyl prednisolone should have less tendency to cause fluid retention than prednisolone (a problem with older asthmatics) but there is no good evidence to support this claim. The rate of metabolism of cortisol and consequent fall in plasma level has been considered to be faster in patients with asthma, but there is no data to support this claim. Previous corticosteroid therapy does not affect the rate of metabolism but concomitant drug therapy with barbiturates, rifampicin and other liver enzyme-inducing drugs will reduce plasma cortisol levels; in patients on rifampicin the dose of corticosteroid needed to produce the same blood level is approximately twice as high.

Additional Therapy and Supportive Measures in Acute Asthma

Additional therapy must be given with corticosteroids as outlined above. Nebulised β_2-stimulants are usually considered standard therapy for severe asthma and unlike theophylline and ipratropium bromide there is some evidence to suggest that the combination of corticosteroids and β_2-stimulant is synergistic (Middleton, 1975). Also, patients who have previously failed to respond to β_2-stimulants, may become responsive in the presence of corticosteroids.

Oxygen

Controlled oxygen therapy should be used in patients who are hypoxic. Concentrations in excess of 50% inspired oxygen, although unlikely to produce carbon dioxide retention in patients with acute asthma, can lead to pneumonitis and, ultimately, a secondary fall in arterial oxygen concentrations. Oxygen therapy may well be needed for some days as, although there may be a dramatic improvement in indices of airflow obstruction, arterial oxygen concentrations may continue to be reduced. This hypoxia is related to small airways obstruction and mucous plugging which leads to ventilation perfusion mismatching. Such mismatching may well be exacerbated by the action of β_2-stimulant therapy.

Rehydration and Potassium Replacement

Patients also require rehydration especially if the attack has been slowly progressive over a few days. During rehydration adequate potassium replacement should be given as the combination of apparent hyperventilation and high inspiratory thoracic pressures leads to marked hypokalaemia.

Complications of Steroid Therapy in Acute Asthma

Metabolic Effects

The side effects of high dose corticosteroid administration are outlined in table 7.5. Hypokalaemia and, after the first day's therapy, fluid retention, are the most commonly seen side effects. An initially low potassium may be made worse by the metabolic alkalosis induced by the corticosteroids and lead to gross hypokalaemia. Potassium replacement requirements are usually most easily monitored by regular estimation of serum potassium. Fluid retention is usually most severe when intravenous hydrocortisone has to be continued for many days and occurs more frequently in the very ill or patients requiring supportive ventilation. Diuretic therapy will usually rapidly clear the retained fluid but with concomitant loss of potassium. Aldosterone antagonists may be useful in this situation. Glycosuria or frank diabetes mellitus, with or without ketoacidosis may occur, especially in the elderly asthmatic or the obese patient. Regular urine testing for glucose rapidly warns the clinician of this problem and if the blood sugar is raised, insulin should be given in the standard fashion. Insulin requirements usually fall dramatically as the corticosteroids are reduced.

Blood Pressure Effects

Hypertension, if it occurs, can be difficult to treat. β-blockers must not be given as even the most 'selective' is likely to worsen bronchoconstriction, especially at the time of an acute attack. Thus the choice of treatment is restricted to diuretics, methyldopa and vasodilators.

Table 7.5. Side effects of corticosteroids, which may be of sudden onset, associated with short term high dose therapy ($\geq$ 40mg prednisolone, 200mg hydrocortisone)

Hypokalaemic alkalosis (exacerbated by hyperventilation)

Clinical diabetes mellitus (exacerbated by parenteral feeding)

Hyperosmolar non-ketotic coma

Hypertension

Sodium and water retention (oedema) – exacerbated by the use of intermittent positive pressure ventilation

Mental disturbances including severe psychoses

Cerebral oedema (especially in young children)

Proximal myopathy

Glaucoma

Pancreatitis

Peptic ulceration and gastrointestinal haemorrhage (not proven side effects)

Gastrointestinal Complications

During any episode of severe stress the incidence of intestinal perforation or intestinal haemorrhage is higher. Whether corticosteroids increase these complications has not been satisfactorily determined, but certainly the clinical signs of perforation may be masked by the use of corticosteroids. It is not universally accepted that antacids and H_2-receptor blockers need be given to all patients during an attack of severe asthma. If the patient recovers rapidly then regular meals are effective in reducing possible gastrointestinal complications. In patients with protracted attacks, or those requiring supportive ventilation, there is a case for regular antacids, and the use of H_2-receptor blockers to reduce gastric acidity. These can be stopped as soon as the patient is eating regularly. It should be borne in mind that cimetidine substantially increases the half-life of theophylline and therefore serum theophylline measurements are essential in patients receiving both drugs; ranitidine, a related H_2-receptor blocker, does not appear to have this drawback (Breen, et al., 1982).

Other Complications

Two important but fortunately less common complications are sudden mental disturbance, usually an acute psychosis in adults, and the development of cerebral oedema in children. In both these conditions treatment is difficult but patients usually respond to the withdrawal of the corticosteroids and appropriate symptomatic treatment. Why cerebral oedema is more frequent in children is not known. Fortunately both these conditions, which can cause subtle changes in personality, often come to the early notice of relatives. Proximal myopathy is uncommon using the doses of corticosteroids recommended here.

Reducing Corticosteroids After an Acute Attack of Asthma

The approach to reducing corticosteroids after an acute attack of asthma will depend upon the response of the patient and the concomitant therapy. Recently there has been an increased interest in the recovery phase of acute asthma, two populations being recognised: a group who tend to return to near normal levels of lung function in less than 3 days, and others who tend to take much longer. The faster responding group are usually children or young adults, or those patients whose attack of asthma developed rapidly, in less than 24 to 48 hours. The more elderly group of asthmatics, and also those who suffered a protracted decline in exercise tolerance before developing the severe acute attack, frequently do not achieve their previous best respiratory function for 10 days. The mechanism for this disparity of response is thought to be the involvement of the smaller airways, with mucous plugging and bronchial casts. However, there appears to be little advice or evidence to guide the clinician as to how rapidly corticosteroids can be safely reduced or whether or not the patient with the less protracted attack requires 10 days of corticosteroid therapy to diminish the irritability of the airway. Reduction of corticosteroids is frequently carried out at the same time as reduction of other therapy.

In the author's unit, any patient requiring admission to hospital for an acute attack of asthma receives prednisolone or its equivalent at a level between 30 to 50mg daily, depending on bodyweight, for at least 7 days after a satisfactory response. This dose of prednisolone is then reduced over a period of 1 to 2 weeks depending on the severity of the asthma, and previous oral steroid requirements. Concomitant therapy, especially nebulised β_2-stimulants, is gradually withdrawn as, in the author's experience, sudden reduction may be associated with a further acute attack of asthma. Patients must not be suddenly changed from doses of β_2-stimulants such as 40mg a day via a nebuliser to 800 μg a day via a pressurised aerosol (dosage as for salbutamol) on the day they are discharged; they will frequently suffer a further acute attack of asthma.

Side effects from severe suppression of the pituitary-adrenal axis appear to be uncommon if these high doses of corticosteroids are maintained only for a few days. The longer intravenous hydrocortisone is given, the greater the degree and duration of adrenal suppression to be expected. Patients who require surgery or have another medical emergency within 2 weeks of withdrawal of oral corticosteroids should have steroid replacement. Some authors (Hugh-Jones et al., 1975) have suggested that patients should receive synthetic ACTH during withdrawal of oral corticosteroids, the theory being that not only can the adrenal axis be assessed in this way, but any adrenal suppression diminished by active stimulation. Although theoretically attractive, this approach has not received general support.

Steroids in Acute Severe Asthma: in Summary

In an acute severe attack of asthma the efficacy of corticosteroids is debated but the author believes they may be life saving and, if used correctly, safe. Intravenous hydrocortisone is the drug and route of choice. There appears to be no justification for massive doses but a dose adequate to ensure a plasma level of 100 to 150 μg/100ml (3-4 mg/kg bodyweight as a loading dose followed either by infusion or injection of 4 mg/kg 6-hourly) is recommended.

Rehydration, potassium replacement, controlled oxygen therapy and inhaled or intravenous bronchodilators should be given simultaneously. Complications should be anticipated rather than awaited and reduction of therapy related to repeated measurements of the indices of severity. Maintenance prophylactic therapy, especially with inhaled corticosteroids, should be introduced before the systemic corticosteroids are completely withdrawn. Oral corticosteroids should be reduced over approximately 2 weeks if the patient has had a protracted attack of severe asthma but very slowly reducing regimens are usually not necessary. There is no place for ACTH or tetracosactrin in the management of patients with a severe attack of asthma.

Worsening Chronic Asthma

Fortunately, in the majority of patients, asthma can be well controlled by regular bronchodilators and prophylactic antiasthma preparations. However, asthma is an unpredictable disease and frequently patients whose symptoms were previously well controlled develop an attack of asthma. The cause of the attack may be infection or a high antigen count, such as grass pollen in the summer, but frequently there is no apparent reason.

Patients usually complain of increasing shortness of breath, tightness of the chest, wheezing, especially at night, and often sleep is disturbed during the early hours of the morning. Patients complain that their β_2-stimulant aerosol is less effective in relieving their symptoms and symptoms recur sooner than normally between inhalations. Fortunately, the majority of patients are aware of the worsening of their asthma but about 15 to 20% would appear to underestimate an increase in the severity of an attack (see p.35).

Indications for Corticosteroid Therapy

Worsening Symptoms

Over recent years in Great Britain self-referral systems have been implemented for patients who suffer from asthma and who are attending outpatient clinics. These self-referral systems allow the patient either telephone- or direct-access to the hospital specialist when their asthma is becoming more severe. One problem associated with this practice is that of ensuring the patient knows exactly when to seek this advice. Only guidelines can be given, but any patient who, previously well controlled, finds his exercise tolerance reduced by a half, or who, previously sleeping well, wakes on two consecutive nights with an acute attack of asthma, probably requires an increase in antiasthma therapy.

Increasing Need for Bronchodilators

Another guideline can be the use of bronchodilator aerosols. Unfortunately, too often patients are inclined to lie to their doctors regarding the use of their aerosol. The cause for this deception is frequently the doctor's reprimanding attitude and the belief that patients may become addicted or tolerant to their β_2-stimulants. There is no good evidence for either tachyphylaxis (in patients with asthma) or addiction to β_2-stimulants. The newer β_2-stimulants would appear to be remarkably safe, even in high oral overdosage (Prior et al., 1981). Rather than admonish the patient perhaps it is better to advise him to increase his β_2-stimulant bronchodilator aerosol if necessary, but to record his usage of the drug. Thus, when a patient who was well controlled on a regimen of prophylactic therapy and '8 puffs' of β_2-stimulant aerosol a day suddenly requires '20 puffs' a day he should be told to seek further advice.

Poor Perceivers of Worsening Asthma

The minority of patients who appear to be less able to appreciate a worsening in the severity of their asthma are more difficult to help. As there appears to be considerable weight to the argument that patients who seek help (and are helped) early during the development of an attack of asthma are less likely to die (Crompton and Grant, 1975) some attempt must be made to identify those patients who have least insight into their illness. Frequently these patients are easy to identify because of their previous medical history of poor compliance, late arrival at emergency departments in a pre-morbid state due to asthma, or because of limited intelligence or a particular ethnic background.

Patients who are poorly able to estimate the severity of an attack of asthma are also unable to assess their response to bronchodilators (unpublished observations) and the author's unit is now studying such patients. Using a visual analogue scale compared to subjective measurement of airflow obstruction (PEFR, FEV_1) patients during the recovery phase from an acute attack of asthma are asked to assess the efficacy of varying doses from active and placebo aerosols. Most patients (80%) can judge improvements using the visual analogue scale in parallel with the objective response as shown by their change in PEFR. However, a minority are unable to do this at all accurately and it is these patients who will be most helped by regular estimations of PEFR at home. They can then be told when to seek advice or alter drug therapy in relationship to changes in their PEFR. See also Chapter III.

Drug Treatment of Worsening Chronic Asthma

Although it is almost universally accepted that steroids should be given to patients with worsening asthma the doses used vary and there is little evidence to support any particular regimen. Where possible any particular cause for the increased symptoms should be identified and in the presence of pyrexia and increased sputum production, broad spectrum antibiotics are probably indicated. An increase in bronchodilator therapy is usually required, but it is the use of oral corticosteroids which may prevent the development of a severe attack.

Prednisolone Regimens

Two basic regimens have been suggested: an adult course of 7 days of oral prednisolone, 40 mg/day (or 0.5 mg/kg bodyweight/day in children) and then stopping abruptly; or a similar dosage initially but reducing, either by 5mg a day or every other day, until the patient has been completely withdrawn from steroids. Both regimens have their advocates. The first is associated with acute hypothalamic-pituitary-adrenal suppression (Webb and Clark, 1981) but this is only likely to be a potential problem in the 2 to 3 days after stopping the corticosteroids, while the second regimen is probably associated with a higher failure rate in preventing an acute attack of asthma developing or continuing. Obviously, the regimen adopted may depend on the precipitating factors: in a patient allergic to house dust who is moving home then the obvious course is to use regular high dose prednisolone during the few days before and after moving, whereas in the patient with an acute upper respiratory tract infection, a reducing regimen associated with a course of antibiotics may be more logical. Whichever approach is used, it is essential to monitor the patient's response to therapy and it is often easier to do this using the 7-day course of 40mg a day of prednisolone. When the patient is reviewed after a week therapy may be continued, intensified or stopped depending on improvement in exercise tolerance, symptoms and respiratory function. Measurement of PEFR at home allows an objective assessment of improvement, diminishing the chances of being misled by any euphoriant effect of the corticosteroids.

ACTH and Depot Preparations

ACTH or synthetic analogues (tetracosactrin) have been used instead of prednisolone but because of variability of response, and possible allergic reactions, they are no longer indicated. Although with their use cortisol levels of 90 μg/100ml can be achieved and maintained in some patients, in patients who have previously received corticosteroids adrenal atrophy may lead to much lower levels. The hoped-for protection of the adreno-cortical response is not a reality as although the adrenal cortex may be preserved, the hypothalamic-pituitary part of the axis will be suppressed; pituitary failure can frequently be more refractory than adrenal failure. Thus, adreno-cortical stimulation cannot be recommended as treatment for a patient whose asthma is worsening.

Depot or slow-release injections of prednisolone have been insufficiently studied in this situation but may have a certain appeal for the patient who is poorly compliant. The author has used them, but only in the recovery phase when the patient has sought discharge before adequate control of symptoms. The dose required is impossible to predict. A recent survey has shown that patients who are suffering from symptoms of asthma are remarkably compliant and usually oral prednisolone therapy is taken as prescribed (James et al., in press).

Complications of Short Courses of Oral Corticosteroids

Metabolic Complications

Obviously care must be taken as, although hypothalamic-pituitary-adrenal suppression may not be profound or prolonged, patients especially the more elderly may develop hypokalaemia, hypertension and fluid retention. Less frequently glycosuria and frank diabetes mellitus may be induced, but this can be anticipated in older, obese patients who should be advised to check their urine for sugar using a simple dipstick method. The evening post-prandial urine, rather than early morning urine, should be tested as any glycosuria is more likely to occur at this time and any serious hyperglycaemia thus prevented.

Gastrointestinal Complications

Prednisolone should be given as a single morning dose, after or with food to diminish any direct gastrointestinal discomfort; if the patient has suffered from gastrointestinal symptoms previously enteric-coated prednisolone is prescribed. The absorption characteristics of regular and enteric-coated prednisolone are similar in most patients and the dose is identical, although there have been occasional reports of diminished bioavailability from enteric-coated prednisolone preparations.

HPA Axis Impairment

The biological half-life (table 7.2) allows for once-daily oral dosing and, unlike maintenance corticosteroid therapy (p.114), there is no advantage in using higher dose alternate-day therapy. Morning dosing possibly diminishes the adrenal cortical depression as it is at this time that the natural diurnal variation of cortisol is at its maximum, whereas evening therapy could further suppress the already low circulating levels. Another argument for morning therapy is that it diminishes the nocturnal euphoria and insomnia corticosteroids may induce when given in the evening.

Steroids in Worsening Asthma: in Summary

Corticosteroids may prevent the development of acute severe asthma if given early in the evolution of an attack. Increasing shortness of breath, tightness in the chest and a documented increase in β_2-stimulant bronchodilator usage are all indications for additional therapy. A course of oral prednisolone (40mg daily for an adult) for either 7 days, or as a rapidly reducing regimen, should be given with other appropriate therapy, such as increased dosage of bronchodilators and antibiotics. Side effects must be anticipated and if the risks warrant it the patient should be admitted to hospital. HPA axis suppression is usually not severe. The effectiveness of the treatment must be monitored, if necessary with PEFR measurements in the home. Patients with least insight into the severity of their disease should be identified, otherwise they are unlikely to seek medical advice early enough; regular monitoring of their PEFR at home will compensate for their poor perception of worsening asthma and encourage them to ask for help earlier. There appears to be little place for ACTH or its synthetic derivatives in the management of worsening asthma, but the use of depot injections of steroids needs to be assessed further.

Long Term Maintenance Therapy

Demonstration of their obvious efficacy in high doses in patients with acute asthma was followed by the use of oral corticosteroids as maintenance therapy, over many years, at a lower dose (reviewed by Walsh and Grant, 1966). It was this long term use which led to corticosteroids being regarded as dangerous, as regular intake of 10mg of prednisolone or more over many months is likely to lead to a number of systemic side effects (table 7.6).

Patient Selection

Recognising patients who require regular oral corticosteroids is usually easy, they form the group who have numerous symptoms and need frequent hospitalisation and time away from work or school. However, every attempt should be made to control their symptoms using other therapy before resorting to oral steroids. With the appropriate use of inhaled steroids (p.148,177) and high doses of β_2-stimulants (Prior et al., 1982) many patients need no longer rely on daily oral steroids.

Maintenance Regimens

Daily Corticosteroid Therapy

The total daily requirement should be given as a single morning dose to coincide with the physiological peak of diurnal steroid secretion. Prednisolone or methyl prednisolone are the most suitable corticosteroids as a shorter half-life is probably associated with fewer metabolic side effects (table 7.6). The longer-acting drugs are also considerably more potent and make the management of dosage regimens more difficult. Their longer half-life appears to increase both the degree of HPA suppression and the incidence of skeletal side effects. Prednisolone is preferred to prednisone which requires conversion by the liver to the pharmacologically active prednisolone.

Alternate-day Therapy

When patients, particularly children, have been stabilised on once-daily therapy an attempt should be made to transfer them to alternate-day therapy. Alternate-day dosage of prednisolone has been accepted as being associated with a lower incidence of side effects, diminishing hypokalaemia, adrenal suppression and growth retardation in children although recently it has been shown that there may be no advantage in alternate-day compared with daily doses where growth effects of steroids are concerned (Chang et al., 1982). Many methods of transferring patients from once-daily to alternate-day dosage have been suggested but once well controlled on a single, morning oral dose of prednisolone with associated

Table 7.6. Side effects of corticosteroids more likely to be associated with long term administration (10-20mg prednisolone or equivalent). Sudden onset side effects may also occur (see table 7.5)

Osteoporosis with vertebral compression and multiple bone fractures
Aseptic necrosis of bone
Cerebral atrophy
Development of latent epilepsy
Variations in mood – depression, anxiety and lability of mood
Posterior sub-capsular cataracts
Hyperlipidaemia with perhaps increased incidence of gallstones
Centripetal obesity (lemon on a tooth pick appearance)
Growth failure in children and adolescents
Secondary amenorrhoea
Suppression of hypothalamic-pituitary-adrenal axis
Impaired wound healing with subcutaneous tissue atrophy
Diminished immune response leading to increased vulnerability from bacterial and opportunistic organisms

bronchodilator therapy this is not usually difficult. The daily dose of prednisolone which will control the symptoms adequately is doubled and then given on alternate days. Occasionally it may be necessary to reduce the dose on one day (e.g. by 5mg) increasing the following dose by the same amount until transfer is complete. No-one knows why many asthma patients can be well controlled on alternate-day corticosteroid therapy. However, some children have increased wheezing on their steroid-free days and the difficult decision has to be made between the disadvantage of this and being symptom-free with the possibility of increased side effects if daily steroids are given. As severe asthma may, of itself, lead to retarded growth a regimen giving the best control of symptoms is probably the correct choice. Alternate-day therapy is of no use when treating an increase in severity of asthma.

Oral plus Inhaled Steroids

As mentioned previously, now alternative, safer treatments are available, few patients, adults or children, need regular oral corticosteroids to control their asthma; unfortunately those who do need them often require them in high doses. Despite using alternate-day therapy side effects can occur and the use of an oral steroid-sparing manoeuvre should be considered. Although the resulting regimen may be complex it is worthwhile attempting as, even in the most chronically ill patient, the use of inhaled corticosteroids may diminish the dose of prednisolone required and be advantageous. The addition of inhaled corticosteroids to alternate-day oral prednisolone may reduce symptoms on the steroid-free day in children.

'Pulsed' Therapy

A few patients appear to have a slow decline in lung function, despite maximal therapy with other drugs, and if not prescribed corticosteroids will develop an acute attack of asthma. In this group of patients, rather than alternate-day oral therapy, 'pulsed' high dose oral corticosteroid therapy (40 mg/day prednisolone for one week) may prevent the development of acute attacks (fig. 7.1). If he has no rapid access to advice, monitoring the PEFR and symptoms may well allow the patient to take such a course of therapy at a predetermined level of PEFR and symptoms.

ACTH and Tetracosactrin Injections

In the past the use of ACTH or tetracosactrin parenterally has been advocated, especially in children. The arguments advanced in their favour were that adreno-cortical function would be preserved and there would be less effect on growth. The latter is no longer considered to be true and the former may, as mentioned earlier, be irrelevant as rather than adrenal suppression from exogenous steroids, pituitary suppression may occur. The side effects encountered are those of the glucocorticoids with the addition of hyperpigmentation, induction of androgen secretion leading to virilisation and allergic reactions. Although severe allergic reactions have been associated mainly with ACTH there are reports of severe reactions (including a fatal reaction) to tetracosactrin. There is no advantage in using stimulants of endogenous corticosteroid production.

Complications of Long Term Oral Steroids

Unlike the short term, high dose use of corticosteroids for acute asthma, when side effects are uncommon (and are usually either reversible or capable of correction) with maintenance treatment side effects occur in the majority of patients. Commonest are suppression of the hypothalamic-pituitary-adrenal axis, centripetal obesity with 'moon' faced appearance and osteoporosis in the elderly, and retarded growth in children and adolescents. Other side effects, listed in table 7.6, are less common but poor wound healing may be a problem in patients requiring surgery, especially of the gastrointestinal tract. Vulnerability to opportunistic infection or recurrence of pulmonary tuberculosis is rarely a problem unless the patient has another concomitant cause of a depressed immune response, such as a neoplasm, or is receiving cytotoxic therapy.

In patients on long term corticosteroids regular measurement of blood pressure, blood glucose and serum electrolytes is mandatory. Obese patients should be observed carefully and weight reduction suggested. Fluid retention or mild hypertension should be treated with diuretics and potassium supplements if indicated. In adults, regular examination of the eye should be carried out yearly. Patients with a history of gastritis or symptoms suggestive of peptic ulceration should be investigated fully and treated with antacids and/or selective H_2-receptor blockers to diminish gastric acid production. Occasionally transferring to enteric-coated prednisolone may reduce symptoms of gastric ulceration. The problems associated with osteoporosis are more difficult to combat and although various regimens have been suggested, their efficacy is in doubt. Most physicians recommend a diet adequate in calcium but do not resort to other treatments.

Patients should be given a card to keep with them at all times stating the dose and frequency of corticosteroid prescribed. In the author's unit patients are not only given a steroid card but one listing all their medications.

Long Term Maintenance Therapy: in Summary

With the availability of inhaled corticosteroids few patients now require long term maintenance therapy with systemic steroids. Those who do should be given oral prednisolone, if possible using an alternate-day regimen. Side effects are common, with suppression of HPA function, change in body shape and osteoporosis in the elderly, and reduced growth rate in children almost without exception. Alternate-day therapy significantly reduces side effects but asthmatic symptoms may occur on the steroid-free day. The addition of inhaled topically active steroids should be considered (p.128,176). Occasional patients may do better by having regular 'pulsed' therapy using short courses of high dose prednisolone at intervals rather than continuous lower doses. ACTH and its synthetic derivatives offer no advantage.

Trial of Corticosteroids in Patients With Chronic Airflow Obstruction

The majority of patients who have asthma, both young and old, are easily recognised by their typical history of variable airflow obstruction. However, a few patients, often the more elderly, give a history of shortness of breath on exertion, wheezing – especially at night – and tightness of the chest, and appear to have chronic bronchitis. Despite the lack of features associated with a diagnosis of asthma a proportion of these patients may respond to corticosteroids. Because of this, almost all patients with chronic airflow

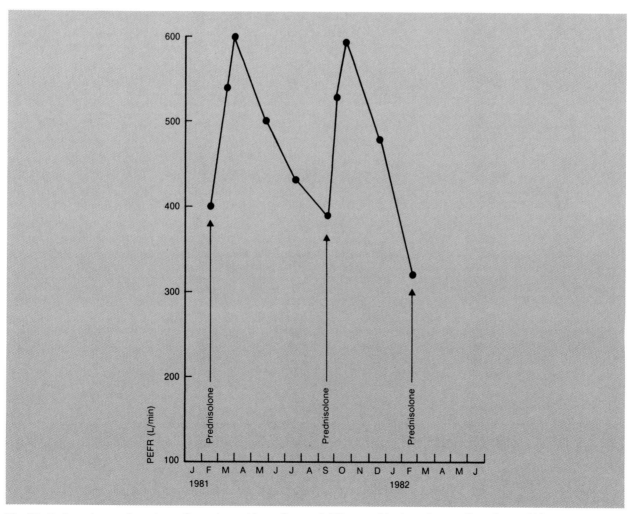

Fig. 7.1. Peak expiratory flow chart of a patient taking salbutamol 400 μg and beclomethasone dipropionate 200 μg (both 4 times daily by pressurised aerosol), who had previously developed severe acute attacks of asthma when his PEFR fell below 300 litres/minute. His workload was high and he was not always able to seek advice easily; he was started on 'pulsed' oral corticosteroids. His response to one week of prednisolone 40mg per day is obvious. At review there was no evidence of any corticosteroid complications.

obstruction should be given a trial of steroids. Features which suggest that the patient is likely to respond to a course of steroids have been mentioned elsewhere (p.111,103). Patients who have documented swings in PEFR of greater than 25% on any day are more likely to respond to corticosteroids but this does not preclude other patients responding, despite a lack of abnormal diurnal variation.

Trial of Corticosteroids

There is no standard regimen for a trial of corticosteroids in patients with chronic airflow obstruction (the description following is of the author's usual protocol, another, with slight variations, is to be found in Chapter XI, p.169). There is evidence to suggest (Webb et al., 1981) that most patients who have not responded to a trial of steroids after 8 days are unlikely to respond at all. In fact the majority will respond by the seventh day. In hospital practice, because of the timing of clinics, there is a tendency to leave corticosteroid trials running for 2 weeks but in general practice assessment after one week is probably most appropriate; however, if there is no response, the course should be continued for a further 7 days. Oral prednisolone 30mg (< 70kg) to 40mg (> 70kg) according to bodyweight as a single dose each morning has been suggested as the most suitable regimen as only a small percentage of patients will respond to higher doses (60 mg/day), and the risks of maintaining a patient on such a high dose outweigh any benefit.

Assessment of Response to Corticosteroids

Monitoring the effect of the trial of steroids is essential but unfortunately not all authors can agree on the best technique. As corticosteroids may have a euphoriant effect it is essential to obtain some objective assessment of the response. Symptom scores and diary card recording may be influenced by any euphoriant effect and a simple exercise test before and after therapy can be a more objective guide. Monitoring PEFR 3 times daily has been widely accepted as a reliable indicator in the majority of patients who are likely to respond significantly to corticosteroids. The closer correlation between FVC and exercise tolerance may explain the occasional difference between the doctor's and patient's assessment of the response to corticosteroids when PEFR is used as the sole criterion. As can be seen from figure 7.2, PEFR monitored at home may show little or no change whereas FVC measurement over the same period of time reveals marked diurnal variations. The introduction of small portable spirometers may well overcome this problem. These and other aspects of patient self-monitoring are discussed in Chapter III.

Patients must be in stable condition before any trial of corticosteroids; for instance they should not be given corticosteroids during an infective episode. Transient responses to corticosteroid therapy occur during acute infective exacerbations but are not an indication for long term corticosteroid therapy as the symptomatic improvement may be associated only with the reduction in the inflammatory response to infection.

Complications

At the end of the trial of corticosteroids therapy may be stopped abruptly with few problems and only transitory compromise of the HPA axis. Other complications have been considered earlier in this chapter. After assessment of the response a decision is made whether or not steroid therapy should be continued. Many

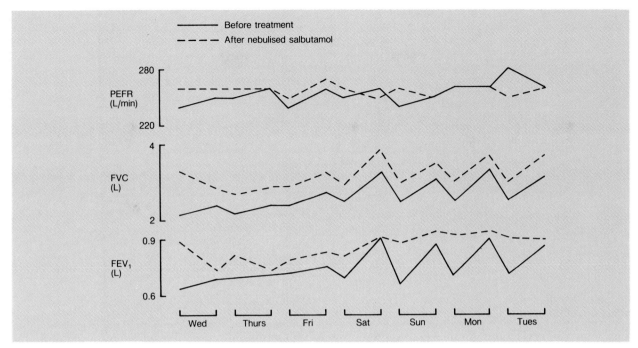

Fig. 7.2. Measurements of PEFR (at home), forced expired volume in one second (FEV$_1$) and forced vital capacity (FVC) in a patient with minimal changes in PEFR but marked diurnal changes in FEV and FVC, and a response to nebulised salbutamol. The patient suffered from considerable reduction in exercise tolerance in the mornings until he had nebulised salbutamol.

patients who have chronic bronchitis and emphysema will be non-responders, showing no change in any objective measurement. The patients who have responded are usually transferred to inhaled corticosteroids although some may need long term oral therapy or a combination of both (see p.171). Some patients respond dramatically to a short course of steroids, maintaining their improvement over months without need of any regular corticosteroid prophylaxis.

A Trial of Steroids: in Summary

All patients who have chronic airflow obstruction and severe symptoms should be given a trial of oral corticosteroids. Doses greater than prednisolone 40 mg/day for longer than 2 weeks will not significantly increase the number of responders. Objective assessment is essential and a simple exercise test and regular at-home PEFR measurements are all that are required in the majority, although FVC, if available, is probably a more accurate method of measurement response. More subtle respiratory function testing is not usually helpful. Further management will vary with the response to steroids but abrupt stopping of the oral steroids is associated with few problems, and those encountered are, only transitory.

References

Breen, K.J.; Bury, R.; Desmond, P.V.; Mashford, M.L.; Morphett, B.; Westwood, B. and Shaw, R.G.: Effects of cimetidine and ranitidine on hepatic drug metabolism. Clinical Pharmacology and Therapeutics 31: 297 (1982).

Hugh-Jones, P.; Pearson, R.B.B. drug metabolism. Clinical Pharmacology and Therapeutics 31: 297 (1982).

Britton, M.G.; Collins, J.V.; Brown, D.; Fairhurst, N.P.A. and Lambert, R.G.: High dose corticosteroids in severe acute asthma. British Medical Journal 2: 73 (1976).

Chang, K.C.; Miklich, D.R.; Barwise, G.; Chai, H. and Miles-Lawrence, R.: Linear growth of chronic asthmatic children: the effects of the disease and various forms of steroid therapy. Clinical Allergy 12: 369 (1982).

Clark, T.J.H.: Acute severe asthma; in Clark and Godfrey (Eds) Asthma, p.303 (Chapman and Hall, London 1977).

Cochrane, G.M.; Prior, J.G. and Wolff, C.B.: Chronic stable asthma and the normal arterial pressure of carbon dioxide in hypoxia. British Medical Journal 281: 705 Advanced Medicine, (1980).

Collins, J.V.; Clark, T.J.H.; Brown, D. and Townsend, J.: The use of corticosteroids in the treatment of acute asthma. Quarterly Journal of Medicine 44: 259 (1975).

Crompton, G.K. and Grant, I.W.B.: Edinburgh emergency asthma admission service. British Medical Journal 4: 680 (1975).

Fanta, C.H.; Rossing, T.H. and McFadden, E.R.: Glucocorticoids in acute asthma. A critical controlled trial. American Review of Respiratory Disease 125(4, past 2): 94 (1982a).

Fanta, C.H.; Rossing, T.H. and McFadden, E.R.: Emergency room treatment of asthma. American Journal of Medicine 72: 416 (1982b).

Grant, I.W.B.: Are corticosteroids necessary in the treatment of severe acute asthma? British Journal of Diseases of the Chest 76: 125 (1982).

Hugh-Jones, P.; Pearson, R.B.B. and Booth, M.: Tetracosactrin for the management of asthmatic patients after long term corticosteroids. Thorax 30: 426 (1975).

James, P.N.E.; Henry, J. and Cochrane, G.M.: Compliance with therapy in patients with diseases of chronic airflow obstruction. In press (1982).

Jones, E. Sherwood: The recognition and management of acute severe asthma; in Bellingham (Ed) p.9 (Pitman Medical, London 1980).

Luksza, A.R.: Acute severe asthma treated with steroids. British Journal of Diseases of the Chest 76: 15 (1982).

McFadden, E.R.; Kiser, R.; de Groot, W.J.; Holmes, B.; T.J.H.: Recovery of plasma corticotrophins and cortisol levels Kiber, R. and Viser, G.: A controlled study of the effects of single doses of hydrocortisone on the resolution of acute attacks of asthma. American Journal of Medicine 60: 52 (1976).

Middleton, E.: Mechanism of action of corticosteroids; in Stein (Ed) New Directions in Asthma, p.433 (American College of Chest Physicians, I-linois 1975).

Morris, M.J.: Asthma – expiratory dyspnoea? British Medical Journal 283: 838 prednisolone in chronic airflow (1981).

MRC: Cortisone acetate in status asthmaticus. Lancet 2: 903 (1956).

Prior, J.G.; Cochrane, G.M.; Raper, S.M.; Ali, C. and Volans, G.N.: Self poisoning with oral salbutamol. British Medical Journal 282: 1932 (1981).

Prior, J.G.; Nowell, R.V. and Cochrane, G.M.: High dose terbutaline in the management of chronic severe asthma: comparison of wet nebulisation and tube spacer delivery. Thorax 37: 300 (1982).

Rossing, T.H.; Fanta, C.H.; Goldstein, D.H.; Snapper, J.R. and McFadden, E.R.: Emergency therapy of asthma: Comparison of acute effecvts of parenteral and inhaled sympathomimetics and infused aminophylline. American Review of Respiratory Disease 122: 365 (1980).

Walsh, S.D. and Grant, I.W.B.: Corticosteroids in the treatment of chronic asthma. British Medical Journal 2: 796 (1966).

Webb, J. and Clark, T.J.H.: Recovery of plasma corticotrophin and cortisol levels after a three-week course of prednisolone. Thorax 36: 22 (1981).

Webb, J.; Clark, T.J.H. and Chilvers, C.: Time course of response to obstruction. Thorax 36: 18 (1981).

Chapter VIII

Inhaled Steroids: Pharmacology and Toxicology

R.N. Brogden

Although several corticosteroids with characteristics likely to make them suitable for use by inhalation (high topical relative to systemic activity) have now been used to treat asthma, the majority of studies have been carried out with beclomethasone dipropionate and, to a lesser extent, betamethasone valerate.

Pharmacology

Topical Anti-inflammatory Activity

Beclomethasone dipropionate is a synthetic chlorinated corticosteroid with a high index of local activity when applied to the skin as an alcoholic solution (Gruvstad and Bengtsson, 1980; Harris, 1975). This activity is demonstrated by the human skin vasoconstriction assay, in which the corticosteroid is applied to the skin as an alcoholic solution or in an ointment base and covered with a plastic film for several hours. The resultant vasoconstriction is manifest as a blanching effect which is assessed visually. On the basis of this method (table 8.1), beclomethasone dipropionate is more active than the potent vasoconstrictors fluocinolone acetonide, triamcinolone acetonide or betamethasone valerate and comparable with budesonide (Gruvstad and Bengtsson, 1980) which latter is also used by inhalation to treat asthma.

Effect on Antigen-induced Asthmatic Reactions

The effect of pre-challenge inhalation of therapeutic doses (200μg) of beclomethasone dipropionate on immediate (type I) and delayed (type III) asthmatic reactions to provocation challenge tests with a range of allergens has been studied by Pepys et al. (1974).

Whereas both immediate and delayed types of asthmatic reaction were inhibited by 20 to 40mg of sodium cromoglycate, only the late (type III) reactions are prevented by beclomethasone dipropionate (Breslin et al., 1973; Pepys et al., 1974). This effect of beclomethasone dipropionate was evident whether the type III reaction occurred alone and was not preceded by the type I reaction, or was part of a dual reaction.

Airways reactivity to inhalation of the parasympathomimetic drug, methacholine was not modified by 4 months' administration of inhaled beclomethasone dipropionate 400μg daily (Easton, 1981). This suggests that a change in airway cholinergic receptor activity is not part of the mechanism of action of inhaled corticosteroids in asthma.

In a recent review (Burge, 1982) it has been suggested that, contrary to popular belief, inhaled corticosteroids can have a protective effect on immediate asthmatic reactions, observable only after several days pre-challenge treatment; paradoxically, late asthmatic reactions are inhibited by single doses whereas inhibition of immediate reactions is demonstrable only after several days pretreatment.

Table 8.1. Topical potency of various corticosteroids as assessed by the vasoconstriction assay on human skin (after Harris, 1975)

Corticosteroid	Relative potency
Betamethasone	0.8
Dexamethasone	0.8
Beclomethasone	0.8
Dexamethasone isonicotinate	8.0
Triamcinolone acetonide	100.0
Fluocinolone acetonide	100.0
Beclomethasone propionate	360.0
Beclomethasone dipropionate	500.0

Effect on Exercise-induced Asthma

Single doses of inhaled steroids do not inhibit exercise-induced asthma in asthmatic patients (e.g. Hills et al., 1974; Hodgson et al., 1974; Yazigi et al., 1978), but some protection against exercise-induced asthma is afforded by 2 to 4 weeks of treatment with usual therapeutic doses (Hartley et al., 1977; Hodgson et al., 1974).

Effect on Immune Mechanisms

Systemically administered corticosteroids induce a prompt, transient decrease in blood concentrations of thymus-dependent lymphocytes, depress lymphocyte proliferation in response to stimulation by haemagglutinin and decrease total eosinophil count.

In contrast, usual doses of beclomethasone dipropionate by inhalation, do not affect total white cell count and lymphocyte count (Schuyler et al., 1981), and do not interfere with the recovery from the transient (< 24 hour) abnormalities of lymphocyte function induced by systemic prednisone (Chiang et al., 1980). However, inhalation of beclomethasone dipropionate at doses which cause systemic effects (e.g. 500 to 1600μg per dose) can produce a significant decrease in lymphocyte and eosinophil count in healthy subjects (Harris, 1975; Blaiss et al., 1982) and in asthmatic patients (Toogood et al., 1977).

Inhalation of beclomethasone dipropionate 400μg daily has been reported to decrease serum immunoglobulin G(IgG), but not other immunoglobulins (De Cotiis and Settipane, 1980). Similarly, local application of beclomethasone dipropionate to the nasal mucosa for a period of 4 weeks appears not to decrease IgA concentrations (Freed et al., 1979).

Effect on Bronchial Tissue

There is a general awareness amongst clinicians that powerful topical corticosteroids may cause dermal atrophy particularly with long term use and when applied under occlusive dressings. This raised the question as to whether prolonged local application of powerful corticosteroids to the respiratory tract, as occurs with inhalation, would result in adverse effects similar to those that occur with the skin. However, histological and electron microscope studies of lung biopsies from patients treated for up to 3 years with usual daily doses of beclomethasone dipropionate, have revealed no important treatment-related changes in lung tissue (table 8.2) Similarly, beclomethasone dipropionate has been shown not to have

Table 8.2. Summary of histological and electron microscope studies of lung biopsies from asthmatic patients treated with beclomethasone dipropionate

Author	No. of patients	Duration of treatment	Control measures	Conclusions
Andersson (1975)	12	6 months	Nil	No adverse changes
Andersson et al. (1977)	11 3	12 months 18 months	Nil	No adverse changes related to treatment
Lundgren (1977)	8	6 months	Pretreatment examination	No evidence of damage to ciliated epithelium
Jorde and Werdermann (1977)	56	≤32 months	180 patients not receiving BDP	No adverse changes related to treatment
Thiringer et al. (1975)	7	4 months	a) Pretreatment examination b) Group (8 patients) on oral steroids	No histopathological changes
Thiringer et al. (1977)	15	36 months	Pretreatment examination	No adverse changes related to treatment

an adverse effect on the nasal mucosa of patients using it intranasally for rhinitis (Mygind, 1977).

Effect on Hypothalamic pituitary-adrenal Function

Resting early morning plasma cortisol concentrations, and those after tetracosactrin (synthetic ACTH) stimulation, provide data on the state of adrenal function, but do not provide information regarding the integrity of the hypothalamic-pituitary portion of the axis. Such information is provided by the insulin stress test. However, this test is unpleasant for the patient and is not without some risk. It is for such reasons that the insulin stress test has seldom been used to study the effects of inhaled corticosteroids on the hypothalamic-pituitary-adrenal axis. See also Appendix 2.

Usual inhaled dosages of beclomethasone dipropionate (British Thoracic and Tuberculosis Association, 1975; Maberly et al., 1973), betamethasone valerate (BTTA, 1975; McAllen et al., 1974), flunisolide (Spangler et al., 1979), triamcinolone acetonide (Bernstein et al., 1982), or budesonide (Willey et al., 1982), seldom cause significant decreases in plasma cortisol concentrations. Nevertheless, it is clear that suppression of endogenous cortisol secretion can occur when the dose is substantially increased. The daily dose at which adrenal suppression has been reported to occur in some adult patients treated with beclomethasone dipropionate has been 400 μg/d (Mygind and Hansen, 1973), 1500 μg/d (Smith and Hodson, 1982) 1600 μg/d (Gaddie et al., 1973) and 2000 μg/d (Choo-Kang et al., 1972; Harris et al., 1973). Others have reported no adrenal suppression at dosages of 400 to 2000 μg/d (Costello and Clark, 1974).

Insulin Stress Test

The relatively few studies that have assessed the response to insulin-induced hypoglycaemia in patients who have been treated for several months with aerosol corticosteroids, have usually found a normal response in most patients. This has been the case whether the patients had had their maintenance systemic corticosteroids replaced by the aerosol, or had not been receiving maintenance systemic steroids prior to the study (table 8.3). In the only study in children, and the only one that included a control group of non-asthmatic patients, Vaz et al. (1982) noted that 5 patients had an abnormal response and that the mean plasma cortisol in patients was lower than in controls (fig. 8.1). However, their plasma cortisol concentrations increased normally after tetracosactin stimulation. Serial insulin stress tests in patients who showed a normal response to tetracosactrin, became normal 4.5 months (mean) after daily administered oral prednisone had been replaced by betamethasone valerate (Roscoe et al., 1975).

Tetracosactrin Stimulation

The short tetracosactrin test, in which the increase in plasma cortisol is measured 30 minutes after injection of synthetic adrenocorticotrophic hormone (ACTH), has been a widely used method of evaluating the effect of inhaled corticosteroids in adrenal function. There has been a general trend for a normal response to ACTH a few months after withdrawal of daily doses of systemic corticosteroids and their replacement with aerosol corticosteroids. Similarly, treatment with inhaled steroids has not usually caused abnormal responsiveness to tetracosactrin stimulation in patients not previously receiving maintenance systemic steroids.

A well conducted study which illustrates the return to normal of adrenal function after withdrawal of systemic corticosteroids in adult patients treated with beclomethasone dipropionate 400 to 600 μg per day, is that of Maberly et al. (1973). This study, in which tetracosactrin tests were conducted before, and at regular intervals during treatment, also illustrates the continued adrenal suppression in patients able to decrease, but not discontinue, sys-

Table 8.3. The effect of aerosol beclomethasone dipropionate and betamethasone valerate on hypothalamic-pituitary-adrenal function as assessed by the insulin stress test

Author	Population (number)[1]	Steroid-dependent	Dosage[2] (μg/d)	No. with normal response[3]	Duration of treatment
Brown et al. (1972)	Adult asthmatics (27)	Yes (13) No (14)	400 BDP	11/13 13/14	≤12 months
Friedman et al. (1974)	Adult volunteers (9)	No	1600 BV	4/9	7 days
McAllen et al. (1974)	Adult asthmatics (5)	No	400-800 BV	5/5	3 months
Roscoe et al. (1975)	Adult asthmatics (11)	Yes	800-1600 BV	9/11	≤12 months
Vaz et al. (1982)	Children asthmatics (16)	No	300-500 BDP	11/16	6-36 months

1 — Number of patients who underwent the insulin stress test.
2 — BDP = beclomethasone dipropionate; BV = betamethasone valerate.
3 — Where a 'normal' response has not been defined in the study, an increment in plasma cortisol of ≥7 μg/100ml (200 nmol/L) and a maximum concentration after stimulation of ≥20 μg/100ml (550 nmol/L) has been taken as 'normal'.

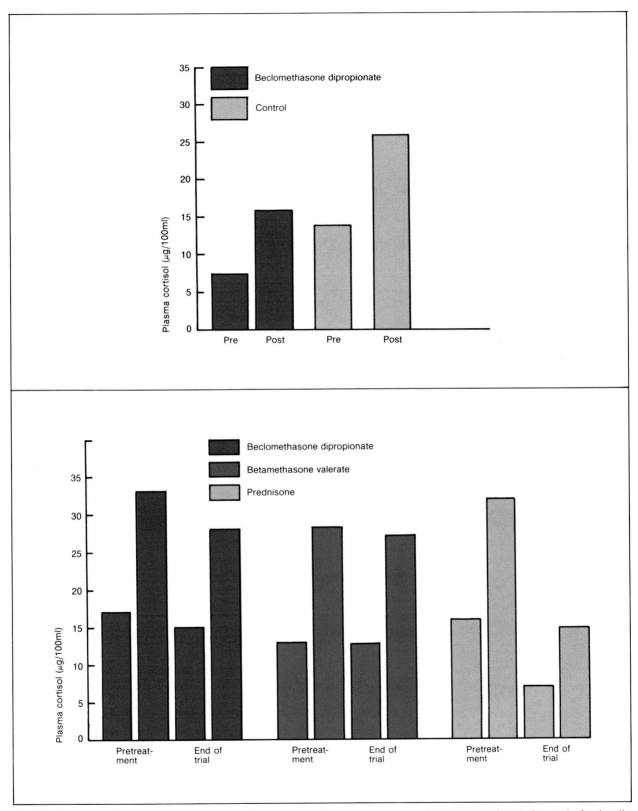

Fig. 8.1. Hypothalamic-pituitary-adrenal axis function as assessed by mean plasma cortisol concentrations before and after insulin-induced hypoglycaemia in 6 children receiving long term treatment with inhaled beclomethasone dipropionate, compared with that in 48 normal children (data from Vaz et al., 1982).

Fig. 8.2. State of adrenal function as judged by plasma cortisol concentrations before and after synthetic ACTH stimulation in asthmatic patients treated with inhaled beclomethasone dipropionate, inhaled betamethasone valerate, or oral prednisone (data from British Thoracic and Tuberculosis Association Study, 1975).

Table 8.4. Results of serial tetracosactrin stimulation tests in steroid-dependent asthmatic patients treated with aerosol beclomethasone dipropionate (data after Maberly et al., 1973)

Prestudy steroid dosage (prednisone mg)	Maintenance regimen (no. of patients)	Proportion of patients with normal[1] tests			
		pretreatment	1 month	2 months	4 months
Group 1 5-15	400-600 µg/d BDP no oral steroids (6)	6/6	3/6	5/6	5/6
Group 2 10-20	400-600 µg/d BDP 5-7.5 mg/d prednisone (4)	0/4	0/4	0/4	NP[2]
Group 3 10-20	400-600 µg/d BDP 10-20 mg/d prednisone (6)	0/6	NP	NP	0/6

1 — A normal response to the short tetracosactrin stimulation test was defined as the presence of at least 2 of the following; a resting plasma-cortisol concentration of >6 µg/100ml (170 nmol/L) a post-stimulation concentration at 30 minutes of >18 µg/100ml (495 nmol/L) and an increment of >7 µg/ml (200 nmol/L) [Greig et al., 1969]. Concentration determined by binding assay.
2 — Tests not performed.

temic steroids (table 8.4). A well designed study conducted by the British Thoracic and Tuberculosis Association in 1975 compared the effect on adrenal function of inhaled beclomethasone dipropionate, inhaled betamethasone valerate and oral daily prednisone, each at doses that controlled asthma equally well (fig. 8.2). Before treatment adrenal function was normal in about 95% of patients in each treatment group. However, after 24 weeks of treatment, adrenal responsiveness was normal in only 36% of patients treated with oral prednisone compared with in 74 to 100% of those treated with inhaled corticosteroids (table 8.5).

Daily Versus Alternate-day Oral Corticosteroids

The normally observed improvement in adrenal function when institution of inhaled corticosteroids enables a substantial decrease, or the complete withdrawal of oral corticosteroid maintenance therapy, has until recently been demonstrated solely in patients receiving daily doses of prednisone or one of the other corticosteroids (e.g. British Thoracic and Tuberculosis Association, 1976; Gaddie et al., 1973; Lal et al., 1972). However, studies from the United States (Kershnar et al., 1978; Nassif et al., 1980; Toogood, 1979; Wyatt et al., 1978) suggest that in children, at least, the substitution of beclomethasone dipropionate inhaler for alternate-day prednisone, is less likely to improve adrenal or HPA function as the degree of adrenal suppression is similar with each regimen.

In the Wyatt study, inhaled beclomethasone dipropionate (mean dose 550 or 576µg daily) was compared with alternate-day prednisone 20 to 40mg (mean 33mg) and with a control group of asthmatics who had not received maintenance oral corticosteroids. The effect of replacing alternate day prednisone with inhaled beclomethasone dipropionate and of combining the two regimens, was also studied. Serum cortisol, urinary free cortisol output (fig. 8.3) and serum 11-desoxycortisol (compound S) after metyrapone (metopirone) stimulation (fig. 8.4), was significantly lower with all corticosteroid regimens than in the control group. There were no significant differences between the single treatment regimens but a greater degree of suppression occurred with the combination. The

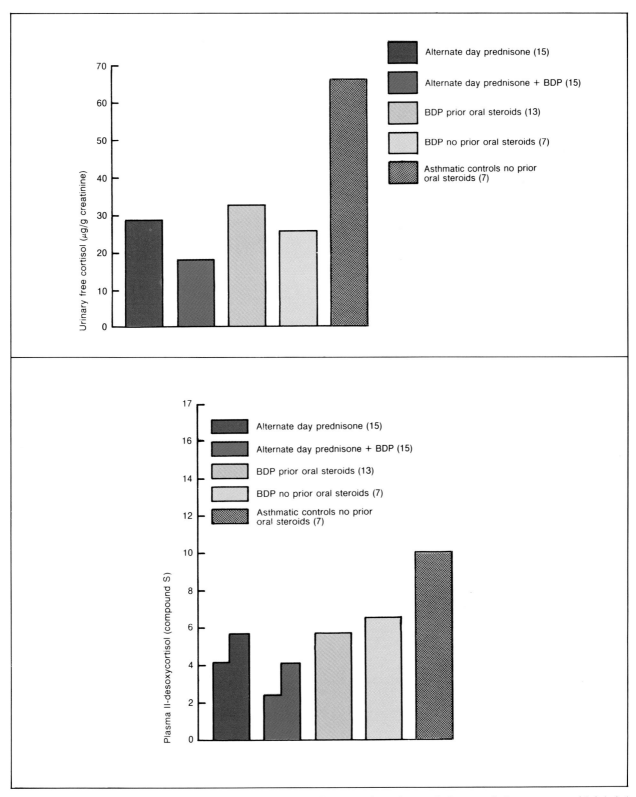

Fig. 8.3. Adrenal function in asthmatic patients assessed by mean 24-hour urinary free cortisol output during treatment with inhaled beclomethasone dipropionate (BDP), alternate-day oral prednisone or both regimens. The effect of BDP was studied in patients who had previously received maintenance corticosteroids and those who had not and in all instances were compared with results in a control group of asthmatics who had not required maintenance corticosteroid therapy (after Wyatt et al., 1978).

Fig. 8.4. Pituitary-adrenal responsiveness as determined by the mean serum concentrations of 11-desoxycortisol (compound-S) after metyrapone stimulation. The split bars indicate the concentrations either 24 hours (left) or 48 hours (right) after a dose of alternate day prednisone (after Wyatt et al., 1978).

dosage of 400 to 800 µg/d of inhaled beclomethasone dipropionate used by Wyatt et al. (1978) is somewhat higher than that usually prescribed in children, but the degree of control of asthma was similar with each of the single treatments. See also p.203 and Appendix 2.

Toogood (1979) compared the effects of inhaled beclomethasone dipropionate with both daily and alternate-day prednisone. The addition of high-dose (about 1500µg/d) inhaled beclomethasone dipropionate to daily prednisone in 17 children resulted in symptom improvement and an additive increase in cortisol suppression. After prednisone dosage had been decreased to the lowest effective dose (final dose 4.8 mg/day) 14 months later, there was a 20% mean rise in morning plasma cortisol. In the 17 patients who had originally received alternate-day prednisone, the increase in plasma cortisol 14 months after beginning beclomethasone di-

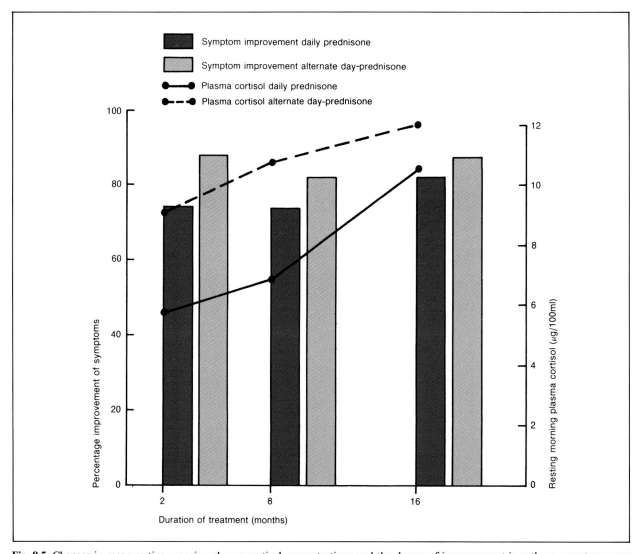

Fig. 8.5. Changes in mean resting morning plasma cortisol concentrations and the degree of improvement in asthma symptoms over a 16 month period after starting treatment with beclomethasone dipropionate (BDP) in 34 patients previously treated with daily (17) or alternate day prednisone (17). The mean daily dose of BDP was 1114µg in the daily prednisone group and 993µg in the alternate day group. The daily prednisone dose at the end of the study was 4.8mg in the daily group and 3.2mg (6.4mg on alternate days) in the alternate day group (data after Toogood, 1979).

Table 8.6. Extent of recovery of pituitary-adrenal function in 34 steroid-dependent asthmatic children treated with inhaled beclomethasone dipropionate (after Kershnar et al., 1978)

Study period	Test		
	diurnal cortisol[1]	tetracosactrin stimulation[2]	metyrapone[3] stimulation (IV)
Pretreatment			
Normal	6	20	4
Abnormal	28	12[4]	30
After Inhaled BDP			
Normal	22	28	12
Abnormal	12	3[4]	22

1 — Normal defined as 8am plasma cortisol concentration of 7.5 μg/100ml (206 nmol/L) with a 4pm decrease.

2 — Normal defined as an increment in plasma cortisol of 7 μg/100ml (200 nmol/L).

3 — Normal defined as a post infusion (4 hours) plasma 11-deoxycortisol concentration greater than 6 μg/100ml (170 nmol/L).

4 — Tests not performed in 3 and 2 patients who previously had anaphylactic reactions to ACTH.

propionate and after a decrease in prednisone (to 3.2 mg/d) was less pronounced than in the daily prednisone group (fig. 8.5).

The findings of Kershnar et al. (1978) [table 8.6] differ from those of Wyatt et al. (1978). Substitution of inhaled beclomethasone dipropionate 400 μg/d for alternate-day prednisone (mean 19mg) resulted in a return to 'normal' of diurnal plasma cortisol in 16 of 28 children and of the response to tetracosactrin in 9 of 12 patients in whom it was abnormal before starting beclomethasone dipropionate. However, the criteria for a normal response to ACTH were less exacting than those of Greig et al. (1969) as the mean maximum plasma cortisol after stimulation was 16.9 μg/100ml (p.227). Also a control group was not included. Despite the improvement in plasma cortisol, the intravenous metyrapone test remained abnormal in 22 of 34 children, having been abnormal in 30 patients before the introduction of inhaled beclomethasone dipropionate into the treatment regimen.

Pharmacokinetics

Pharmacokinetic studies of corticosteroids used topically to treat bronchial asthma have been confronted with explaining the reason for the difference between the glucocorticoid potency of the drug when administered intravenously (fig. 8.6) and when given orally or by inhalation (fig. 8.7).

As less than 25% of an inhaled dose is deposited in the respiratory tract, and animal studies indicate rapid pulmonary absorption of flunisolide (Chaplin et al., 1980a) and beclomethasone dipropionate (Martin et al., 1975), metabolic inactivation in the lung is not the reason for the low glucocorticoid potency of the inhaled drugs. Likewise, poor gastrointestinal absorption is not responsible (Chaplin et al., 1980a,b; Martin et al., 1974). However, absorption of beclomethasone dipropionate from the gastrointestinal tract is slow. The low systemic bioavailability suggests that most of the absorbed drug is probably metabolised during its first passage through the liver (Chaplin et al., 1980b; Martin et al., 1974).

Also as the dose of oral beclomethasone dipropionate needed to suppress plasma cortisol concentrations is greater than that required by inhalation (fig. 8.7), it is the portion absorbed from the lungs that is mainly responsible for any systemic effects (Harris, 1975).

Absorption

Studies to determine the pharmacokinetics of orally administered beclomethasone dipropionate were conducted by Martin et al. (1974, 1975) using tritium-labelled drug and similar studies with flunisolide were performed by Chaplin et al. (1980b). It was estimated that 90% of a 4mg dose of beclomethasone dipropionate given as a microfine suspension and 61 to 76% of that administered as capsules was absorbed. The rate of absorption of beclomethasone dipropionate is slow, with peak plasma concentrations of 9.5 to 15.2 ng/ml (capsules) and 20 ng/ml (suspension) being attained 3 to 5 hours after ingestion. Absorption of flunisolide is more rapid, peak plasma concentrations being reached about 1 hour after oral administration.

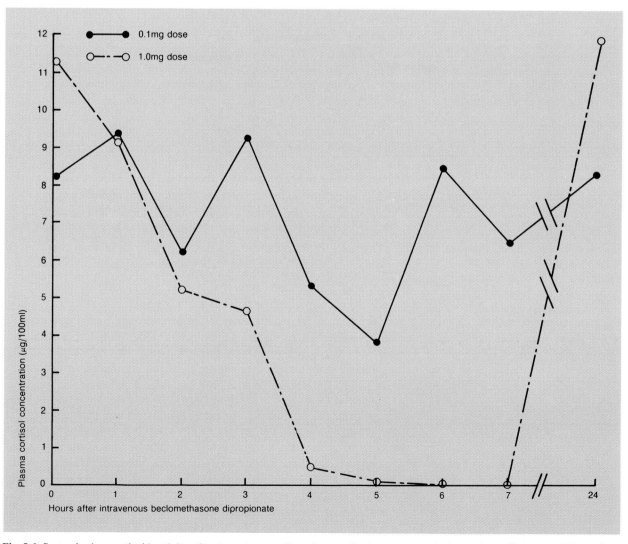

Fig. 8.6. Systemic glucocorticoid activity of beclomethasone dipropionate after intravenous administration of 0.1mg and 1.0mg doses (after Harris, 1975).

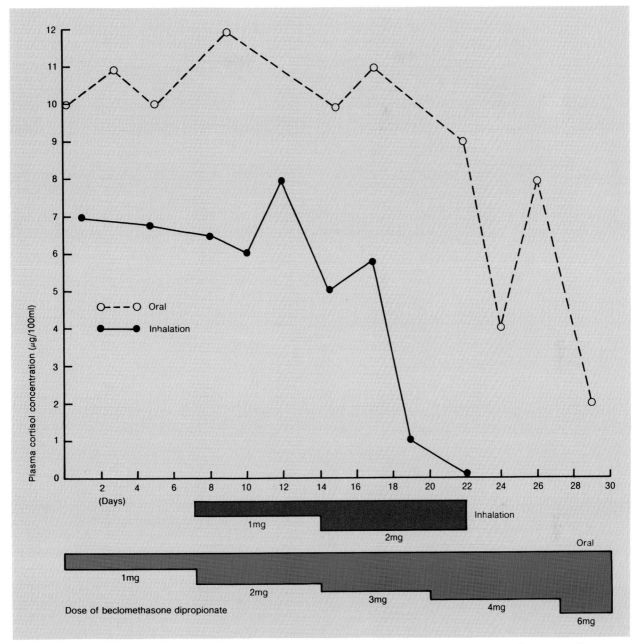

Fig. 8.7. Relative systemic glucocorticoid activity of increasing doses of oral and inhaled beclomethasone dipropionate in the same subject (after Harris, 1975).

Excretion and Metabolism

The specific activity of tritium-labelled beclomethasone dipropionate was not high enough to study pulmonary absorption and metabolism by man of inhaled therapeutic doses. However, as the portion of the inhaled dose that is absorbed directly from the lung into the blood stream will be cleared and metabolised in the same manner as intravenously administered drug, the pharmacokinetics of an intravenous dose have been studied (Martin et al., 1975).

Ten to 15% of the administered radioactivity after oral or intravenous administration of tritiated beclomethasone dipropionate was recovered in the urine as metabolites over a period of 72 to 96 hours. Corresponding values for flunisolide are about 10 to 20% (Chaplin et al., 1980b).

Faecal radioactivity accounted for 37 to 47% of a 4mg oral dose given as microfine suspension and 50 to 67% of that given as capsules (Martin et al., 1974, 1975). 64% and 40% of an intravenous dose of beclomethasone dipropionate and flunisolide respectively was excreted in the faeces during a 96-hour period after injection and is present almost entirely as free and conjugated metabolites. Biliary excretion studies of beclomethasone dipropionate in rats confirmed that the polar metabolites are excreted via the bile. Beclomethasone monopropionate and beclomethasone dipropionate are present in faeces after oral administration. As beclomethasone dipropionate is hydrolysed by tissue and faecal esterases *in vitro* (Martin et al., 1974), it is probable that the beclomethasone monopropionate and beclomethasone dipropionate present in faeces after oral administration result from hydrolysis of unabsorbed drug by gut esterases.

Results of these studies suggest that one of the reasons for lack of systemic glucocorticoid effect of inhaled therapeutic doses of flunisolide and beclomethasone dipropionate is most likely that the absorbed steroid is converted to pharmacologically inactive metabolites during its passage through the liver.

Half-life

After intravenous injection of tritiated beclomethasone dipropionate there is a rapid removal of radioactivity from the plasma and then residual radioactivity is removed more slowly. The half-life of the second phase was about 15 hours for beclomethasone dipropionate (Martin et al., 1975) and 1.7 hours for flunisolide (Chaplin et al., 1980a).

In summary

The characteristics typical of corticosteroids with high topical relative to systemic activity make them candidates for use by inhalation in the treatment of asthma. Beclomethasone dipropionate, the most extensively studied of the group has been shown to be without unwanted effects on bronchial tissue or pituitary-adrenal function, its substitution for oral steroid therapy being frequently followed by full recovery of a previously suppressed axis. Increasing doses of inhaled steroids have an increasing effect on tests of HPA function; the results of some studies suggest even at normally used doses they may cause subtle biochemical changes in the response to some tests.

References

Andersson, E.: An investigation of the bronchial mucous membrane after long-term treatment with beclomethasone dipropionate. Postgraduate Medical Journal 51 (Suppl. 4): 32 (1975).

Andersson, E.; Smidt, C.M.; Sikjaer, B.; Hinge, G. and Poynter, D.: Bronchial biopsies after beclomethasone dipropionate aerosol. British Journal of Diseases of the Chest 77: 35 (1977).

Bernstein, I.L.; Chervinsky, P. and Felliers, C.J.: Efficacy and safety of triamcinolone aerosol in chronic asthma. Chest 81: 20 (1982).

Blaiss, M.S.; Herrod, H.G.; Crawford, L.V. and Lieberman, P.L.: Beclomethasone dipropionate aerosol: Haematologic and immunologic effects. Annals of Allergy 48: 210 (1982).

Breslin, A.B.X.; Pepys, J.; Davies, R.J. and Hendrick, D.J.: Effect of beclomethasone dipropionate on antigen bronchial challenge in asthmatic patients. Australian lymphocyte and New Zealand Journal of Medicine 3: 324 (1973).

British Thoracic and Tuberculosis Association: Inhaled corticosteroids compared with oral prednisone in patients starting long term corticosteroid therapy for asthma. Lancet 2: 469 (1975).

British Thoracic and Tuberculosis Association: A controlled trial of inhaled corticosteroids in patients receiving prednisone tables for asthma. British Journal of Diseases of the Chest 70: 95 (1976).

Brown, H.M.; Storey, G. and George, W.H.S.: Beclomethasone dipropionate: A new steroid aerosol for the treatment of allergic asthma. British Medical Journal 1: 585 (1972).

Burge, P.S.: The effects of corticosteroids on the immediate asthmatic reaction. European Journal of Respiratory Diseases 63: 163 (1982).

Chaplin, M.D.; Cooper, W.C.; Segre, E.J.; Jones, E.R. and Nerenberg, C.: Correlation of flunisolide plasma levels to eosinopenic response in humans. Journal of Allergy and Clinical Immunology 65: 445 (1980a).

Chaplin, M.D. Rooks, W.; Swenson, E.W.; Cooper, W.C.; Nerenberg, C. and Chu, N.I.: Flunisolide metabolism and dynamics of a metabolite. Clinical Pharmacology and Therapeutics 27: 402 (1980b).

Chiang, J.L.; Patterson, R.; McGillen, J.J.; Phair, J.P.; Roberts, M.; Harris, K.E. and Riesing, K.S.: Long term corticosteroid effect on and polymorphonuclear cell function in asthmatics. Journal of Allergy and Clinical Immunology 65: 263 (1980).

Choo-Kang, Y.F.J.; Cooper, E.J.; Tribe, A.E. and Grant, I.W.B.: Beclomethasone by inhalation in the treatment of airways obstruction. British Journal of Diseases of the Chest 66: 101 (1972).

Costello, J.F. and Clark, T.J.: Response of patients receiving high dose beclomethasone dipropionate. Thorax 29: 571 (1974).

De Cotiis, B.A. and Settipane, G.A.: The effect of inhaled beclomethasone on serum immunoglobulins. Abstract. Journal of Allergy and Clinical Immunology 65: 218 (1980).

Easton, J.G.: Effect of an inhaled corticosteroid on methacholine airway reactivity. Journal of Allergy and Clinical Immunology 67: 338 (1981).

Freed, D.L.J.; Sinclair, T.; Topper, R.; Brenchley, P. and Taylor, G.: IgA levels in rhinitic nasal secretion during short term therapy with sodium cromoglycate, beclomethasone and antihistamine; in Pepys and Edwards (Eds) The Mast Cell its Role in Health and Disease p.795 (Pitman, London 1979).

Friedman, M.; Frears, J. and Crowley, M.F.: The effect of betamethasone valerate on the hypothalamic-pituitary-adrenal axis of normal adults. Postgraduate Medical Journal 50 (Sept. Suppl.): 11 (1974).

Gaddie, J.; Petrie, G.R.; Reid, I.W.; Sinclair, D.J.M.; Skinner, C. and Palmer, K.N.V.: Aerosol beclomethasone dipropionate: A dose-response study in chronic bronchial asthma. Lancet 2: 280 (1973).

Greig, W.R.; Maxwell, J.D.; Boyle, J.A.; Lindsay, R.M. and Browning, G.M.C.K.: Criteria for distinguishing normal from subnormal adrenocortical function using the synacthen test. Postgraduate Medical Journal 45: 307 (1969).

Gruvstad, E. and Bengtsson, B.: A comparison of a new steroid, budesonide, with other topical corticosteroids in the vasoconstriction assay. Drugs in Experimental and Clinical Research 6: 385 (1980).

Harris, D.M.: Some properties of beclomethasone dipropionate and related steroids in man. Postgraduate Medical Journal 51 (Suppl. 4) : 20 (1975).

Harris, D.M.; Martin, L.E.; Harrison, C. and Jack, D.: The effect of oral and inhaled beclomethasone dipropionate on adrenal function. Clinical Allergy 3: 243 (1973).

Hills, E.A.; Davies, S. and Geary, M.: The effect of betamethasone valerate aerosol in exercise-induced asthma. Postgraduate Medical Journal 50 (Sept. Suppl.): 67 (1974).

Hartley, J.P.R.; Charles, T.J. and Seaton, A.: Betamethasone valerate inhalation and exercise-induced asthma in adults. British Journal of Diseases of the Chest 71: 253 (1977).

Hodgson, S.V.; McPherson, A. and Friedman, M.: The effect of betamethasone valerate aerosol on exercise-induced asthma in children. Postgraduate Medical Journal 50 (Sept. Suppl.): 69 (1974).

Jorde, W. and Werdermann, K.; Etride de la cytologie bronchique apres traitment prolonge par le dipropionate de beclomethasone. La Nouvelle Presse Medicale 6 (15): 1281 (1977).

Kershnar, H.; Klein, R.; Waldman, D.; Berger, W.; Rachelefsky, G.; Katz, R. and Siegel, S.: Treatment of chronic childhood asthma with beclomethasone dipropionate aerosols. II. Effect on pituitary-adrenal function after substitution for oral corticosteroids. Pediatrics 62: 189 (1978).

Lal, S.; Harris, D.M.; Bhalla, K.K.; Singhal, S.N. and Butler, A.G.: Comparison of beclomethasone dipropionate aerosol and prednisolone in reversible airways obstruction. British Medical Journal 3: 314 (1972).

Lundgren, R.: Scanning electron microscopic studies of bronchial mucosa before and during treatment with beclomethasone dipropionate inhalations. Scandinavian Journal of Respiratory Diseases (Suppl. 101): 179 (1977).

Maberly, D.J.; Gibson, G.J. and Butler, A.G.: Recovery of adrenal function after substitution of beclomethasone dipropionate for oral corticosteroids. British Medical Journal 1: 778 (1973).

McAllen, M.K.; Kochanowski, S.J. and Shaw, K.M.: Steroid aerosols in asthma: An assessment of betamethasone valerate and a 12-month study of patients on maintenance. British Medical Journal 1: 171 (1974).

Martin, L.E.: Harrison, C. and Tanner, R.J.N.; Metabolism of beclomethasone dipropionate by animals and man. Postgraduate Medical Journal 51 (Suppl. 4): 11 (1975).

Martin, L.E.; Tanner, R.J.N.; Clark, T.J.H. and Cochrane, G.M.: Absorption and metabolism of orally administered beclomethasone dipropionate. Clinical Pharmacology and Therapeutics 15: 267 (1974).

Mygind, N.: Effects of beclomethasone dipropionate aerosol on nasal mucosa. British Journal of Clinical Pharmacology 4: 2875 (1977).

Mygind, N. and Hansen, I.U: Beclomethasone dipropionate aerosol effect on the adrenal in normal persons. Acta Allergologica 28: 211 (1973).

Nassif, E.; Weinberger, M.; Thompson, R. and Sherman, B.: Effects of continuous corticosteroid therapy on children with chronic asthma. Journal of Allergy and Clinical Immunology 65: 219 (1980).

Pepys, J.; Davies, R.J. Breslin, A.B.X.; Hendrick, D.J. and Hutchcroft, B.J.: The effect of inhaled beclomethasone dipropionate (Becotide) and sodium cromoglycate on asthmatic reactions to provocation tests. Clinical Allergy 4: 13 (1974).

Roscoe, P.; Choo-Kang, Y.F.J. and Horne, N.W.: Betamethasone valerate in corticosteroid-dependent asthmatics. British Journal of Diseases of the Chest 69: 240 (1975).

Schuyler, M.R.; Bondarevsky, E.; Schmartz, H.J. and Schmitt, D.: Corticosteroid-sensitive lymphocytes are normal in atopic asthma. Journal of Allergy and Clinical Immunology 68: 72 (1981).

Smith, M.J. and Hodson, M.L.: The effects of long term inhaled high dose beclomethasone dipropionate on adrenal function. Lancet 2: in press (1982).

Spangler, D.L.; Bloom, F.L.; Brestel, E.P. and Wittig, H.J.: One year trial of aerosolized flunisolide in severe steroid-dependent asthmatics. Abst. 186. Annals of Allergy 39 (1): 70 (1979).

Thiringer, G.; Eriksson, N.; Malinberg, R.; Svedmyr, N. and Zettergren, L.: Bronchoscopic biopsies of bronchial mucosa before and after beclomethasone dipropionate therapy. Postgraduate Medical Journal 51 (Suppl. 4): 30 (1975).

Thiringer, G.; Ericksson, N.; Malmberg, N.; Svedmyr, N. and Zettergren, L.: Bronchoscopic biopsies of bronchial mucosa before and after beclomethasone dipropionate therapy. Scandinavian Journal of Respiratory Diseases (Suppl. 101): 173 (1977).

Toogood, J.H.: Steroids in Asthma. Letter. Lancet 2: 1185 (1979).

Toogood, J.H.; Lefcoe, N.M.; Haines, D.S.M.; Jennings, B.; Errington, N.; Baksh, L. and Chuang, L.: A graded-dose assessment of the efficacy of beclomethasone aerosol for severe chronic asthma. Journal of Allergy and Clinical Immunology 59: 298 (1977).

Vaz, R.; Senior, B.; Morris, M. and Binkiewicz, A.: Adrenal effects of beclomethasone inhalation therapy in asthmatic children. Journal of Pediatrics 100: 660 (1982).

Willey, R.F.; Godden, D.J.; Carmichael, J.; Preston, P.; Frame, M. and Crompton, G.K.: Comparison of twice daily administration of a new corticosteroid budesonide with beclomethasone dipropionate four times daily in the treatment of Chronic asthma. British Journal of Diseases of the Chest 76: 61 (1982).

Wyatt, R.; Waschek, J.; Weinberger, M. and Sherman, B.; Effects of inhaled beclomethasone dipropionate and alternate-day prednisone on pituitary-adrenal function in children with chronic asthma. New England Journal of Medicine 299: 1387 (1978).

Yazigi, R.; Sly, M. and Frazer, M.: Effect of triamcinolone acetonide aerosol upon exercise-induced asthma. Annals of Allergy 40: 322 (1978).

Chapter IX

Inhaled Steroids: Studies in Adult and Childhood Asthma

R.N. Brogden

Inhaled Steroids in Steroid-dependent Adult Asthmatics

Short Term Studies

Inhaled corticosteroids are now well established in the management of asthma in steroid-dependent patients. It is generally accepted that inhaled corticosteroids can reduce the need for oral corticosteroids in the majority of such patients and enable their complete withdrawal in many.

Numerous uncontrolled studies have reported the efficacy of beclomethasone dipropionate 300 to 600 μg/d (e.g. Brown and Storey, 1975; Chatterjee et al., 1972; Clark, 1972) triamcinolone acetonide 400 to 1400 μg/d (Falliers, 1976; Golub, 1980), betamethasone valerate (Arora and Maher-Loughnan, 1974) and flunisolide 2000 μg/d (Webb et al., 1979), in decreasing the need for oral corticosteroids. However, with no placebo control, it cannot be certain that the oral steroid dosage could not have been decreased to some extent without the inhaled steroid.

Placebo controlled studies have clearly shown, however, that treatment with inhaled corticosteroids generally permits the withdrawal of maintenance oral corticosteroids in the majority of patients studied for short (table 9.1) or long periods (see page 137).

Withdrawal of systemic corticosteroids after starting treatment with inhaled steroids does not usually result in deterioration of asthma (table 9.2) as evidenced by salbutamol consumption (Cameron et al., 1973) lung function studies (Chervinsky, 1977; Grieco et al., 1978; Hodson et al., 1974; Vilsvik and Schaanning, 1974) or asthmatic symptoms (Chervinsky, 1977; Grieco et al., 1978; Hodson et al., 1974). As illustrated in table 9.2, there was an improvement in symptoms and lung function in the inhaled steroid group, despite a 77% decrease in the dose of oral maintenance corticosteroids. In contrast, asthma control deteriorated in the control group despite a minimal decrease in oral steroid dosage.

Inhaled Steroids Compared with Oral Steroids

Inhaled beclomethasone dipropionate and betamethasone valerate have been directly compared with daily doses of oral prednisolone or prednisone in asthmatic patients who had either been maintained on stable doses of systemic corticosteroids (Eriksson et al., 1975; Lal et al., 1972), or were considered to be in need of long term corticosteroid treatment (British Thoracic and Tuberculosis Association Study, 1975; Prakesh et al., 1976). In all studies the aim was to determine the dose-equivalence of the different corticosteroids.

In the best designed of the studies (British Thoracic and Tuberculosis Association Study, 1975), inhaled beclomethasone dipropionate or betamethasone valerate at a mean dose of about 400 μg/d was equivalent to 7 to 8mg of prednisone over a 6 month study period (table 9.3). Other studies (all of cross-over design) have reported a similar ratio, each 100μg of beclomethasone di-

Table 9.1. Efficacy of inhaled corticosteroids relative to placebo in allowing a decrease in the dosage of maintenance oral steroids in steroid-dependent adult asthmatics

Author	No. of patients	Dose (μg/d)	Percentage of patients able to discontinue oral corticosteroids	
			inhaled steroid	placebo
Beclomethasone dipropionate				
Cameron et al. (1973)	20	400	20	0
Webb et al. (1977)	28	400	75	8
Hodson et al. (1974)	22	400	91	0
Vilsvik and Schaanning (1974)	27	400	100	15
Triamcinolone acetonide				
Chervinsky (1977)	32	800	81	19
Grieco et al. (1978)	60	800	64	10
Betamethasone valerate				
El-Shaboury and Williams (1974)	19	400	67	30

Table 9.2. Effect of substitution of inhaled triamcinolone acetonide for oral corticosteroids on the control of asthma (after Chervinsky, 1977)

Criteria	Triamcinolone		Placebo	
	baseline	week 12	baseline	week 12
Oral steroid dose[1] (mg)	8.3	1.88	9.1	7.65
Forced expiratory volume (litres)	1.19	1.72	1.00	0.98
Nights awakened	4.63	2.19	3.47	4.76
Shortness of breath[2]	1.88	1.33	2.29	2.41
Wheeze	1.94	1.38	2.18	2.41
Tightness	2.00	1.25	2.12	2.35
Cough	1.81	1.25	2.06	2.24

1 — Prednisone equivalent (mean value).

2 — Symptons scored on a 5-point scale; 1 = no symptons, 5 = very severe.

propionate being equivalent to about 2mg of oral prednisolone (Eriksson et al., 1975; Lal et al., 1972; Prakesh et al., 1976).

A finding common to all of these studies was that the inhaled corticosteroids caused less suppression of adrenal function than a therapeutically equivalent daily dose of oral corticosteroid, as evidenced by changes in resting and stimulated plasma cortisol. An example of the relative effects on plasma cortisol is shown in figure 9.1.

Thus, although there may be little difference between the efficacy of inhaled beclomethasone dipropionate or betamethasone valerate 400μg/d and oral prednisone 7 to 8mg daily in the management of asthma in steroid-dependent patients, systemic side effects are less of a problem with the inhaled drugs.

Long Term Controlled Trials

Because of organisational difficulties and ethical considerations, most medium or long term trials of inhaled corticosteroids in chronic steroid-dependent asthma are of open design. Nevertheless, there have been a few well designed placebo-controlled trials conducted over periods of up to 12 months (British Thoracic and Tuberculosis Association 1975, 1976; Brompton Hospital/MRC Trial 1974, 1979). These studies have provided much data on the usefulness of inhaled corticosteroids, particularly beclomethasone dipropionate, in the treatment of chronic asthma in steroid-dependent patients.

The main criterion of efficacy in the Brompton Hospital/MRC Trials was the decrease in maintenance oral corticosteroid requirements after starting inhaled beclomethasone dipropionate. There was no difference between the 400 and 800μg daily dosages with respect to the decrease in prednisone dose where the initial dose was 5 to 9 or 10 to 15mg daily, but in patients who had required more than 16mg daily of prednisone, the 800μg dose was better than the lower dose (fig. 9.2). In the trial conducted by the British Thoracic and Tuberculosis Association (1976) the 800μg dose was better than the 400μg dose in enabling patients to remain off oral steroids over a 6 to 12 month period (fig. 9.3). The improvement observed at the end of the oral steroid dose adjustment phase was maintained for 1 year in the patients treated with beclomethasone

Table 9.3. Control of asthma by beclomethasone dipropionate or betamethasone valerate aerosol and by oral prednisone over a period of 24 weeks (after British Thoracic and Tuberculosis Association Study 1975)

Criteria	Treatment group		
	beclomethasone dipropionate (mean dose 432 μg/d)	prednisone (mean dose 8.3 mg/d)	betamethasone valerate (mean 392 μg/d)
Percentage of patients requiring oral prednisone to control exacerbation	5	4	10
Percentage of patients requiring increase in stable dose	16	26	14
Number of failure days[1] per patient	4	5	5
Percentage of maximum[2] possible score in last period of the study	74	80	74
Mean monthly peak flow (L/min)	300	302	270

1 — A 'failure day' was one on which more than 4 double-puffs (2 discharges taken singly) of salbutamol were needed or the dose of tablets plus aerosol was increased by the patient.
2 — The maximum score represented excellent control of asthma.

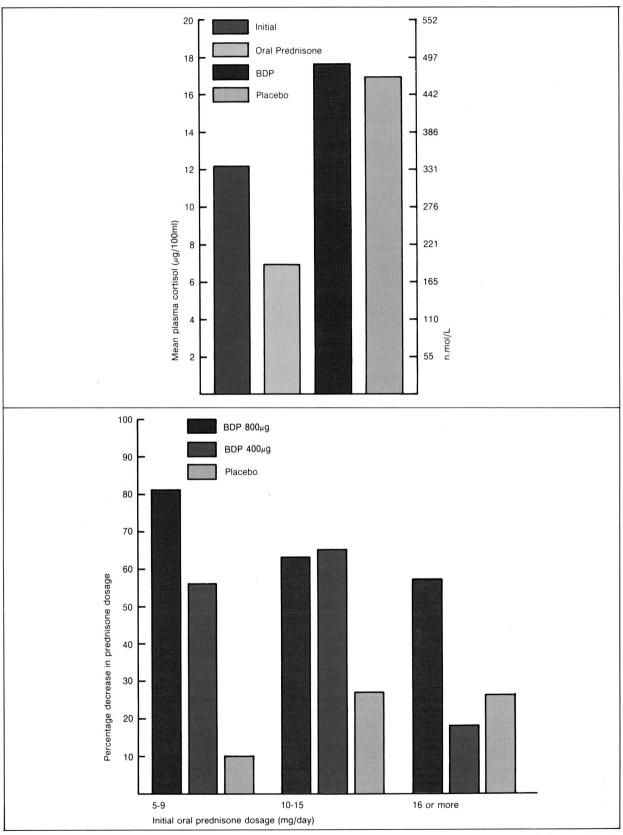

Fig. 9.1. Mean resting plasma cortisol after 4 weeks' treatment with inhaled beclomethasone dipropionate, oral prednisolone or placebo. All patients had been maintained on oral prednisolone prior to the study (data after Lal et al., 1972).

Fig. 9.2. Mean percentage decrease in oral prednisone dosage in steroid-dependent asthmatic patients treated with beclomethasone dipropionate aerosol 800μg daily or 400μg daily or with placebo for 28 weeks (after Brompton Hospital/MRC Trial, 1974).

800µg daily irrespective of whether they had originally received up to 9 or 15mg daily of prednisone. However, the 400µg dosage was less satisfactory in those patients who had required 10 to 15mg daily of prednisone when admitted to the trial 1 year earlier. Although there was no significant difference between beclomethasone dipropionate 400 and 800µg daily and betamethasone valerate 800µg daily at the end of the first phase of the BTTA (1976) trial, the higher dosage of beclomethasone dipropionate was more effective than the low dose after another 24 weeks treatment.

The rather high response to placebo in the BTTA (1976) study, points to the desirability of carefully establishing the minimum effective dose of oral maintenance steroids before starting a trial which uses the decrease in oral steroid dosage as the principal criterion of efficacy of an inhaled steroid. It also emphasises the importance of regularly reviewing the dose of oral corticosteroid needed by patients with chronic asthma.

The important finding of these long term controlled studies is that the substitution of inhaled corticosteroids for oral steroids is achieved without deterioration in lung function (table 9.4).

It is studies such as these, that have provided the basis for the 'standard' 400 to 800µg daily dosage of beclomethasone dipropionate aerosol used by most clinicians to treat adult asthma. A case for increasing the dosage of beclomethasone to higher levels in severe chronic asthma has been presented by the investigations

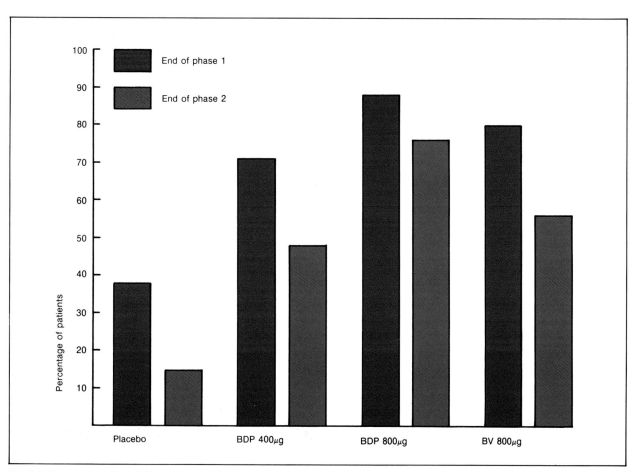

Fig. 9.3. Percentage of steroid-dependent patients receiving inhaled beclomethasone dipropionate (BDP) or betamethasone valerate (BV) able to discontinue oral maintenance corticosteroids at the end of phase 1 and the percentage who remained off prednisone 24 weeks later (phase 2) [after British Thoracic and Tuberculosis Association Study 1976].

Table 9.4. The effect of substituting inhaled beclomethasone dipropionate for oral prednisone as reflected in the changes in percentage FEV$_1$ at 28 weeks in all patients (Brompton Hospital/MRC Trial, 1974) and in those who continued with their allocated treatment for a further 24 weeks (Brompton Hospital/MRC, 1979)

Prednisone on admission (mg/day)	Decrease in prednisone at 28 weeks (%)	No. of patients	Mean FEV$_1$ (% predicted)[1]		No. of patients on same treatment[2]	Mean FEV$_1$ (% predicted)	
			on admission	at 28 weeks		at 28 weeks	at 52 weeks
5-9	0-49	19	72	75	5	87	86
	50-99	7	76	82	6	80	76
	100	15	68	81	15	81	84
10-15	0-49	18	62	58	3	64	58
	50-99	15	68	69	15	69	73
	100	4	56	60	4	60	71
≥16	0-49	12	45	45	0	-	-
	50-99	5	56	51	3	65	79

1 — FEV$_1$ determined at 4-weekly intervals.
2 — The main criterion for allowing patients to continue with their allocated 'blind' treatment was that oral prednisone dosage was decreased to half or less of that needed on admission.

of Toogood et al. (1977, 1978). The median minimum effective maintenance dose, determined after carefully adjusting the dose over a period of 30 weeks, was 1050µg daily. An unusual approach to determining this dosage was adopted by these investigators, who added beclomethasone dipropionate at increasing doses up to 1600µg daily to an unchanged dosage of oral prednisone. The dosage of prednisone was then progressively decreased and was withdrawn completely in 15 of 34 patients over a period of 24 weeks. Subsequently, the minimum effective maintenance dosage of beclomethasone dipropionate was determined while the new dosage of prednisone was maintained. The effective dosage of beclomethasone ranged from 200 to 1800µg daily, with only 12% of patients being satisfactorily controlled on 400µg daily or less.

The high doses in this study probably arise from the difference in therapeutic goal compared with that in some other studies. Toogood and his colleagues aimed to improve control of asthma and to eliminate disability. Withdrawal of prednisone or normalisation of plasma cortisol concentrations were secondary considerations. More frequently, the aim has been to withdraw prednisone and improve plasma cortisol, without permitting deterioration in asthma control. Nevertheless improved control of asthma has also sometimes been achieved (e.g. Brown and Storey, 1975).

Long Term Open Studies

Many short term studies conducted over the last 10 years have conclusively demonstrated the superiority of the inhaled corticosteroids over placebo in maintaining corticosteroid-dependent asthmatics in whom oral maintenance corticosteroids have been reduced or withdrawn. Many longer term trials have now been reported and adequately show that improvement can be maintained for long periods in most patients who experience a good initial response.

In a 10 year follow-up of 100 patients, Kennedy et al. (1981) found that the response to beclomethasone dipropionate aerosol achieved after 3 years (Kennedy et al., 1975) was largely maintained (fig. 9.4). There were 8 deaths over the 10-year period, but none was related to beclomethasone dipropionate treatment or due to asthma. As would be expected, the overall response was better in non-steroid-dependent patients than in those initially on long term oral corticosteroids (fig. 9.5). However, in only about 5% of patients was it necessary to reintroduce oral maintenance steroids by 1980. 92 patients continued to use sodium cromoglycate or inhale salbutamol or other β-adrenergic stimulants before each inhalation of beclomethasone dipropionate. In this, as in shorter controlled studies (e.g. Brompton Hospital/MRC Trial, 1979), about 30% of patients did not respond to usual dosages of inhaled beclomethasone dipropionate. Over the 10-year study, oropharyngeal candidiasis occurred in a total of 23 patients. Withdrawal of treatment was necessary in 2 patients because of persistent fungal infection. There was no clinical evidence of adrenal suppression as a result of long term treatment of patients not initially steroid-dependent.

Other studies of up to 20 months duration have consistently shown that the initial response to inhaled corticosteroids can be maintained in most patients treated with betamethasone valerate 400 to 800mg daily (Arora and Maher-Loughnan, 1974; El-Shaboury and Williams, 1974) triamcinolone acetonide 400 to 2000μg daily (Bone et al., 1977; Kriz et al., 1977; Williams, 1975) or beclomethasone dipropionate (Brown and Storey, 1975; Brown et al., 1972; Epstein and Thompson, 1976; Kass et al., 1977; Pines, 1973;

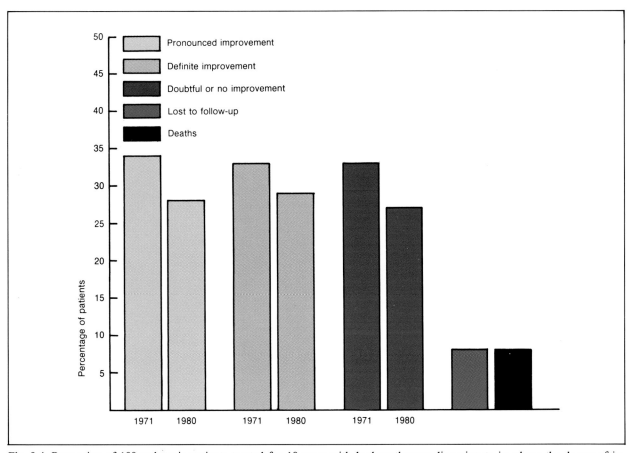

Fig. 9.4. Proportion of 100 asthmatic patients treated for 10 years with beclomethasone dipropionate in whom the degree of improvement in the first year was maintained (data after Kennedy et al., 1981).

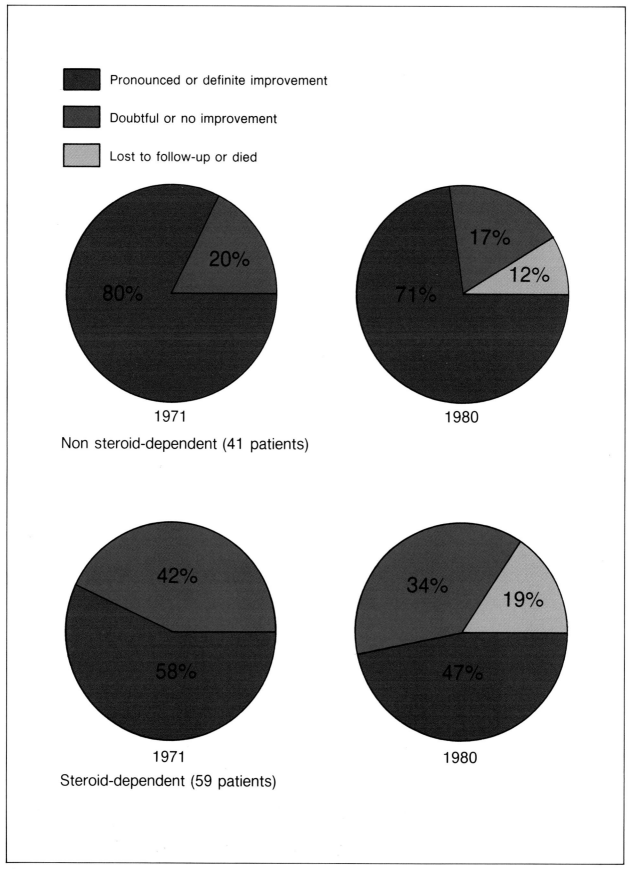

Fig. 9.5. Response to treatment with inhaled beclomethasone dipropionate in non-steroid-dependent and steroid-dependent asthmatics treated for 10 years (data after Kennedy et al., 1981).

Toogood et al., 1978). There has been a general trend towards improved symptomatic control and lung function in many patients after substitution of inhaled corticosteroids for oral steroids, and for this degree of response to be maintained. However, a variable proportion of patients who are able to discontinue oral maintenance steroids after a few months' treatment with an inhaled corticosteroid, subsequently require one or more brief courses of oral steroids to control exacerbations of their asthma over the next year or so.

Where studied, adrenal function has tended to return towards normal in many patients who have had daily oral steroids completely or partially replaced by inhaled corticosteroids (e.g. Brown et al., 1972; Epstein and Thompson, 1976; Kass et al., 1977). The lesser systemic effect of the inhaled steroids has frequently been evidenced by the presence of corticosteroid withdrawal effects and the exacerbation of underlying atopic conditions formerly controlled by the systemic steroid.

In a study in geriatric patients (61-78 years), institution of inhaled beclomethasone dipropionate 400 to 1200μg daily enabled complete withdrawal of oral steroids in 19 of 27 patients and conversion to alternate day oral steroids in a further 4 patients over a 6 month period. A moderate improvement in lung function was also noted (Fein, 1981).

Studies Comparing Inhaled Corticosteroids

As the great majority of the published work and clinical experience with inhaled corticosteroids concerns beclomethasone dipropionate, as would be expected it has been the standard against which the efficacy of other inhaled steroids is assessed (table 9.5).

In a dose-finding study (BTTA, 1975), beclomethasone dipropionate and betamethasone valerate were equipotent in controlling non-steroid-dependent asthma, about 400μg daily of each drug being equivalent to 7 to 8mg of oral prednisone (table 9.3). In a later study (BTTA, 1976) 800μg daily of beclomethasone dipropionate was superior to 400μg daily and comparable with betamethasone valerate 800μg daily in allowing patients to remain off prednisone (fig. 9.3). Little difference between beclomethasone dipropionate 400 μg/d and 800μg daily of betamethasone valerate was found by Loudon (1974) and Riordan et al. (1974) in double-blind cross-over studies of short duration. Neither drug caused adrenal suppression.

Comparisons between beclomethasone dipropionate and dexamethasone isonicotinate suggest that 200μg daily of beclomethasone dipropionate is equivalent to 500μg daily of dexamethasone isonicotinate, but that dexamethasone isonicotinate is associated with a greater degree of adrenal suppression (Girard et al., 1975; Salorinne and Klemetti, 1979).

Budesonide 400μg daily (200μg twice daily) was found to be similar in efficacy to the same daily dose of beclomethasone dipropionate given in 4 doses of 100μg (Willey et al., 1982).

Inhaled Corticosteroids in Steroid-dependent Asthmatic Children

Double-blind and single-blind studies have clearly shown beclomethasone dipropionate 300 to 400μg/d (Godfrey and Konig, 1973; Richards et al., 1978; Smith, 1973), betamethasone valerate 800μg/d (Frears et al., 1975; Howard and Jacoby, 1974), flunisolide 1000μg/d (Shapiro et al., 1982) and triamcinolone acetonide 400

Table 9.5. Relative efficacy of inhaled corticosteroids in the treatment of chronic asthma

Author	No. of patients	Dosage[1]	Duration[2]	Results	Adrenal suppression
Non-steroid-dependent patients					
BTTA (1975)	75	BDP 432 BV 390	>24 wks	BDP=BV[3]	BDP=BV[4]
Girard et al. (1975)	20	BDP 600 DI 1500	4 wks	BDP=DI	DI>BDP[5]
Salorinne and Klemetti (1979)	8	BDP 200-400 DI 500-1000	1 wk	BDP=DI	-[6]
Willey et al. (1982)	30	BDP 400 Bud 400	4 wks	BDP=Bud	BDP=Bud[4]
Steroid-dependent patients					
BTTA (1976)	158	BDP 400 BDP 800 BV 800 Placebo	>24 wks	BDP>placebo BV>placebo BDP 800> 400 BDP=BV	BDP=BV[4]
Loudon (1974)	14	BDP 400 BV 800	4 wks	BDP=BV	-[6]

1 — BDP = beclomethasone dipropionate; BV = betamethasone valerate; DI = dexamethasone isonicotinate; Bud = budesonide.
2 — Duration on each drug.
3 — In the BTTA (1975) study dosage was adjusted to provide the same degree of asthma control.
4 — Neither drug caused adrenal suppression.
5 — DI suppressed adrenal function but BDP did not.
6 — Not studied.

μg/d (Sly et al., 1978) to be superior to placebo in enabling a decrease in systemic corticosteroid dosage, and often also in the frequency of bronchodilator use, whilst maintaining or improving the quality of control of severe asthma (figs. 9.6 and 9.7). Generally, children respond particularly well to inhaled steroids with few side effects and seldom any evidence of adrenal suppression at usual therapeutic dosages.

Numerous long term open studies of up to 8 years duration (Brown et al., 1980) have demonstrated that once an inhaled steroid has been carefully substituted for oral maintenance corticosteroids over several months, it is seldom necessary to revert to regular oral steroids (e.g. Godfrey et al., 1978; Gwynn and Smith, 1974; Scherr et al., 1980) [table 9.6]. However, as with adults, some children subsequently require short courses of oral steroids to control exacerbations of asthma (Godfrey and Konig, 1974; Gwynn and Smith, 1974). It has been suggested that about 3% of asthmatic children cannot be satisfactorily controlled by inhaled steroids (Jacoby, 1977) and require oral steroids as well. However, failure to replace oral steroids with inhaled steroids in up to 25 to 45% have been noted occasionally (Dickson et al., 1973; Francis, 1976; Rao et al., 1982) in steroid-dependent asthmatics.

Systemic corticosteroid withdrawal symptoms, other than ex-

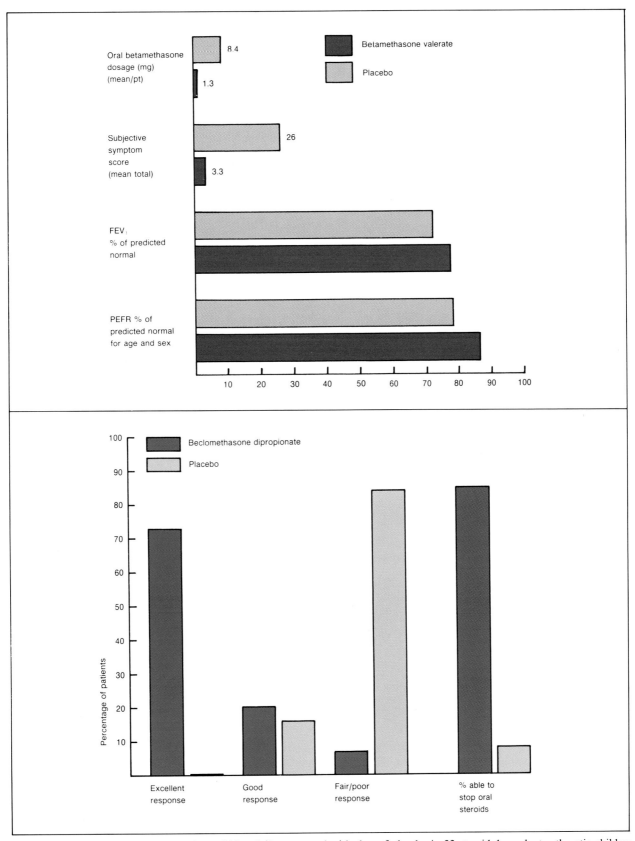

Fig. 9.6. Efficacy of betamethasone valerate 800μg daily compared with that of placebo in 22 steroid-dependent asthmatic children studied under double-blind conditions (after Howard and Jacoby, 1974).

Fig. 9.7. Relative efficacy of inhaled beclomethasone dipropionate and placebo in a double-blind study in 27 steroid-dependent asthmatic children, as evidenced by the physicians' evaluation and the withdrawal of corticosteroids (after Richards et al., 1978).

Table 9.6. Efficacy in open studies of long term inhaled beclomethasone dipropionate in enabling withdrawal of oral corticosteroids in children with steroid-dependent asthma

Author	No. of patients[1]	Dose (μg/d)	Duration (months)	Percentage ceasing oral steroids[2]	Effect on lung function[3]
Apold and Djoseland (1975)	10	200-400	8	80	slight decrease
Brown and Storey (1973)	15	300-600	$\leqslant$19	94	increase in 93%
Dickson et al. (1973)	21	200-400	4	62	increase in 64%
Francis (1976)	15	100-300	$\leqslant$36	-	increase in 64%
Godfrey and Konig (1974)	26	100-800	$\leqslant$20	94	-
Gwynn and Smith (1974)	53	100-400	12	75	increased
Manicatide et al. (1978)	29	400	14-26	100	increased
Rao et al. (1982)	9	400-800	36	55	-
Scherr et al. (1980)	56	384 (mean)	4	94	increased

1 — Number of steroid-dependent asthmatics.
2 — Percentage of patients able to remain off regular oral corticosteroids throughout the study.
3 — Lung function after substitution of beclomethasone aerosol relative to that before treatment with the inhaled steroid.

acerbation of atopic conditions, appear to have been less of a problem in children than in adults. Similarly, oropharyngeal candidiasis has occurred less frequently in children receiving inhaled corticosteroids than in adults treated with these drugs.

Inhaled Steroids in Patients not Receiving Systemic Corticosteroids

Inhaled corticosteroids have proved to be particularly effective in patients with moderately severe asthma who are candidates for treatment for the first time with maintenance doses of oral corticosteroids. In such patients, beclomethasone dipropionate 200 to 400μg daily (Brown et al., 1972; Chambers and Malfitan, 1979; Clark, 1972; Gaddie et al., 1973; Johannessen et al., 1979; Lovera et al., 1975; Smith et al., 1973), flunisolide 1000μg daily (Meltzer et al., 1982; Webb et al., 1979), betamethasone valerate 400 to 800μg daily (McAllen et al., 1974; Taylor and Norman, 1975; Vernon et al., 1976), triamcinolone acetonide 800 to 1600 μg/day (Bernstein et al., 1982) and budesonide 400 μg/day (Willey et al., 1982) have generally provided effective control of asthma in about three-quarters or more of adults or children.

In studies which have included both steroid-dependent and and non steroid-dependent asthmatics, the improvement in pulmonary function and symptoms and the decrease in bronchodilator use, has tended to be more pronounced in patients not requiring oral maintenance corticosteroids (e.g. Apold and Djoseland, 1975; Brown et al., 1972; Clark, 1972; Lovera et al., 1975).

In placebo-controlled studies, the inhaled steroids have invariably been superior to placebo in decreasing symptoms and bronchodilator use and in improving pulmonary function (fig. 9.8).

Long term open and placebo-controlled trials have demonstrated that the initial improvement can largely be maintained (fig. 9.9) with betamethasone valerate 800 μg/day and beclomethasone dipropionate 100 to 400μg daily.

Inhaled Steroids Compared with Other Antiasthmatic Drugs

Aerosol preparations of betamethasone valerate and beclomethasone dipropionate have generally been shown to be more effective than sodium cromoglycate in non-steroid dependent asthmatics on the basis of both subjective and objective criteria. This has been noted with betamethasone valerate in adults (Couch et al., 1977) and in children (Hiller and Milner, 1975; Kuzemko et al., 1974; Ng et al., 1977), although Mitchell et al. (1976) found no

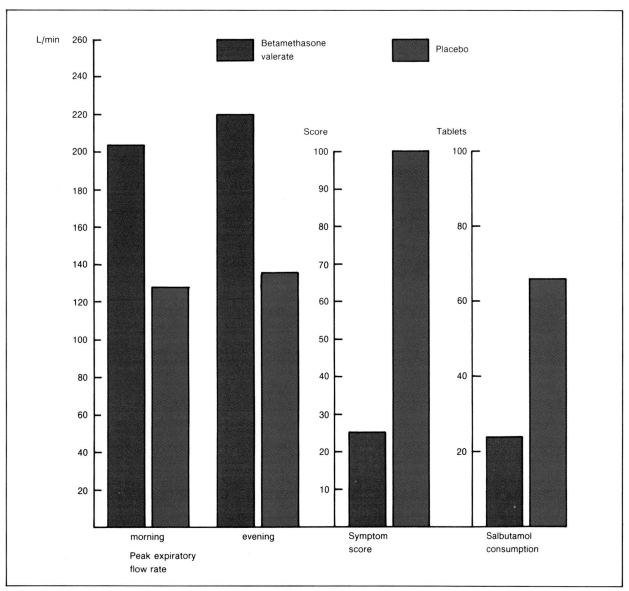

Fig. 9.8. Relative efficacy of inhaled betamethasone valerate and placebo in non-steroid-dependent children, as evidenced by the twice daily mean peak expiratory flow rate, symptom score and consumption of salbutamol tablets (after Taylor and Norman, 1974).

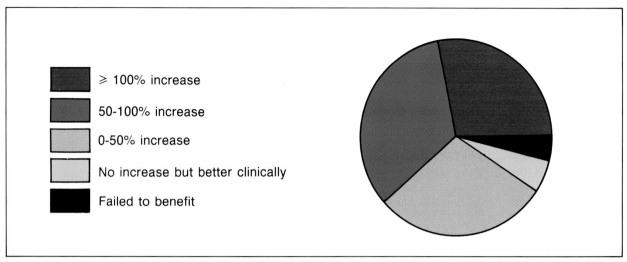

Fig. 9.9. Changes in mean peak expiratory flow observed in 109 asthmatics (32 children, 77 adults) not requiring maintenance systemic corticosteroids, when treated for up to 4 years with beclomethasone dipropionate aerosol (after Brown and Storey, 1975).

significant difference between beclomethasone dipropionate and sodium cromoglycate in a study involving only 14 children. The comparison between betamethasone valerate and sodium cromoglycate in the study of Hiller and Milner (1975) was invalid, as all 11 children were selected because they were unresponsive to cromoglycate.

Alternative Formulations of Steroids for Inhalation

Aerosol delivery devices have become widely accepted by most patients who require inhaled corticosteroid therapy. However, some patients, particularly the elderly and young children, have difficulty in synchronising inspiration and activation of the pressurised aerosol, and these patients may benefit from a breath-actuated device that delivers the drug as a dry powder.

Dry-powder Inhalation

Double-blind studies comparing beclomethasone dipropionate by aerosol and dry-powder inhalation have found 400 µg daily of the aerosol to be similar in efficacy to 400 to 800 µg daily of the powder (Carmichael et al., 1978; Chatterjee and Butler, 1980; Edmunds et al., 1979; Lal et al., 1980). There is little formal evidence that the dry-powder inhalation is more effective than the aerosol in those patients with a mediocre or poor technique with the conventional aerosol (Campbell et al., 1980; Finnegan et al., 1982). However, Edmunds et al. (1979) reported that children aged 5 to 7 years preferred the dry-powder inhalation while older children preferred the aerosol. Smith and Gwynn (1978) considered 22 of 37 children to be better controlled on the powder than on the aerosol, but there were no differences between the 2 preparations as assessed by other criteria. (See also Chapter XII and Appendix 1). Short term tolerability appears to be similar with both preparations.

High Dose Beclomethasone Dipropionate Aerosol

Some severely affected asthmatic patients, particularly those who have required long term maintenance doses of oral corticosteroids, or are unresponsive to 400µg daily, may require higher than usual dosages of inhaled corticosteroids to control their symptoms once oral steroids have been decreased to the lowest possible maintenance dose. There is a need to individualise inhaled steroid dosage in these patients as has previously been done with oral corticosteroids. In such patients, an inhaler delivering 250µg per actuation, as opposed to the usual 50µg per actuation, offers advantages in terms of compliance, accuracy of daily dosage and patient convenience.

Clinical and spirometric benefit from increasing the daily dosage of inhaled beclomethasone dipropionate from 400µg to 800µg or more has been demonstrated in controlled trials (BTTA, 1976), in partially controlled trials (Toogood et al., 1977) and in uncontrolled trials (Costello and Clark, 1974). A clear dose-response was demonstrated by Toogood et al, (1977) who aimed to improve asthma control in 34 patients unable to increase their oral corticosteroid dosage because of side effects. A dose-related improvement was evident as beclomethasone dosage increased from 400 to 1600 µg/d at 14-day intervals. A mean dose of 1050µg daily of inhaled beclomethasone dipropionate was required to maintain the desired level of control of symptoms once oral corticosteroids were decreased to the lowest dosage consistent with good control (Toogood et al., 1978). Attack frequency was decreased relative to baseline in 29 out of 34 patients. Addition of sodium cromoglycate 80mg daily did not permit a further decrease in inhaled beclomethasone dipropionate dosage. Biochemical evidence of partial adrenal suppression was evident in some patients, but plasma cortisol had improved in 13 patients, 11 of whom had experienced a 40 to 100% decrease in attack frequency relative to that at the beginning of the 2-year trial.

In a retrospective study of 293 asthmatic patients not adequately controlled with standard doses of inhaled beclomethasone dipropionate (Smith and Hodson, 1982) doses ranging from 500 to 2000 µg/day by high dose (250µg per actuation) pressurised aerosol lead to overall improvement in asthma control in 62%; 27% of patients were able to stop their oral steroids altogether and the mean daily prednisolone requirements for the group fell from 11.5mg (on standard dose therapy) to 6.0mg on high dose therapy. Attack frequency was reduced and lung function increased with high dose inhalations.

Nebuliser Suspension of Beclomethasone Dipropionate

Recently an aqueous suspension of beclomethasone dipropionate (50µg/ml) for use with a respirator or nebuliser has been developed. Its use is indicated in patients who are unable to operate a pressurised aerosol or breath-actuated inhaler, such as the very young and those with a very low inspiratory flow. Preliminary data suggest that the nebulised suspension has been beneficial in doses of 100µg 3 or 4 times daily in adults and children over 1 year of age.

References

Apold, J. and Djoseland, O.: Inhaled beclomethasone dipropionate in the treatment of childhood asthma. Postgraduate Medical Journal 51 (Suppl. 4): 104 (1975).

Arora, N.S. and Maher-Loughnan, G.P.: The substitution of betamethasone valerate for systemic steroids in chronic asthmatics. Postgraduate Medical Journal 50 (Sept. Suppl.): 20 (1974).

Bernstein, I.L.; Chervinsky, P. and Falliers, C.J.: Efficacy and safety of triamcinolone acetonide aerosol in chronic asthma. Results of a multicenter, short-term controlled and long-term open study. Chest 81: 20 (1982).

Bone, R.C.; Pingelton, W.W.; Kerby, G.R. and Ruth, W.E.: Early pulmonary function response as a predictor of long term benefit from triamcinolone acetonide aerosol. American Review of Respiratory Disease 115: 89 (1979).

British Thoracic and Tuberculosis Association: Inhaled corticosteroids compared with oral prednisone in patients starting long-term corticosteroid therapy for asthma. Lancet 2: 7933 (1975)..

British Thoracic and Tuberculosis Association: A trial of inhaled corticosteroids in patients receiving prednisone Journal of Diseases of the Chest 70: 95 (1976).

Brompton Hospital/Medical Research Council Collaborative Trial: Double-blind trial comparing two dosage schedules of beclomethasone dipropionate aerosol in the treatment of chronic bronchial asthma. Lancet 2: 303 (1974).

Brompton Hospital/Medical Research Council Collaborative Trial: Double-blind trial comparing two dosage schedules of beclomethasone dipropionate aerosol with a placebo in chronic bronchial asthma. British Journal of Diseases of the Chest 73: 121 (1979).

Brown, H.M. and Storey, G.: Treatment of allergy of the respiratory tract with beclomethasone dipropionate steroid aerosol. Postgraduate Medical Journal 51 (Suppl. 4): 59 (1975).

Brown, H.M.: Storey, G. and George, W.H.S.: Beclomethasone dipropionate: A new steroid aerosol for the treatment of allergic asthma. British Medical Journal 1: 585 (1972).

Brown, H.M.; Bhowmik, M.; Jackson, F.A. and Thantrey, N.: Beclomethasone dipropionate aerosols in the treatment of asthma in childhood. The Practitioner 224: 847 (1980).

Cameron, S.J.; Cooper, J.; Crompton, G.K.; Hoare, M.V. and Grant, I.W.B.: Substitution of beclomethasone aerosol for oral prednisolone in the treatment of chronic asthma. British Medical Journal 4: 205 (1973).

Campbell, I.A.; Finnegan, O.C.; Todd, J. and Smith, D.: A comparison of aerosol and powder inhalation of beclomethasone. British Journal of Diseases of the Chest 74: 419 (1980).

Carmichael, J.; Duncan, D. and Crompton, G.K.: Beclomethasone dipropionate drypowder inhalation compared with conventional aerosol in chronic asthma. British Medical Journal 2: 657 (1978).

Chambers, W.B. and Malfitan, V.A.: Beclomethasone dipropionate aerosol in the treatment of asthma in steroid-independent children. Journal of International Medical Research 7: 415 (1979).

Chatterjee, S.S. and Butler, A.G.: Beclomethasone dipropionate in asthma: A comparison of two methods of administration. British Journal of Diseases of the Chest 74: 175 (1980).

Chatterjee, S.S.; Ross, A.E.; Carroll, K.; Harris, D.M. and Butler, A.G.: Respiratory function in asthmatic patients using beclomethasone dipropionate administered by pressurised aerosol. Current Medical Research and Opinion 1: 173 (1972).

Chervinsky, P.: Treatment of steroid-dependent asthma with trimacinolone acetonide aerosol. Annals of Allergy 38: 192 (1977).

Clark, T.J.H.: Effect of beclomethasone dipropionate delivered by aerosol in patients with asthma. Lancet 1: 1361 (1972).

Costello, J.F. and Clark, T.J.: Response of patients receiving high dose beclomethasone dipropionate. Thorax 29: 571 (1974).

Couch, A.H.C.; Sutton, P.H. and Walker, S.R.: A 12-month double-blind clinical comparison of betamethasone valerate and sodium cromoglycate in the treatment of asthma. The Practitioner 219: 751 (1977).

Dickson, W.; Hall, C.E.; Ellis, M. and Horrocks, R.H.: Beclomethasone dipropionate aerosol in childhood asthma. Archives of Disease in Childhood 48: 671 (1973).

Edmunds, A.T.; McKenzie, S.; Tooley, M. and Godfrey, S.: A clinical comparison of beclomethasone dipropionate delivered by pressurised aerosol and as a powder from a rotahaler. Archives of Disease in Children 54: 233 (1979).

El-Shaboury, A.H. and Williams, D.A.: Betamethasone valerate aerosol in asthmatic patients receiving long-term oral steroid therapy: A double-blind controlled trial and follow-up of patients for 20 months. Postgraduate Medical Journal 50 (Sept. Suppl.): 15 (1974).

Epstein, S.W. and Thompson, G.L.: A study of inhaled beclomethasone dipropionate therapy in asthma. Canadian Family Physician 22: 274 (1976).

Eriksson, N.E.; Lindgren, S. and Lindholm, N.: A double-blind comparison of beclomethasone dipropionate aerosol and prednisolone in asthmatic patients. Postgraduate Medical Journal 51 (Suppl 4.): 67 (1975).

Falliers, C.J.: Triamcinolone acetonide aerosols for asthma. I. Effective replacement of systemic corticosteroid therapy. The Journal of Allergy and Clinical Immunology 57: 1 (1976).

Fein, B.T.: Geriatric asthma: Treatment with beclomethasone dipropionate aerosol. Southern Medical Journal 74: 1186 (1981).

Finnegan, O.C.; Campbell, I.A.; Dennison, J. and Smith, D.: Management of asthma with beclomethasone dipropionate. A comparison of pressurized aerosol and rotahaler powder inhalation. The Practitioner 226: 1588 (1982).

Francis, R.S.: Long-term beclomethasone dipropionate aerosol therapy in juvenile asthma. Thorax 31: 309 (1976).

Frears, J.; Hodgson, S. and Friedman, M.: Effect of placebo substitution during long-term betamethasone valerate aerosol treatment in asthmatic children. Archives of Disease in Childhood 50: 387 (1975).

Gaddie, J.; Petrie, G.R.; Reid, I.W.; Sinclair, D.J.M.; Skinner, C. and Palmer, K.N.V.: Aerosol beclomethasone dipropionate in chronic bronchial asthma. Lancet 1: 691 (1973).

Girard, J.P.; Vonlanthen, M.C. and Heimlich, E.M.: Therapeutic index of steroid aerosols in asthma. A single-blind comparative trial of beclomethasone dipropionate vs dexamethasone isonicotinate. Acta Allergologica 30: 363 (1975).

Godfrey, S. and Konig, P.: Beclomethasone aerosol in childhood asthma. Archives of Disease in Childhood 48: 665 (1973).

Godfrey, S. and Konig, P.: Treatment of childhood asthma for 13 months and longer with beclomethasone dipropionate aerosol. Archives of Disease in Childhood 49: 591 (1974).

Godfrey, S.; Balfour-Lynn, L. and Tooley, M.: A three- to five-year follow-up of the use of the aerosol steroid, beclomethasone dipropionate, in childhood asthma. Journal of Allergy and Clinical Immunology 62: 335 (1978).

Golub, J.R.: Long-term triamcinolone acetonide aerosol treatment in adult patients with chronic bronchial asthma. Annals of Allergy 44: 131 (1980).

Grieco, M.H.; Dwek, J.; Larsen, K. and Rammohan, G.: Clinical effect of aerosol triamcinolone acetonide in bronchial asthma. Archives of Internal Medicine 138: 1337 (1978).

Gwynn, C.M. and Smith, J.M.: A 1 year follow-up of children and adolescents receiving regular beclomethasone dipropionate. Clinical Allergy 4: 325 (1974).

Hiller, E.J. and Milner, A.D.: Betamethasone 17 valerate aerosol and disodium cromoglycate in severe childhood asthma. British Journal of Diseases of the Chest 69: 103 (1975).

Hodson, M.E.; Batten, J.C.; Clarke, S.W. and Gregg, I.: Beclomethasone dipropionate aerosol in asthma. Transfer of steroid-dependent asthmatic patients from oral prednisone to beclomethasone dipropionate aerosol. American Review of Respiratory Diseases 110: 403 (1974).

Howard, K. and Jacoby, N.M.: Betamethasone valerate treatment of steroid dependent children. Postgraduate Medical Journal 50 (Sept. Suppl.): 41 (1974).

Jacoby, N.M.: The routine treatment of asthmatic children with betamethasone valerate aerosol. The Practitioner 218: 856 (1977).

Johannessen, H.; Halvorsen, F.J. and Kommedal, T.M.: Long-term treatment of patients with perennial bronchial asthma with beclomethasone dipropionate aerosol: A 24-month follow-up study. Current Therapeutic Research 26: 592 (1979).

Kass, I.; Vijayachandran Nair, S. and Patil, K.D.: Beclomethasone dipropionate aerosol in the treatment of steroid-dependent asthmatic patients. An assessment of 18 months of therapy. Chest 71: 703 (1977).

Kennedy, M.C.S.; Posner, E. and Thursby-Pelham, D.C.: Long-term treatment of asthma with beclomethasone dipropionate. Postgraduate Medical Journal 51 (Suppl. 4): 84 (1975).

Kennedy, M.C.S.; Haslock, M.R. and Thursby-Pelham, D.C.: Aerosol therapy for asthma: A 10-year follow-up of treatment with beclomethasone dipropionate in 100 asthmatic patients. Pharmatherapeutica 2: 648 (1981).

Kriz, R.J.; Chmelik, F.; doPico, G. and Reed, C.E.: A one-year trial of triamcinolone acetonide aerosol in severe steroid-dependent asthma. Chest 72: 36 (1977).

Kuzemko, J.A.; Bedford, S.; Wilson, L. and Walker, S.R.: A comparison of betamethasone valerate aerosol and sodium cromoglycate in children with reversible airways obstruction. Postgraduate Medical Journal 50 (Sept. Suppl.): 53 (1974).

Lal, S.; Harris, D.M.; Bhalia, K.K.; Singhal, S.N. and Butler, A.G.: Comparison of beclomethasone dipropionate aerosol and prednisolone in reversible airways obstruction. British Medical Journal 3: 314 (1972).

Lal, S.; Malhotra, S.M.; Gribben, M.D. and Butler, A.G.: Beclomethasone dipropionate aerosol compared with dry powder in the treatment of asthma. Clinical Allergy 10: 259 (1980).

Loudon, H.W.G.: Betamethasone valerate and beclomethasone dipropionate aerosols in patients with asthma. Postgraduate Medical Journal 50 (Suppl.) 65 (1974).

Lovera, J.; Collins-Williams, C. and Bailey, J.: Beclomethasone dipropionate by aerosol in the treatment of asthmatic children. Postgraduate Medical Journal 51 (Suppl. 4): 96 (1975).

McAllen, M.K.; Kochanowski, S.J. and Shaw, K.M.: Steroid aerosols in asthma: An assessment of betamethasone valerate and a 12-month study of patients on maintenance. British Medical Journal 1: 171 (1974).

Meltzer, E.O.; Kemp, J.P.; Orgel, H.A. and Izu, A.E.: Flunisolide aerosol for treatment of severe, chronic asthma in steroid-independent children. Pediatrics 69: 340 (1982).

Mitchell, I.; Paterson, I.C.; Cameron, S.J. and Grant, I.W.B.: Treatment of childhood asthma with sodium cromoglycate and beclomethasone dipropionate aerosol singly and in combination. British Medical Journal 2: 457 (1976).

Ng, S.H.; Dash, C.H. and Savage, S.J.: Betamethasone valerate compared with sodium cromoglycate in asthmatic children. Postgraduate Medical Journal 53: 315 (1977).

Pines, A.: Beclomethasone dipropionate used as an aerosol in the treatment of asthma. The Practitioner 211: 86 (1973).

Prakesh, C.; Chopra, J.S. and Chugh, V.K.: Double blind cross over trial of beclomethasone dipropionate aerosol and oral prednisolone in bronchial asthma. Journal of the Association of Physicians of India 24: 3 (1976).

Rao, M.; Steiner, P.; Maraya, R.; Victoria, M.S.; Jabar, H. and Hunt, J.: Beclomethasone dipropionate for chronic asthma in children: The Kings County Hospital experience. Journal of Asthma 19: 21 (1982).

Richards, W.; Platzker, A.; Church, J.A.; Yamamoto, F. and Foster, S.: Steroid-dependent asthma treated with inhaled beclomethasone dipropionate in children. Annals of Allergy 41: 274 (1978).

Riorden, J.F.; Dash, C.H.; Stillett, R.W. and McNichol, M.W.: A comparison of betamethasone valerate, beclomethasone dipropionate and placebo by inhalation for the treatment of chronic asthma. Postgraduate Medical Journal 50 (Sept. Suppl.): 61 (1974).

Salorinne, Y. and Klemetti, L.: Dexamethasone-21-isonicotinate and beclomethasone dipropionate in the treatment of patients with asthma. IRCS Medical Science: Clinical Pharmacology and Therapeutics 7: 109 (1979).

Scherr, M.S.; Scherr, L.B. and Morton, J.L.: Use of inhaled beclomethasone dipropionate and optimized theophylline doses in asthmatic children at camp bronco junction, 1977-1978. Annals of Allergy 44: 82 (1980).

Shapiro, G.G.; Izu, A.E.; Furukawa, C.T.; Pierson, W.E. and Bierman, C.W.: Short-term double-blind evaluation of flunisolide aerosol for steroid-dependent asthmatic children and adolescents. Chest 80: 671 (1981).

Sly, R.M.; Imseis, M.; Frazer, M. and Joseph, F.: Treatment of asthma in children with triamcinolone acetonide aerosol. Journal of Allergy and Clinical Immunology 62: 76 (1978).

Smith, J. Morrison: A clinical trial of beclomethasone dipropionate aerosol in children and adolescents with asthma. Clinical Allergy 3: 249 (1973).

Smith, J. Morrison, and Gwynn, C.M.: A clinical comparison of aerosol and powder administration of beclomethasone dipropionate in asthma. Clinical Allergy 8: 479 (1978).

Smith, M.J. and Hodson, M.E.: High dose beclomethasone inhaler in the treatment of asthma. Lancet 2: in press (1982).

Taylor, B. and Norman, A.P.: Betamethasone 17-valerate in childhood asthma. Acta Paediatrica Scandinavica 64: 234 (1975).

Toogood, J.H.; Lefcoe, N.M.; Haines, D.S.M.; Jennings, B.; Errington, N. and Chuang, L.: A graded dose assessment of the efficacy of beclomethasone dipropionate aerosol for severe chronic asthma. Journal of Allergy and Clinical Immunology 59: 298 (1977).

Toogood, J.H.; Lefcoe, N.M.; Haines, D.S.M.; Chuang, L.; Jennings, B.; Errington, N.; Baksh, L. and Cauchi, M.: Minimum dose requirements of steroid-dependent asthmatic patients for aerosol beclomethasone and oral prednisone. Journal of Allergy and Clinical Immunology 61: 355 (1978).

Toogood, J.H.; Jennings, B. and Lefcoe, N.M.: Clinical trial of combined cromolyn/beclomethasone treatment for chronic asthma. Journal of Allergy and Clinical Immunology 67: 317 (1981).

Vernon, D.R.H.; MacLeod, J.M. and Kerr, J.W.: A 12-month double-blind assessment of betamethasone valerate aerosol in the management of asthma. Clinical Allergy 6: 261 (1976).

Vilsvik, J.S. and Schaanning, J.: Beclomethasone dipropionate aerosol in adult steroid-dependent obstructive lung disease. Scandinavian Journal of Respiratory Diseases 55: 169 (1974).

Webb, D.R.; Mullarkey, M.F. and Freeman, M.I.: Flunisolide in chronic bronchial asthma. Annals of Allergy 42: 80 (1979).

Willey, R.F.; Godden, D.J.; Carmichael, J.; Preston, P.; Frame, M. and Crompton, G.K.: Comparison of twice daily administration of a new corticosteroid budesonide with beclomethasone dipropionate four times daily in the treatment of chronic asthma. British Journal of Diseases of the Chest 76: 61 (1982).

Williams, M.H.: Treatment of asthma with triamcinolone acetonide aerosol. Chest 68: 765 (1975).

Chapter X

Factors which may Affect the Response to Inhaled Steroids; Side Effects

R.N. Brogden

Factors Influencing Reponse to Inhaled Corticosteroids

Various factors, such as pretreatment oral steroid dosage, presence of allergy, age, pulmonary function and adrenal function, have been considered by many investigators to determine their influence on the response to inhaled corticosteroids.

In nearly all published studies that have considered the possible importance of the various determinants, analyses have been based on the response to beclomethasone dipropionate 400 to 800 µg/day or an equivalent dosage of one of the other inhaled corticosteroids. The determinants of response to dosages of up to 1600µg daily of beclomethasone dipropionate aerosol have been reported by Toogood et al. (1977b), as these investigators found that most of their patients needed more than 400µg daily, and this study is the most extensive examination of this aspect so far published. The problem with most analyses of determinants, with the exception of that conducted by Toogood et al. (1977b), is that the possible determinants have been considered in isolation.

Initial Dose of Oral Maintenance Corticosteroid

Several studies have noted that withdrawal of oral corticosteroids in steroid-dependent asthmatics treated with inhaled corticosteroids has been easier when the daily dose has been less than 10mg of prednisone or its equivalent (Brompton Hospital/MRC Trial, 1974, 1979; BTTA, 1976; Bacal and Patterson, 1978; Gwynn and Smith, 1974; Holst and O'Donnell, 1974; Kennedy et al., 1981; McAllen et al., 1974; Mackay, 1975; Vandenberg, 1974; Vandenberg et al., 1975). The relationship between initial maintenance dosages of prednisone and their ease of replacement by inhaled beclomethasone is clearly illustrated in children in the study of Gwynn and Smith (1974) [table 10.1] and in adults by Bacal and Patterson (1978) [fig. 10.1]. Contrary findings have, however, been reported occasionally (Kass et al., 1977; Imbeau and Geller, 1978), finding no relationship between initial oral steroid maintenance dose and clinical response or the ease of completely withdrawing oral cortcosteroids.

In the study of Toogood et al. (1977b) there was no correlation between the change in asthma attack frequency and the pre-beclomethasone dipropionate dose of oral corticosteroids.

Presence of Allergy

An elevated serum IgE has been reported to be a favourable factor in influencing the response to inhaled beclomethasone dipropionate (Kennedy et al., 1981; Smith, 1973; Vandenberg et al., 1975). A tendency for oral steroids to be withdrawn more often or a more consistent improvement in pulmonary function in 'extrinsic' rather than in 'intrinsic' asthmatics, was noted by Bülow and Kalén (1974), Maberly et al. (1973) and Manicatide et al. (1978), whilst El-Shaboury and Williams (1974) noted a tendency for a poor response to betamethasone valerate occurred in patients with negative skin tests for common allergens.

Table 10.1. Response to beclomethasone dipropionate inhaler as evidenced by reduction in maintenance corticosteroid requirements in asthmatic children originally controlled on daily systemic corticosteroids (after Gwynn and Smith, 1974)

Initial steroid dosage	No. of patients	Effect on systemic steroid requirements (%)		
		stopped	reduced	unchanged
10mg or more prednisolone daily	8	3 (37)	3 (37)	2 (25)
5 to 10mg prednisolone daily	26[1]	15 (58)	1 (3.8)	7 (27)
2.5mg or less prednisolone daily	15	14 (93)	-	1 (6)
Prednisolone + tetracosactrin × 2 weekly	2[2]	-	1	-
Tetracosactrin × 2 weekly	2	2	-	-

1 — 1 patient discontinued beclomethasone dipropionate, and no data are given for the remaining 2 patients.
2 — No data are given for the other patient.

However, in some studies there was no association between response and the different types of asthma (Smith et al., 1973 and p.195) or results of skin reactions to common allergens (Kuzemko et al., 1974). Contrary to other investigations, Toogood et al. (1977b) found that an elevated serum IgE was not a favourable factor influencing response.

Respiratory Function

Although a positive association between the initial FEV_1 and subsequent response to beclomethasone dipropionate has been reported by Vandenberg et al. (1975), a lack of correlation between response and initial FEV_1 has been noted by Bülow and Kalén (1974), Gaddie et al. (1973) and Maberly et al. (1973). Imbeau and Geller (1978) noted a greater increase in post-treatment FEV_1 in those patients with a low FEV_1/FVC percent ratio.

The degree of reversibility of airways obstruction appears to influence the response to beclomethasone dipropionate inhaler. Kennedy et al. (1981) noted that most non-responders (fig. 10.2) had what was described as grade 4 asthma, in which ventilatory capacity remains impaired between attacks and cannot be brought within normal limits with treatment. The failure to reverse part of the obstruction may indicate the presence of an element of irreversible chronic obstructive lung disease. In the comprehensive analysis of Toogood et al. (1977b), those patients who responded poorly despite treatment with 1600 μg daily of inhaled beclomethasone dipropionate, differed from the responsive patients mainly in the greater degree of chronic obstructive lung disease associated with their asthma.

The influence of sputum production on response to inhaled corticosteroids is unclear. Toogood et al. (1977b) reported that recurrent mucopurulent bronchitis was a limiting factor in symptom response at the highest (1600μg) and lowest (400μg) doses of beclomethasone dipropionate. Brown and Storey (1975) found that frequent bronchial infection before and after introduction of be-

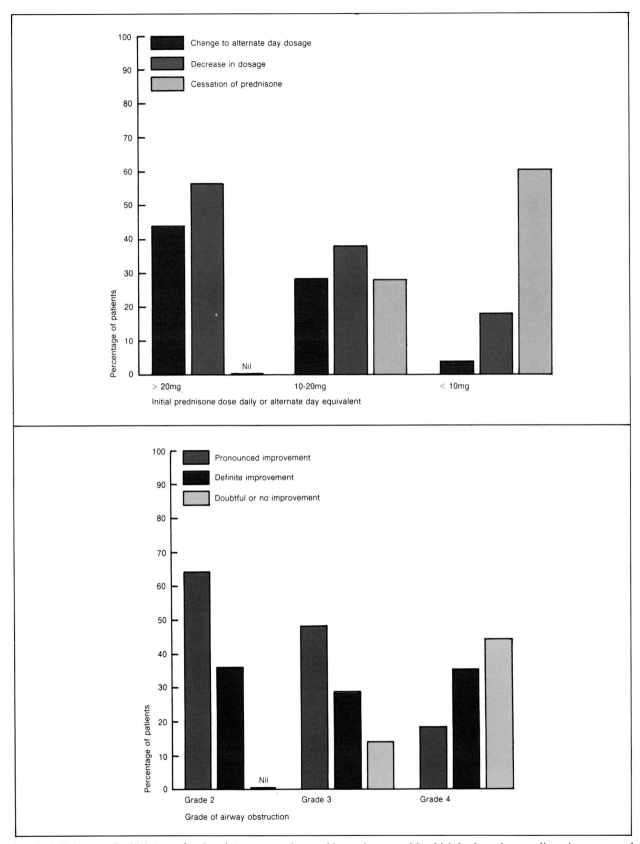

Fig. 10.1. Influence of initial dose of oral maintenance corticosteroids on the ease with which beclomethasone dipropionate aerosol could be substituted for the oral drug (after Bacal and Patterson, 1978).

Fig. 10.2. Degree of improvement in asthma symptoms during long term treatment with inhaled beclomethasone dipropionate, according to the grade of airway obstruction (after Kennedy et al., 1981).

Table 10.2 Efficacy of high (1600µg) and low (400µg) dosages of inhaled beclomethasone dipropionate in 34 steroid-dependent asthmatics (after Toogood et al., 1977a)

Assessment criteria[1]	Percentage of patients attaining a normal (or zero) score		ED_{50}[2] ($\mu g/d$)
	400 $\mu g/d$	1600 $\mu g/d$	
MMFR	3	5	>1600
Bronchodilator (oral) use	29	50	1600
Asthma attack frequency	26	60	1050
Inhaled bronchodilator use	45	77	500
Asthma disability score by patient	72	95	<200
Asthma disability score by physician	76	98	<200

1 — MMFR = maximum midexpiratory flow rate.
2 — Dosage required to achieve a normal value in 50% of the treatment group.

clomethasone dipropionate aerosol was the cause of the treatment failure in 11 of 25 steroid-dependent patients, but no association between sputum production and response to beclomethasone dipropionate was found in the British Thoracic and Tuberculosis Association Trials (1975, 1976). A possible influence of sputum production on response to betamethasone valerate was recorded by El-Shaboury and Williams (1974) and McAllen et al. (1974).

Age

There is no clear association between age and the response to treatment with inhaled corticosteroids. Although a trend towards a better result in younger than older patients was noted by some investigators (Brown and Storey, 1975; Kennedy et al., 1981; Vandenberg et al., 1975), and there is a general clinical impression of better overall response in children than in adults, other workers have found no such tendency (Bülow and Kalén, 1974; Maberly et al., 1973; Toogood et al., 1977b), or have reported good results in patients aged 61 to 78 years (Fein, 1981).

Dose of Inhaled Corticosteroid

In many instances, the influence on response of the dosage of an inhaled corticosteroid has been studied over a narrow range of dosages, usually up to a maximum of 800µg daily. Under these circumstances a daily dose of 800µg of beclomethasone dipropionate has been found better than 400µg daily in enabling the withdrawal of oral corticosteroids in patients whose initial daily dose was 16mg or more (Brompton Hospital/MRC Trial, 1974), in maintaining improvement in patients whose pretreatment oral corticosteroid requirement was 10mg or more daily (Brompton Hospital/MRC Trial, 1979) and in permitting patients to remain off oral corticosteroids over a 6-month period (BTTA, 1976). Evidence of improvement in FEV_1 in patients whose dose of beclomethasone dipropionate was increased from 400 to 1000 µg/day was reported by Costello and Clark (1974) and in 293 patients increasing standard doses to 500 to 2000 µg/day resulted in better symptomatic response and a decrease in oral steroid requirement (Smith and Hodson, 1982). Although there was no clear dose-related effect in mildly affected asthmatic children, in those with moderate to severe asthma, 400µg daily appeared to be more beneficial than lower dosages on the basis of physicians' overall rating (Chambers and Malfitan, 1979).

A statistically significant and dose-related improvement in asthma symptoms and disability (table 10.2) occurred in 34 adult steroid-dependent asthmatics given beclomethasone dipropionate in increasing dosages of 200 to 1600μg daily (Toogood et al., 1977a). The clear dose-response seen in this, but not in other studies, may be related to the fact that the baseline dose of oral corticosteroids remained constant while the beclomethasone dipropionate dose was increased. No dose-related response was found by Gaddie et al. (1973) in non-steroid-dependent adult asthmatics whose dose of beclomethasone dipropionate was increased from 400 to 1600μg daily at 28-day intervals, but these patients had not been shown to be unresponsive to the lower dose.

Increasingly patients are being treated with the much more convenient twice-daily dosage regimen of inhaled steroid, rather than the previously used four times a day, with evidence of comparable control in most (Munch et al., 1982).

Worsening asthma in a patient previously well controlled on inhaled steroids is not an indication for increasing the inhaled dose but for a course of oral steroids (p.111) which patients should always have by them for use in emergency.

Method of Use

In some patients, failure to respond to inhaled corticosteroids has been associated with poor technique in using the inhaler (Brown et al., 1972; Gwynn and Smith, 1977; Kennedy et al., 1975; Maberly et al., 1973) or misunderstanding of its prophylactic purpose (Gregg, 1977). Thus, it is clearly important that patients be instructed in the correct use of the inhaler (Appendix 1).

Table 10.3. Incidence of oropharyngeal candidiasis (thrush) in adult asthmatics treated with inhaled corticosteroids for 6 months or more

Author	Drug[1]	Dose (μg/d)	No. of patients	Incidence of candidiasis (%)	Treatment duration	Diagnostic criteria
Brompton Hosp/ MRC, 1974	BDP	400 800	33 31	45[2] 77	6 months	white patches, colony counts
Brompton Hosp/ MRC, 1979	BDP	400 800	349 samples 544 samples	10 20	12 months	white patches, colony counts
BTTA, 1976	BDP BV	400-800 800	105	6-10	6 months	visual, + culture in most
McAllen et al. (1974)	BDP BV	200-800	120	13	12 months	white patches, + culture
Milne and Crompton (1974)	BDP	≤400	510	5.5[3]	variable	symptoms, + culture
Willey et al. (1976)	BDP	≤400	400	4.5[3]	1-75 months (mean 19)	white patches, + culture
Chervinsky and Petraco (1979)	TA	400-800	568	3	≥6m	visual, + cultures

1 — BDP = beclomethasone dipropionate; BV = betamethasone valerate; TA = triamcinolone acetonide.
2 — Cumulative incidence in the Brompton Hospital/MRC Trial (1974).
3 — Based on findings from a single examination.

Side Effects

Oropharyngeal
Candidiasis

The most common side effects associated with the long term use of inhaled corticosteroids have been oropharyngeal candidiasis, caused by *Candida albicans*, hoarseness and sore throat. The reported incidence of *Candida* infections varies greatly, having ranged from 0 to 77%, the high figure being a cumulative incidence (Brompton Hospital/MRC Trial, 1974). The large variation in the incidence of thrush may be accounted for in part by the variations in the criteria for the diagnosis and methods used. A summary of the findings in adults treated with inhaled corticosteroids for 6 months or more is shown in table 10.3. The incidence of oral candidiasis appears to be similar with each of the inhaled corticosteroids, although most of the published data are concerned with beclomethasone dipropionate. The frequency of asymptomatic oral yeast infections in asthmatic or other outpatients not receiving inhaled or oral corticosteroids has varied between studies (e.g. Milne and Crompton, 1974; Sahay et al., 1979; Toogood et al., 1977a), but results of studies that have incorporated a control group clearly indicate that inhaled steroids increase oral candidiasis in adults (Brompton Hospital/MRC Trial, 1974; Milne and Crompton, 1974).

Well conducted studies (e.g. Brompton Hospital/MRC Trials, 1974, 1979; McAllen et al., 1974; Milne and Crompton, 1974; Toogood et al., 1980) indicated that the incidence of oral candidiasis is dose-related, becoming higher as dosage is increased, although there is some evidence that frequency of inhaler use, rather than acutal total daily dose of steroid inhaled may be important (Smith and Hodson, 1982). However, clinical thrush has seldom become a major problem. It has usually been readily controlled with topical nystatin or amphotericin B or a decrease in dosage, and has seldom necessitated the withdrawal of inhaled therapy (Milne and Crompton, 1974; Brompton Hospital/MRC Trial, 1979; Kennedy et al., 1981). In general, the reported incidence of oropharyngeal candidiasis among children treated with inhaled corticosteroids is less than that in adults (Brown and Storey, 1973; Chambers and Malfitan, 1979; Francis, 1976; Godfrey et al., 1978; Meltzer et al., 1982; Ng et al., 1977). The lower incidence in children may be, in part, a function of the generally lower dosage in children, but other as yet unidentified factors appear to be involved also.

It has been suggested, but seldom supported by appropriate data, that the concomitant administration of oral and inhaled corticosteroids increases the incidence of oral candidiasis (Brown et al., 1977; Kershnar et al., 1978). However, studies in relatively large numbers of patients indicate that combined oral and inhaled treatment does not necessarily lead to an increased incidence of oral candidiasis (McAllen et al., 1974; Milne and Crompton, 1974; Willey et al., 1976). Also the lack of influence of oral corticosteroid withdrawal on the frequency of thrush during a constant dosage of inhaled steroid in the study of Toogood et al. (1980), tends to confirm this.

It has been suggested by several investigators that rinsing out the mouth with tap water immediately after inhalation of aerosol corticosteroid, may decrease the frequency of thrush and other effects on the throat (Brown et al., 1977; Chatterjee, 1977; McAllen et al., 1974; Toogood et al., 1980). In a formal study, however, there appeared to be no clear benefit resulting from the mouthwash procedure (Sahay et al., 1979).

Published studies have not detected any difference in the incidence of oropharyngeal candidiasis in adult patients treated with either beclomethasone dipropionate aerosol or dry-powder inhalation of the same drug (Chatterjee and Butler, 1980; Lal et al., 1980). See also p.181.

Sore Throat and Hoarseness

A commonly reported side effect of inhaled corticosteroids has been sore throat and/or hoarseness, which has been reported in one study in up to 50 to 81% of patients (Brompton Hospital/ MRC Trial, 1974; Toogood et al., 1980; Pingleton et al., 1977). Hoarseness may occur in patients without thrush (Pingleton et al., 1977; Toogood et al., 1980; Willey et al., 1976) and despite suggestions incriminating the propellant (Kriz et al., 1975, 1976), appears to be due to the steroid rather than placebo (BTTA, 1976; Toogood et al., 1980). As with oral candidiasis, the incidence of hoarseness has varied considerably between studies and may be a function of the care with which it was sought, a checklist being

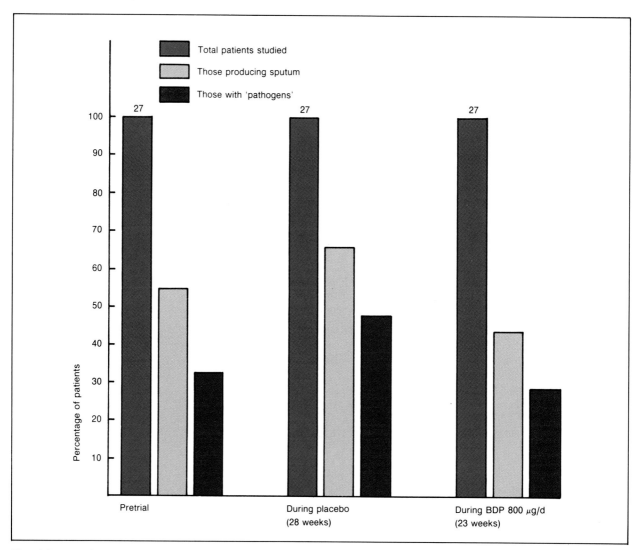

Fig. 10.3A. Relative frequency of isolation of bacteria from the sputum of patients who received inert propellant for 28 weeks then 800 μg/d of inhaled beclomethasone dipropionate for the next 23 weeks (data from Brompton Hospital/MRC Trial, 1979).

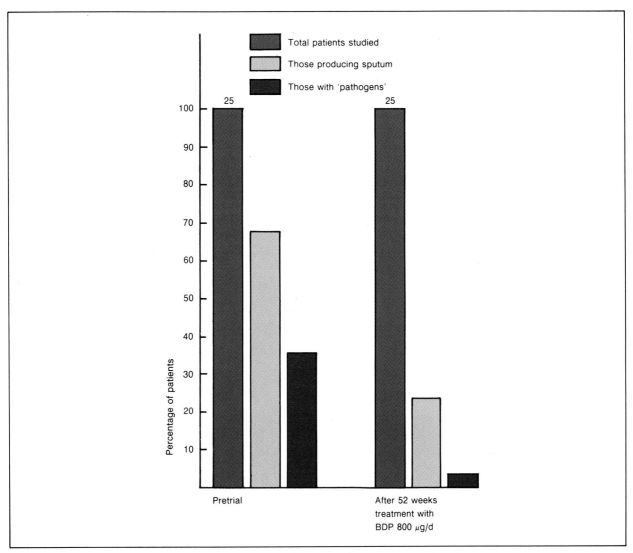

Fig. 10.3B. Relative frequency of isolation of bacteria from the sputum of patients who received inhaled beclomethasone dipropionate 800 µg/d throughout the study (data from Brompton Hospital/MRC Trial, 1979).

used by Toogood et al., (1980) and direct questioning by Pingleton et al. (1977). See also p.182.

There is no evidence that inhaled steroids damage the trachcobronchial lining (p.122).

Chest Infection

When inhaled corticosteroids were first introduced, there was anxiety about the possibility of increased susceptibility to bronchial infection (e.g. McAllen et al., 1974). A few observers have alluded to a possible increased frequency of respiratory infections after starting treatment with beclomethasone dipropionate inhaler (Brown and Storey, 1975; Hodson et al., 1974). However, these studies did not record pretrial data. Regular examination of sputum for possible pathogens, revealed no evidence that pathogens occur more frequently in asthmatics treated with inhaled beclomethasone (Brompton Hospital/MRC Trial, 1979) [fig. 10.3]. As evidenced by the prescription of antibiotics before and after institution of beclomethasone aerosol (Toogood et al., 1977a) and during treatment (BTTA, 1975), no increase in respiratory infection rate occurred during long term treatment. There has been no conclusive evidence of tuberculosis or respiratory tract infection due to *Candida albicans* during treatment with inhaled corticosteroids.

Systemic Corticosteroid Withdrawal Effects

During or after the withdrawal of systemic corticosteroids under the cover of inhaled corticosteroids, symptoms suggestive of steroid withdrawal such as nausea, vomiting, anorexia, tiredness, lassitude, headache, muscle and joint pains and mental depression, have been reported in many studies. The frequency of such symptoms has been greater in studies in which the systemic corticosteroids have been withdrawn rapidly (e.g. Brown et al., 1972; Maberly et al., 1973) than in those in which they have been withdrawn over a much longer period (e.g. Cameron et al., 1973).

A frequently reported problem has been the exacerbation of underlying diseases formerly controlled by systemic corticosteroids. Worsening of eczema, allergic rhinitis and other atopic conditions and reactivation of nasal polyposis have occurred. Reinstitution of oral corticosteroids to control these problems has been necessary only occasionally. In most instances nasal symptoms have been controlled by intranasal beclomethasone dipropionate, and other atopic conditions have been controlled with appropriate topical treatment.

The appearance of withdrawal effects on substituting inhaled for oral corticosteroids, attests to the lack of systemic effect of the inhaled drug. Other indirect evidence of the lack of systemic effect of inhaled corticosteroids when given in usual therapeutic dosages is afforded by reports of disappearance of systemic corticosteroid effects such as moon face (p.206) and dyspepsia (e.g. Brown and Storey, 1975; Pines, 1973).

Although the substitution of inhaled for oral corticosteroid in steroid-dependent asthmatics generally results in an improvement in resting and stimulated plasma cortisol concentrations (page 124), recovery from impaired adrenocortical function caused by prolonged systemic corticosteroid therapy is usually slow. Thus, special care is necessary for the first 9 to 12 months after transfer, until the HPA axis has sufficiently recovered to enable the patient to cope with emergencies such as trauma, surgery, severe infections, or an acute attack of asthma.

In summary

There is no clearly identifiable group of asthmatics unlikely to respond to inhaled steroids. The presence or absence of allergy does not seem to be a determinant and good responses are seen regardless of age. Lung function *per se* is not an indication of likely response but, as might be expected, patients with a degree of irreversibility are likely to respond less completely. Recent studies have confirmed the efficacy of twice-daily dose regimens and the dose-response relationship, higher doses being found effective in the previously unresponsive.

Side effects of inhaled steroids have been confined to oral thrush, sore throat and hoarseness, not generally requiring discontinuation of therapy.

References

Bacal, E. and Patterson, R.: Long-term effects of beclomethasone dipropionate on prednisone dosage in the corticosteroid-dependent asthmatic. Journal of Allergy and Clinical Immunology 62: 72 (1978).

British Thoracic and Tuberculosis Association: Inhaled corticosteroids compared with oral prednisone in patients starting long-term corticosteroid therapy for asthma. Lancet 2: 7933 (1975).

British Thoracic and Tuberculosis Association: A controlled trial of inhaled corticosteroids in patients receiving prednisone tablets for asthma. British Journal of Diseases of the Chest 70: 95 (1976).

Brompton Hospital/Medical Research Council Collaborative Trial: Double-blind trial comparing two dosage schedules of beclomethasone dipropionate aerosol in the treatment of chronic bronchial asthma. Lancet 2: 303 (1974).

Brompton Hospital/Medical Research Council Collaborative Trial: Double-blind trial comparing two dosage schedules of beclomethasone dipropionate aerosol with a placebo in chronic bronchial asthma. British Journal of Diseases of the Chest 73: 121 (1979).

Brown, H. Morrow and Storey, G.: Beclomethasone dipropionate steroid aerosol in treatment of perennial allergic asthma in children. British Medical Journal 3: 161 (1973).

Brown, H. Morrow and Storey, G.: Treatment of allergy of the respiratory tract with beclomethasone dipropionate steroid aerosol. Postgraduate Medical Journal 51 (Suppl. 4): 59 (1975).

Brown, H. Morrow; Storey, G. and George, W.H.S.: Beclomethasone dipropionate: A new steroid aerosol for the treatment of allergic asthma. British Medical Journal 1: 585 (1972).

Brown, H. Morrow; Storey, G. and Jackson, F.A.: Beclomethasone dipropionate aerosol in long-term treatment of perennial and seasonal asthma in children and adults: A report of five-and-half years' experience in 600 asthmatic patients. British Journal of Clinical Pharmacology 4: 259S (1977).

Bülow, K.B. and Kalén, N.: Local and systemic effects of beclomethasone inhalation in steroid-dependent asthmatic patients. Current Therapeutic Research 16: 1110 (1974).

Cameron, S.J.; Cooper, J.; Crompton, G.K.; Hoare, M.V. and Grant, I.W.B.: Substitution of beclomethasone aerosol for oral prednisolone in the treatment of chronic asthma. British Medical Journal 4: 205 (1973).

Chambers, W.B. and Malfitan, V.A.: Beclomethasone dipropionate aerosol in the treatment of asthma in steroid-dependent children. Journal of International Medical Research 7: 415 (1979).

Chatterjee, S.S.: Experience with the use of corticosteroid aerosol. British Journal of Clinical Pharmacology 4: 255S (1977).

Chatterjee, S.S. and Butler, A.G.: Beclomethasone dipropionate in asthma: A comparison of two methods of administration. British Journal of Diseases of the Chest 74: 175 (1980).

Chervinsky, P. and Petraco, A.J.: Incidence of oral candidiasis during therapy with triamcinolone acetonide aerosol. Annals of Allergy 43: 80 (1979).

Costello, J.F. and Clark, T.J.: Response of patients receiving high dose beclomethasone dipropionate. Thorax 29: 571 (1974).

El-Shaboury, A.H. and Williams, D.A.: Betamethasone valerate aerosol in asthmatic patients receiving long-term oral steroid therapy: A double-blind controlled trial and follow-up of patients for 20 months. Postgraduate Medical Journal 50 (Sept. Suppl.): 15 (1974).

Fein, B.T.: Geriatric asthma: Treatment with beclomethasone dipropionate aerosol. Southern Medical Journal 74: 1186 (1981).

Francis, R.S.: Long-term beclomethasone dipropionate aerosol therapy in juvenile asthma. Thorax 31: 309 (1976).

Gaddie, J.; Petrie, G.R.; Reid, I.W.; Sinclair, D.J.M.; Skinner, C. and Palmer, K.N.V.: Aerosol beclomethasone dipropionate: A dose-response study in chronic bronchial asthma. Lancet 2: 280 (1973).

Godfrey, S.; Balfour-Lynn, L. and Tooley, M.: A three- to five-year follow-up of the use of the aerosol steroid, beclomethasone dipropionate, in childhood asthma. Journal of Allergy and Clinical Immunology 62: 335 (1978).

Gregg, I.: Experience of the use of beclomethasone dipropionate aerosol in general practice. British Journal of Clinical Pharmacology 4: 275S (1977).

Gwynn, C.M. and Smith, J.M.: A 1 year follow-up of children and adolescents receiving regular beclomethasone dipropionate. Clinical Allergy 4: 325 (1974).

Gwynn, C.M. and Smith, J. Morrison: Long-term results with beclomethasone dipropionate aerosol in children with bronchial asthma: Why does it sometimes fail? British Journal of Clinical Pharmacology 4: 269S (1977).

Hodson, M.E.; Batten, J.C.; Clarke, S.W. and Gregg, I.: Beclomethasone dipropionate aerosol in asthma. Transfer of steroid-dependent asthmatic patients from oral prednisone to beclomethasone dipropionate aerosol. American Review of Respiratory Diseases 110: 403 (1974).

Holst, P.E. and O'Donnell, T.V.: A controlled trial of beclomethasone dipropionate in asthma. New Zealand Medical Journal 79: 769 (1974).

Imbeau, S.A. and Geller, M.: Aerosol beclomethasone treatment of chronic severe asthma. Journal of the American Medical Association 240: 1260 (1978).

Kass, I.; Nair, S.V. and Patil, K.D.: Beclomethasone dipropionate aerosol in the treatment of steroid-dependent asthmatic patients. An assessment of 18 months of therapy. Chest 71: 703 (1977).

Kennedy, M.C.S.; Haslock, M.R. and Thursby-Pelham, D.C.: Aerosol therapy for asthma: A 10-year follow-up of treatment with beclomethasone dipropionate in 100 asthmatic patients. Pharmatherapeutica 2: 648 (1981).

Kennedy, M.C.S.; Posner, E. and Thursby-Pelham, D.C.: Long-term treatment of asthma with beclomethasone dipropionate. Postgraduate Medical Journal 51 (Suppl. 4): 84 (1975).

Kershnar, H.; Klein, R.; Waldman, D.; Berger, W.; Rachelefsky, G.; Katz, R. and Siegel, S.: Treatment of chronic childhood asthma with beclomethasone dipropionate aerosols: II. Effect on pituitary-adrenal function after substitution for oral corticosteroids. Pediatrics 62: 189 (1978).

Kriz, R.J.; Chmelik, F. and Reed, C.E.: A short-term double-blind evaluation of triamcinolone acetonide aerosol in severe steroid-dependent asthma. Journal of Allergy and Clinical Immunology 55: 122 (1975).

Kriz, R.J.; Chmelik, F.; doPico, G. and Reed, C.E.: A short-term double-blind trial of aerosol triamcinolone acetonide in steroid-dependent patients with severe asthma. Chest 69: 455 (1976).

Kuzemko, J.A.; Bedford, S.; Wilson, L. and Walker, S.R.: A comparison of betamethasone valerate aerosol and sodium cromoglycate in children with reversible airways obstruction. Postgraduate Medical Journal 50 (Sept. Suppl.): 53 (1974).

Lal, S.; Malhotra, M.; Gribben, M.D. and Butler, A.G.: Beclomethasone dipropionate aerosol compared with dry powder in the treatment of asthma. Clinical Allergy 10: 259 (1980).

Maberly, D.J.; Gibson, G.J. and Butler, A.G.: Recovery of adrenal function after substitution of beclomethasone dipropionate for oral corticosteroids. British Medical Journal 1: 778 (1973).

Manicatide, M.A.; Nicholaescu, V.V.; Voiculescu, M.; Racoveanu, C.L. and Stroescu, V.: Long-term corticosteroid aerosol therapy in childhood asthma. Revue Roumaine de Medecine - Serie Medecine Interne 16: 417 (1978).

McAllen, M.K.; Kochanowski, S.J. and Shaw, K.M.: Steroid aerosols in asthma: An assessment of betamethasone valerate and a 12-month study of patients on maintenance. British Medical Journal 1: 171 (1974).

MacKay, J.B.: The impact of beclomethasone dipropionate aerosol on patients with reversible airways obstruction attending a chest clinic. Postgraduate Medical Journal 51 (Suppl. 4): 37 (1975).

Meltzer, E.O.; Kemp, J.P.; Orgel, H.A. and Izu, A.E.: Flunisolide aerosol for treatment of severe, chronic asthma in steroid-dependent children. Pediatrics 69: 340 (1982).

Milne, L.J.R. and Crompton, G.K.: Beclomethasone dipropionate and oropharyngeal candidiasis. British Medical Journal 3: 397 (1974).

Munch, E.P.; Taudorf, E.P. and Weeke, B.: Dose frequency in the treatment of asthmatics with inhaled topical steroid. European Journal of Respiratory Diseases 63: 143 (1982).

Ng, S.H.; Dash, C.H. and Savage, S.J.: Betamethasone valerate compared with sodium cromoglycate in asthmatic children. Postgraduate Medical Journal 53: 315 (1977).

Pines, A.: Beclomethasone dipropionate used as an aerosol in the treatment of asthma. The Practitioner 211: 86 (1973).

Pingleton, W.W.; Bone, R.C.; Kerby, G.R. and Ruth, W.E.: Oropharyngeal candidiasis in patients treated with triamcinolone acetonide aerosol. Journal of Allergy and Clinical Immunology 60: 254 (1977).

Sahay, J.N.; Chatterjee, S.S. and Stanbridge, T.N.: Inhaled corticosteroid aerosols and candidiasis. British Journal of Diseases of the Chest 73: 164 (1979).

Smith, A.P.; Booth, M. and Davey, A.J.: A controlled trial of beclomethasone dipropionate for asthma. British Journal of Diseases of the Chest 67: 208 (1973).

Smith, J. Morrison: A clinical trial of beclomethasone dipropionate aerosol in children and adolescents with asthma. Clinical Allergy 3: 249 (1973).

Smith, M.J. and Hodson, M.J.: High dose beclomethasone inhaler in the treatment of asthma. Lancet 2: 000 (1982).

Toogood, J.H.; Lefcoe, N.M.; Haines, D.S.M.; Jennings, B.; Errington, N.; Baksh, L. and Chuang, L.: A graded dose assessment of the efficacy of beclomethasone dipropionate aerosol for severe chronic asthma. Journal of Allergy and Clinical Immunology 59: 298 (1977a).

Toogood, J.H.; Baskerville, J.; Errington, N.; Jennings, B.; Chuang, L. and Lefcoe, N.: Determinants of the reponse to beclomethasone aerosol at various dosage levels: A multiple regression analysis to identify clinically useful predictors. Journal of Allergy and Clinical Immunology 60: 367 (1977b).

Toogood, J.H.; Jennings, B.; Greenway, R.W. and Chuang, L.: Candidiasis and dysphonia complicating beclomethasone treatment of asthma. Journal of Allergy and Clinical Immunology 65: 145 (1980).

Vandenberg, R.A.: Experience with beclomethasone dipropionate inhaler in the treatment of steroid-dependent chronic asthmatics. Current Therapeutics (Dec. Suppl.): 7 (1974).

Vandenberg, R.; Tovey, E.; Love, I.; Russell, P.; Tidmarsh, J.; Wilson, P. and Geddes, B.: A trial of a new inhalational steroid preparation in treatment of steroid-dependent chronic asthmatics. Medical Journal of Australia 1: 189 (1975).

Willey, R.F.; Milne, L.J.R.; Crompton, G.K. and Grant, I.W.B.: Beclomethasone dipropionate aerosol and oropharyngeal candidiasis. British Journal of Diseases of the Chest 70: 32 (1976).

Chapter XI

The Use of Inhaled Steroids in the Management of Asthma

G.K. Crompton

Since the introduction of inhaled corticosteroid therapy there has been a much welcomed improvement in the quality of life for many thousands of patients with asthma. Soon after it became obvious that systemic corticosteroid treatment improved the symptoms of chronic asthma they were widely used in severe cases. Unfortunately, the doses needed to maintain adequate control of symptoms were often relatively large (e.g. in excess of 10mg prednisolone daily) and side effects ensued. In spite of efforts to withdraw treatment, or to reduce the dose to an absolute minimum, few patients were able to lead anything approaching normal lives because of side effects, poorly controlled asthma or a combination of the two. Frequent contact with these disfigured, wheezy patients often made supervising an asthma clinic a distressing ordeal and one wondered whether the treatment was worse than the disease.

In the last decade there has been a remarkable change in the appearance, performance and attitude of patients in the asthma clinic, since few now require prednisolone in doses large enough to cause side effects. This is, in the main, due to substitution of inhaled corticosteroid therapy for oral treatment. There remain, of course, some patients whose disease is poorly controlled in spite of a combination of inhaled and oral steroids, but these unfortunate 'corticosteroid-resistant' (Carmichael et al., 1981) patients make up less than 5% of the hospital population of patients with severe asthma. Not only have corticosteroid side effects been dramatically reduced since the introduction of inhaled steroids, but control of asthma in the community overall has been improved since these drugs are now being prescribed, with benefit, for patients who would previously have been denied corticosteroid therapy because of the fear of side effects.

Selection of Patients for Inhaled Corticosteroid Therapy

Many patients with chronic asthma and rapidly recurring episodic symptoms benefit from treatment with inhaled corticosteroids. Those for whom this form of therapy is most likely to be of value are listed in table 11.1.

Chronic Asthma Requiring Long Term Treatment with Systemic Corticosteroids, ACTH or Tetracosactrin

It should be assumed that if a patient's asthmatic symptoms respond to systemic steroids, ACTH or tetracosactrin some therapeutic response can be expected from an inhaled corticosteroid. Hence the addition of an inhaled drug to the treatment regimen should be expected to achieve at least a reduction in dose of the non-inhaled corticosteroid preparation or ACTH/tetracosactrin. In some it will be possible to withdraw treatment with the oral or parenteral drug completely after regular treatment with an inhaled corticosteroid has been established. The early studies performed soon after the introduction of beclomethasone dipropionate, the first commercially available inhaled corticosteroid, showed that,

Table 11.1. Patients for whom inhaled corticosteroid therapy is most likely to be of value

- Patients with chronic asthma requiring long term treatment with a systemic corticosteroid preparation, ACTH or tetracosactrin
- Patients with chronic asthma whose symptoms have misled their medical advisers into making an incorrect diagnosis of chronic obstructive bronchitis
- Patients with chronic or rapidly recurring episodic asthmatic symptoms not adequately controlled by conventional treatment but not being treated with corticosteroids
- Patients with usually mild chronic symptoms at times of increased bronchial reactivity
- Patients with seasonal asthma to cover the period of symptoms e.g. pollen asthma

Other indications for considering inhaled corticosteroid therapy are:
- As an alternative treatment to oral methylxanthine drugs
- As an alternative treatment to sodium cromoglycate (cromolyn)

in a dose of 400 μg daily, it could be substituted for between 5 and 10mg of daily oral prednisolone (Brown et al., 1972; Clark, 1972; Maberly et al., 1973; Cameron et al., 1973; Gwynn and Smith, 1974). In other words, beclomethasone dipropionate in a dose of 400μg daily, usually 100μg 4 times daily, given to patients with chronic asthma requiring oral prednisolone for its control allowed a mean withdrawal of 5 to 10mg prednisolone. The amount of prednisolone withdrawn under cover of beclomethasone dipropionate varied from study to study and there was also considerable variation between patients in individual studies. However, the mean prednisolone-sparing effect of beclomethasone dipropionate can be estimated at about 7.5mg. That is to say that a group of patients treated with this inhaled steroid in a dose of 400μg daily, would have the same control of their asthmatic symptoms as they would have if they were being treated with a daily dose of 7.5mg prednisolone. As already stated, however, this prednisolone: beclomethasone equivalent of 7.5mg:400μg has been calculated by amalgamating the mean results of several studies, and the actual range of the prednisolone-sparing effect of beclomethasone dipropionate is quite large. Hence, the ability of an inhaled corticosteroid preparation to allow withdrawal of an oral or injected drug must be determined in each individual patient. However, it can be assumed that an inhaled corticosteroid will, in most cases, allow reduction in the dose of the systemic treatment. Therefore, inhaled therapy should be given to all patients requiring long term corticosteroids in an attempt to reduce the dose of, or withdraw completely, treatment from which side effects can be expected. Complete withdrawal of systemic treatment is, of course, the aim whenever this can be achieved without significantly decreasing the quality of life.

Chronic Asthma Incorrectly Diagnosed as Chronic Obstructive Bronchitis

The symptoms of chronic asthma are often mistaken for those of chronic bronchitis and, unfortunately, once an incorrect diagnostic label has been given to a patient it is rarely questioned, unless that patient changes his doctor, or is referred to hospital. The number of patients referred to hospital with a diagnosis of chronic bronchitis who are subsequently found, after investigation, to have chronic asthma suggests that there are many thousands of patients all over the world being inappropriately treated for chronic bronchitis, and suffering unnecessarily because of this incorrect diagnosis. Many could have their lives transformed if it were known that they had chronic asthma, since the treatment for asthma is generally effective, whereas treatment of chronic bronchitis is not, and drugs commonly prescribed for the bronchitics rarely help the patient with asthma. Antibiotic treatment, so often used in bronchitis, is of little or no value in the treatment of asthma.

Cough and Sputum in Asthma

The symptoms of chronic asthma which most often mislead doctors into making the assumption that the diagnosis must be chronic bronchitis are cough and sputum. It is not widely appreciated that cough can be the major, and sometimes the only, symptom of asthma. This is frequently the case in children and many doctors are now becoming aware of this, but cough as the presenting symptom of asthma in the adult still leads to confusion. Cough in asthma is, of course, predominantly nocturnal but also tends to be troublesome after exercise. Sputum production also appears to suggest a diagnosis of chronic bronchitis rather than asthma to many doctors. However, patients with chronic asthma often produce sputum, particularly when their disease is not adequately controlled. Sputum in chronic asthma is usually mucoid, except during acute episodes and very occasionally when it appears to be purulent because of the presence of large numbers of eosinophil leucocytes. Medical practitioners are deceived by the fact that purulent sputum is usually produced at some time during an acute episode of asthma. It is assumed that bronchial infection has been responsible for the exacerbation and hence, a diagnosis of bronchitis rather than asthma is made and treatment with an antibiotic prescribed. However, when one examines in detail the sequence of events in most exacerbations of asthma it soon becomes apparent that bronchoconstriction is the primary event and purulent sputum a secondary phenomenon. The trigger of the airways narrowing is often unknown but even when it is an infection it is almost always viral and not, therefore, associated with purulent sputum (p.61). The airways narrowing causes retention of bronchial mucus, which may then become infected, or infiltrated with eosinophils. When the acute episode subsides retained bronchial secretions are released and expectorated. Thus sputum is often purulent, but an assumption that bacterial infection has been responsible for the acute episode is wrong in most cases. Bronchoconstriction leads to sputum infection more often than bacterial infection leads to bronchoconstriction. There are, of course, a few patients in whom bacterial infection triggers episodes of asthma, but in these patients there is a clear temporal relationship of purulent sputum preceding symptoms of wheeze and breathlessness. In most cases wheeze and breathlessness come first and during the recovery phase purulent sputum is produced. Support for this hypothesis is the observation that when patients, previously thought to have chronic bronchitis, are given appropriate treatment for their chronic asthma, they very rarely cough up purulent sputum, even after insults such as virus infections which would previously have always been associated with an exacerbation of their asthma and the production of purulent sputum.

Table 11.2. Distinguishing features of chronic asthma and chronic bronchitis

Chronic asthma	Chronic bronchitis
Common in children	Unknown in children
Cough during the night	Cough on going to bed
Symptoms interrupt sleep	Good sleep
Worse at night	Worse in the mornings
Few smoke	Almost all smoke
Family history especially in the young	Family history uncommon
Exercise brings on wheeze	Exercise causes breathlessness
Cough and sputum in some	Cough and sputum in all
Wheeze in all	Wheeze in many
Breathlessness	Breathlessness
Most respond to corticosteroids	Few respond to corticosteroids
Majority have good bronchodilator reversibility	Minority have good bronchodilator reversibility

Smoking and Sleep in Asthma

There are some helpful generalisations about the symptoms of chronic asthma and chronic bronchitis which can be of diagnostic help (table 11.2). For instance, asthmatic patients almost always have symptoms in the middle of the night which disturb sleep, whereas the patient with chronic bronchitis usually has a good night's sleep but is distressed by symptoms on waking in the morning at a normal time. Another helpful pointer is that asthmatic patients are often upset by cigarette smoke and, therefore, do not smoke or try to stop smoking. Sometimes they even go to great lengths to avoid secondary smoking, which can lead to social and domestic friction (p.67). This is in complete contrast to the patient with chronic bronchitis whose disease has, more often than not, been caused by smoking, and who can rarely give up the habit, often because he believes that the first smoke in the morning is good for him since it helps to clear his bronchi. Hence, beware of the 'bronchitic' patient who has never smoked since it is possible that he has asthma, and seek out the non-smoking 'bronchitic' patient with predominantly nocturnal symptoms because it is almost certain that he has asthma.

The Corticosteroid Assessment

Formal demonstration that a wheezy patient's airflow obstruction objectively improves during treatment with a corticosteroid, usually oral prednisolone, is the only reliable method by which patients with steroid-responsive airflow obstruction can be distinguished from those with non-responsive disease. Patients with steroid-responsive airways disease can, for clinical and therapeutic purposes, be regarded as asthmatic, and although it cannot necessarily be assumed that all steroid non-responders have chronic bronchitis, rational therapeutic decisions concerning corticosteroid therapy can only be made after some form of objective assessment of corticosteroid response has been made. Corticosteroid 'trials' are discussed in Chapter VII (p.117). By extending the investigation as described here an early decision can be made on the most appropriate type of steroid maintenance (inhaled or inhaled plus oral) for those who respond.

A decision to treat patients with long term corticosteroids should, whenever possible, be taken only after objective evidence of response has been demonstrated. This was, of course, mandatory before the advent of inhaled corticosteroids because long term treatment with all available systemic drugs carried the risk of many serious side effects. Even though inhaled corticosteroids are infinitely safer, it is still desirable for objective improvement to be demonstrated before long term therapy is started. In those patients whose symptoms are not adequately controlled by treatment with bronchodilators and an inhaled corticosteroid, demonstration that there is response to prednisolone should always precede a decision to start long term treatment with this drug (see Chapter VII, p.67).

Figure 11.1 shows graphically an approach to objective assessment which has been used for many years and has proved to be of great value. This kind of assessment can be performed on inpatients or by outpatients, but of course, it is much more convenient for outpatients to record peak expiratory flow (PEF) with a portable meter or gauge. Daily measurements of ventilatory function [forced expiratory volume in one second (FEV_1) or PEF] are made preferably at the same time(s) of each day. In patients admitted to hospital it is useful to give a few days treatment with placebo prednisolone initially, and during this time bronchodilator reversibility tests can be performed. It is often of value to assess the bronchodilator response to a large dose of salbutamol or terbutaline (2.5–5.0mg) delivered by nebuliser or intermittent positive pressure breathing (IPPB), and to compare this response with that achieved by a smaller dose of the same drug from a conventional

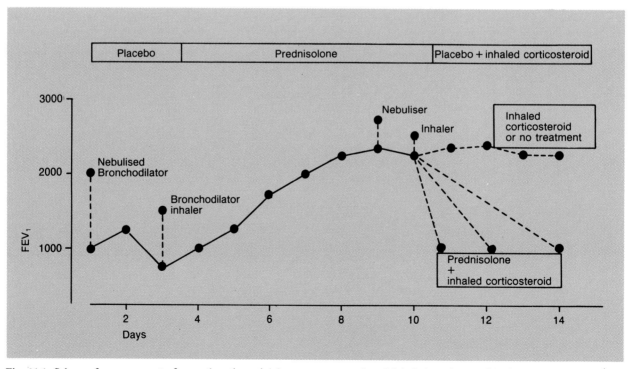

Fig. 11.1. Schema for assessment of an asthmatic patient's response to oral and inhaled corticosteroids. See text for explanation. (Adapted from Crompton, G.K. Diagnosis and Management of Respiratory Diseases, Blackwell Scientific Publications, Oxford 1980.)

pressurised inhaler. The larger doses of salbutamol and terbutaline, used in nebuliser or IPPB reversibility tests, can achieve a greater degree of bronchodilatation than the conventional inhaler (Choo-Kang and Grant, 1975). Since it is always helpful to know the maximum degree of improvement a patient is capable of, a large dose bronchodilator reversibility test should be chosen if only one test is performed. There may, however, be little or no broncho-dilator reversibility, but a subsequent response to prednisolone, and thereafter further improvement when the bronchodilator reversibility test is repeated. In most cases, however, there is bronchodilator reversibility, and this often gives the maximum ventilatory function test value, which is useful for predictive purposes. The therapeutic aim in all patients should be to maintain ventilatory function at a level as close as possible to the maximum response as demonstrated by the bronchodilator reversibility test. If during the period of placebo prednisolone treatment there is spontaneous improvement in ventilatory function, active treatment should not be started unless there is a subsequent plateau of recordings which are still considerably below the patient's predicted normal value. Spontaneous improvement during placebo treatment is not often observed, and when it is it usually reflects the 'therapeutic' effect of removing the patient from the home environment by admission to hospital. There is no need to include the placebo period in outpatient assessments. Active prednisolone tablets are given in a dose of 20 to 40mg daily for 7 to 10 days.

Patients with corticosteroid responsive disease record improvement within a few days and usually achieve a maximum within 7 days. However, whenever there is doubt about response, prednisolone in a dose of 40mg daily should be given for 10 days. When FEV_1 or PEF improvement has reached a plateau, or after treatment has been given for 10 days, active prednisolone is replaced by placebo tablets and at the same time an inhaled corticosteroid drug is started. Bronchodilator reversibility tests can be repeated at this stage to give an indication of the maximum possible FEV_1 or PEF for an individual patient. Maintenance of improved ventilatory function indicates that an inhaled corticosteroid drug should control symptoms, whereas relapse shows that a combination of oral prednisolone and an inhaled corticosteroid is necessary to maintain control of the disease. An improvement in FEV_1 or PEF of 25% or more is usually accepted as a positive response, indicating that the patient should be treated as an asthmatic. In most patients with chronic bronchitis and in the few patients with corticosteroid-resistant asthma, there is usually little or no improvement in FEV_1 or PEF during the period of treatment with prednisolone.

Chronic or Rapidly Recurring Episodic Symptoms Not Controlled by Conventional Non-steroidal Treatments

Over a decade of clinical experience allows us to assume, with a considerable degree of confidence, that inhaled corticosteroid therapy is safe; there is no question about its efficacy. We can, therefore, consider prescribing inhaled beclomethasone dipropionate or one of the similar inhaled corticosteroid preparations, for patients whose symptoms are not being adequately controlled by conventional non-corticosteroid drugs such as selective β_2-sympathomimetics, methylxanthines and sodium cromoglycate. There is little doubt that the therapeutic decision threshold for the prescription of an inhaled corticosteroid can be lowered to allow better control of asthma in patients in whom symptoms are causing inconvenience, but who cannot be classified as having severe chronic asthma. The writer would accept any of the following as rational indications for inhaled corticosteroid therapy, provided important points such as the patient's ability to use an inhaler if on treatment with an inhaled bronchodilator preparation, and serum theophylline levels in the patient on a methylxanthine drug, had been checked:

1) Nocturnal asthmatic symptoms causing sleep disturbance on more than 1 or 2 nights per week
2) Frequent daily use of a bronchodilator inhaler
3) Troublesome exercise-induced asthma in spite of optimal treatment with sodium cromoglycate and β-agonists
4) Sub-optimal ventilatory function in a young patient, irrespective of symptoms.

Nocturnal Asthmatic Symptoms

Sleep interrupted by asthmatic symptoms on more than 1 or 2 nights per week is a reliable indication of poorly controlled disease. In some patients it is not possible to iron out the 'morning dip' phenomenon completely but in all patients with regular nocturnal asthma an attempt to provide them with a full night's sleep should be made by giving an inhaled corticosteroid. A large number of patients have had nocturnal asthmatic exacerbations for so long that they regard them as their norm and will not spontaneously complain of sleep disturbance. Specific questioning about sleep and nocturnal symptoms should, therefore, be part of the routine clinical assessment of every asthmatic patient.

Frequent Daily Bronchodilator Use

Frequent use of a bronchodilator inhaler is a good indicator of poor asthma control. It is often thought that some patients use inhalers frequently out of habit, or because of dependence on the device or the drug, but this is very rarely the case. However, frequent use may be a consequence of poor inhaler technique. Regular excessive use of a bronchodilator inhaler should always be assumed to be a reflection of poor inhalation technique or inadequately controlled asthma. When technique is not at fault an inhaled corticosteroid should be tried in this large group of patients.

Troublesome Exercise-induced Asthma

Exercise-induced asthma is an extremely common and frequently overlooked problem. This is especially so in children and young adults because they indulge in vigorous prolonged exercise more often than older patients. Unfortunately, patients often consider that becoming wheezy after exercise is their norm and avoid sports etc. or, although taking part, are considered to be unfit or unwilling by their sports teachers and colleagues. Specific questioning about exercise-induced symptoms should be a routine with all patients, and exercise or hyperventilation tests (Tweeddale et al., 1981) should be used more often in the assessment of new patients. Much can be done to improve the lives of patients with exercise-induced symptoms, but only when these problems have been recognised. For instance, a bronchodilator inhaler can be used before exercise and many patients get some degree of protection against post-exercise bronchoconstriction by pre-treatment with sodium cromoglycate. However, whenever bronchodilators, including the methylxanthines, and cromoglycate are not effective inhaled corticosteroid should be tried as better overall control of asthma may lead to an improvement in exercise-induced attacks.

Sub-optimal Ventilatory Function in the Young

Patients with chronic asthma, like those with any chronic disease, learn to live with symptoms which become 'normal' for them. They tend to seek medical advice only during exacerbations and the diagnosis of chronic asthma may be long delayed. These patients often deny symptoms between exacerbations, even though tests of ventilatory function clearly demonstrate airflow obstruction. Attempts should be made to detect these patients as early as possible as some develop fixed, or irreversible, airways obstruction, which could perhaps have been prevented by aggressive treatment at an earlier stage. Early diagnosis is dependent upon much more widespread screening of ventilatory function by general practitioners and hospital doctors. A routine medical examination should be considered to be incomplete without a measurement of PEF or FEV_1, just as it would if blood pressure were not recorded.

Patients with sub-optimal ventilatory function should be considered for treatment with an inhaled corticosteroid in an attempt to improve their quality of life, and also to try to prevent gradual deterioration of symptoms and the development of fixed airflow obstruction. These patients should, of course, be given a corticosteroid assessment (p.169) but even if they do not improve their ventilatory function by 25% or more they should still be considered candidates for inhaled therapy.

Usually Mild Chronic Symptoms at Times of Increased Bronchial Reactivity

There are many patients who normally have mild symptoms, but at times, such as after viral infections, and on other occasions perhaps related to exposure to allergens, have much more troublesome symptoms. Even so their asthma is rarely bad enough to be considered for short course prednisolone treatment, and either no extra treatment is given or an antibiotic is prescribed, even though there is rarely any evidence of bronchial infection. These patients, during times of increased symptoms, can benefit from inhaled corticosteroid treatment for short periods of 3 to 4 weeks. Without this form of treatment their symptoms tend to linger for many weeks. They do not, however, need long term treatment with an inhaled corticosteroid.

Seasonal Asthma

There is a small group of patients who develop symptoms only in response to a specific allergen. In some instances it is possible for contact with the offending allergen to be avoided, such as with animal hypersensitivity, although this advice is often taken with very great reluctance. In others, however, it is impossible to avoid allergen contact, e.g. grass pollen asthma. Unfortunately, hyposensitisation is rarely effective in improving the asthma, although associated symptoms of allergic rhinitis (hay fever) may be helped. An inhaled corticosteroid, started a couple of weeks before the pollen season and continued until allergen challenge has subsided, can greatly benefit these patients. Inhalation of a corticosteroid will not, of course, control nasal and conjunctival symptoms, which often require additional topical treatment.

Inhaled Steroids as an Alternative to Methylxanthines

The development of slow release preparations has undoubtedly given new life to these old drugs, which in Britain had almost been discarded because of side effects (Chapter VI, p. 91-95). To produce a worthwhile therapeutic effect, a serum theophylline level of between 5 to 15 μg/ml has to be achieved; unfortunately, methylxanthines have a low therapeutic index and drug toxicity can be a problem with serum levels of over 20 μg/ml (fig. 11.2). Sustained release methylxanthine preparations have revitalised therapy with these drugs; therapeutic efficacy has been improved and drug toxicity decreased. Although they can be used effectively in the treatment of mild to moderate asthma, metabolism of the methylxanthines can be influenced by many factors and in all patients blood sampling is necessary, initially to establish the correct dose, and regularly thereafter to ensure that serum levels remain within the therapeutic range.

There is an inexplicable tendency for paediatricians to favour the use of methylxanthines, but many clinicians now accept that an inhaled corticosteroid, perhaps in low dosage, is preferable because repeated blood tests are not necessary and unpleasant side effects are avoided.

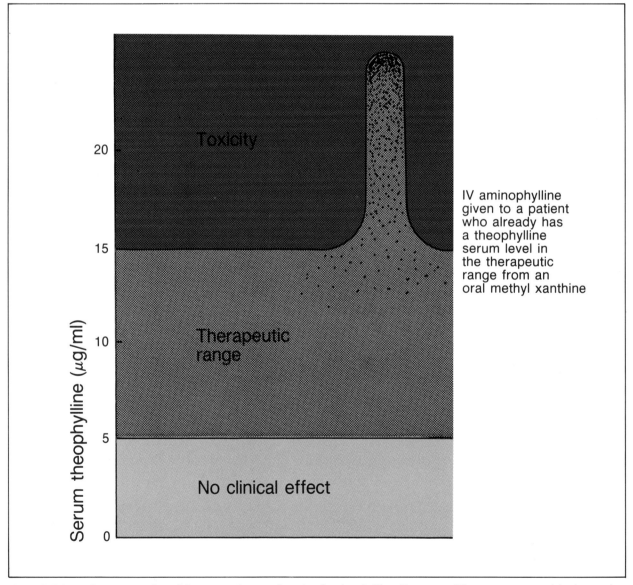

IV aminophylline given to a patient who already has a theophylline serum level in the therapeutic range from an oral methyl xanthine

Fig. 11.2. Schematic representation of the narrow therapeutic ratio of aminophylline. Emergency IV use can cause toxicity in a patient not known to be already on maintenance treatment.

Inhaled Steroids as an Alternative to Sodium Cromoglycate

Sodium cromoglycate has gained the reputation of being most effective in young atopic asthmatics, although there is evidence that it is effective in older patients, and also in non-atopic individuals (Brompton Hospital/MRC Collaborative Trial, 1972). However, many doctors confine their prescribing of cromoglycate to atopic children or teenagers, and are prepared to change treatment to an inhaled corticosteroid at an early stage if there is a less than good response. A combination of sodium cromoglycate and an inhaled corticosteroid has not been shown to offer any advantage.

Delivery Systems for Inhaled Corticosteroid Therapy

The Pressurised Metered Dose Aerosol

This is the most commonly used delivery device. It is essential to ensure that the patient is capable of using an aerosol inhaler properly (see Appendix 1). Initially, corticosteroid aerosols were designed to release a relatively small dose per actuation suitable for 4 times daily treatment. Because of the trend towards twice-daily regimens and the tendency to use higher doses than originally recommended, pressurised aerosols with relatively large doses per valve actuation (e.g. beclomethasone dipropionate 250µg) are now available.

Dry-powder Inhalers

Beclomethasone dipropionate is available for inhalation from 'Rotacaps' using a dry-powder inhaler ('Becotide Rotahaler'[1]). This delivery system should be chosen for all patients not able to use a pressurised aerosol. The present dry-powder device is simple to operate but, used correctly (p.223), the delivery system is probably slightly less efficient than the pressurised aerosol and it is generally recommended that the dose of inhaled steroid given by dry-powder inhaler should be approximately twice that used with the pressurised aerosol.

Respirator Solution

Some young children unable to use the pressurised aerosol or the dry-powder delivery system benefit from inhaled corticosteroid administered via a nebuliser. This form of therapy has been used in a limited number of centres in the United Kingdom and will soon be available for more widespread use. Nebulised corticosteroids could be of value in the treatment of adults unable to use a more conventional and cheaper delivery system.

Future Developments

It is likely that other devices such as spacer attachments to the pressurised aerosol will be available for inhalation of corticosteroid aerosols in the near future (p.213).

Dosage

Conventional 'Safe' Dose

The concept of administering topically active corticosteroids by inhalation for asthma was the achievement of a therapeutic response with little or no risk of systemic side effects. Hence, when beclomethasone dipropionate was introduced the dose chosen was well below that which caused suppression of the hypothalamic-pituitary-adrenal (HPA) axis: 400µg daily in 4 divided doses of 100µg. This was chosen because it had been shown that daily doses of 1600µg or more had to be given to cause HPA suppression in a significant number of patients (Gaddie et al., 1973). However, in the early studies, HPA function was most often assessed by plasma cortisol levels, often in conjunction with short tetracosactrin tests. Using plasma cortisol estimations it was assumed that

---

1 'Becotide Rotahaler' Allen and Hanburys Limited

HPA function was not influenced by beclomethasone dipropionate in a daily dose of 400µg, and that with this dose there was a large margin of safety, since it was considerably below levels which produced plasma cortisol abnormalities. Subsequently, the use of more sensitive tests of HPA function indicated that an effect can be shown with doses of beclomethasone dipropionate which do not significantly affect plasma cortisol (p.123). However, proof that this steroid in a daily dose of 400µg has no clinically significant effect on HPA function is the observation that when patients with proven HPA suppression are weaned off prednisolone, under cover of beclomethasone dipropionate, normal HPA function returns (Clark, 1972; Maberly et al., 1973; Cameron et al., 1973) as assessed by plasma cortisol levels, short tetracosactrin and insulin stress tests. Hence, there can be no doubt that the 'safe' dose of beclomethasone dipropionate is free from clinically significant systemic absorption. The recommended 'safe' dose of betamethasone valerate is 800µg daily.

There is conflicting evidence concerning the benefits of increasing the dose of an inhaled corticosteroid above the 'safe' dose but there is no doubt that increasing the dose increases efficacy. However, in most patients there is no need to exceed the 'safe' dose and in some a smaller dose can be used while still maintaining good symptomatic control. The hospital population of asthmatic patients does, however, include those with the most severe disease who often cannot be controlled by conventional 'safe' doses. It is in this group that the decision about 'safe' versus 'high' dose therapy has to be made. In virtually all adult patients the 'safe' dose of beclomethasone dipropionate can be assumed to be at least twice the originally recommended dose i.e. 800µg daily. If the 'safe' dose of an inhaled drug does not control symptoms adequately there are two alternatives: to continue the 'safe' dose and to add oral prednisolone or to give 'high' doses of the inhaled corticosteroid.

'Safe' Dose Inhaled Corticosteroid plus Oral Prednisolone

Many clinicians prefer to keep within the 'safe' dose and if this is not effective to add oral prednisolone. The rationale behind this is the belief that, with this combination, the likelihood of development of corticosteroid side effects can be assessed, or predicted, with much more certainty than if high doses of the inhaled drug are used. It is assumed that the 'safe' dose of the inhaled drug will not lead to any side effects and, therefore, any which do occur will be attributable to the oral prednisolone; however, Wyatt et al. (1978) have recorded an additive effect on biochemical measures of hypothalamic-pituitary-adrenal function in children receiving both inhaled and oral corticosteroid, as might be expected. See also Appendix 2. Since there has been a considerable experience of long term prednisolone treatment of many diseases, including asthma, the likelihood of a particular dose of prednisolone giving rise to side effects can be predicted with a fair degree of accuracy. For instance long term treatment with prednisolone in a daily dose in excess of 10mg is likely to cause side effects in most patients, whereas doses of 7.5mg daily or less are comparatively safe.

Determining the Maintenance Dose of Prednisolone

In order to reduce the risk of side effects to a minimum the long term maintenance dose of prednisolone in patients needing this additional therapy must, of course, be the smallest effective dose. Finding this dose for individual patients is best achieved by initially gaining control of symptoms with a large dose of prednisolone (20-40mg daily) for 5 to 10 days, and then suddenly reducing the daily dose to 10mg. If good control of symptoms is maintained on prednisolone 10mg daily, plus the 'safe' dose of the inhaled corticosteroid, prednisolone is then slowly reduced. Decreasing the daily dose by 1mg stages each month has been found to be a suitable rate of reduction in most patients. When asthmatic symptoms break through, control is again achieved with a large dose of prednisolone, and the dose is then reduced to the determined maintenance dose which is 1 or 2mg above that at which breakthrough occurred. By titration of dose to symptoms it is usually possible to discover a maintenance dose for each patient with a reasonable degree of accuracy. There will, of course, be times when this dose is not sufficient and breakthrough episodes of asthma have to be treated with short 'booster' courses of prednisolone for 5 to 10 days. As a general rule the 'booster' dose should be at least 4 times the maintenance dose, e.g. maintenance dose of 10mg equals 'booster' dose of 40mg. If, on the other hand, there are prolonged periods of weeks or months during which control of symptoms is excellent an attempt to reduce the maintenance dose should be made.

'High' Dose Inhaled Corticosteroid Therapy

It can be argued that if asthmatic symptoms are not controlled by 'safe' doses of an inhaled corticosteroid that it is rational to increase the dose in order to achieve control (Toogood et al., 1977). This is certainly less confusing to the patient than adding oral prednisolone, and drug compliance may, therefore, be improved. The fact that there will be sufficient systemic absorption to lead to side effects if treatment is prolonged is accepted. At present few clinicians use doses of beclomethasone dipropionate in excess of 1600µg daily, but there has been a gradual tendency over the last few years to increase the dose rather than add oral prednisolone. A major objection to this practice is the fear that inhaled corticosteroids, such as beclomethasone dipropionate, betamethasone valerate and budesonide, may have worse systemic side effects than prednisolone. It cannot be assumed that all corticosteroids have the same side effects: for instance, in the early days of oral therapy some were found to be associated with a higher incidence of myopathy than is prednisolone (or prednisone). Another objection to 'high' dose inhaled therapy is the possibility that increasing the dose still further may encourage patients and medical practitioners to assume this to be a rational treatment of an episode of acute severe asthma – which is certainly not the case. Even when this 'high' dose inhaled therapy is used, acute severe episodes of asthma must be treated with systemic corticosteroids and not by a further increase in the dose of the inhaled drug.

The case for 'high' dose inhaled therapy appears to be reasonably sound, provided that good control of symptoms is achieved and Smith and Hodson (1982) have described its use in a large series of patients in whom increasing the inhaled dose enabled some to stop their oral steroids altogether and many more to reduce the dose needed when only conventional doses were given by inhalation.

'Steroid Cards' for Patients

Whenever a decision is made to treat a patient with an inhaled corticosteroid in a dose which could give rise to HPA suppression, it should be routine for that patient to be warned of this danger and he should be asked to carry a 'steroid card'. There should be no difference in this respect between the management of a patient on 'high' dose inhaled corticosteroids and one taking long term oral prednisolone. Unfortunately, not all patients on regular prednisolone are given steroid cards and there is less chance of one being issued to the patient who gradually drifts from 'safe' to 'high' dose inhaled treatment. This is a dangerous omission since surgeons and anaesthetists, and indeed most medical and dental practitioners, do not associate inhaled corticosteroid with the possibility of HPA suppression.

Dose Frequency

Originally it was recommended that inhaled corticosteroids be taken in 4 divided doses daily, but it soon became apparent to many clinicians that treatment failures were often occurring because patients could not remember to use their inhalers so frequently. Keeping the total 24-hour dose approximately the same while reducing the frequency was tried. Thrice daily treatment was found to be more acceptable than the originally recommended 6-hourly schedule, particularly for children as this meant that they did not have to have treatment at school. Twice daily therapy then evolved as an even more convenient regimen, allowing use of the inhalation device just in the morning and at night, and making it unnecessary for patients to take the inhaler out of the house. It was also of help to clinicians in their vital educational role since the corticosteroid inhaler could now be distinguished from the bronchodilator device; one to be used only twice daily and left at home, the other to be carried and used as necessary. Thus, from the originally recommended 4 times daily dose schedule there evolved thrice and twice daily regimens in order to improve patient compliance. Long after clinicians had discovered for themselves that less frequent dose regimens were effective came confirmation of this fact from clinical trials (Willey et al., 1982; Munch et al., 1982).

It is obvious that if a drug is equally effective in a twice, thrice or 4 times daily schedule, that the twice daily regimen is likely to be the most convenient. Hence, it is likely that this will be adopted as routine for most patients in the future. In the past many asthmatics have been denied the full therapeutic properties of inhaled corticosteroid therapy, simply because they have found it difficult to comply with a 4 times daily regimen.

Although it is likely that twice daily treatment will be used for the majority of patients when 'safe' dose therapy is prescribed, it would probably be wise, in poorly controlled patients, to try the effect of more frequent doses, before resorting to 'high' dose twice daily therapy or adding oral prednisolone. At present there is only evidence in patients with mild to moderate chronic asthma to support the claim that twice daily treatment is as effective as the same total daily dose taken in 4 divided doses. It is possible that in patients with severe chronic asthma twice daily therapy might be less effective than more frequent inhalations. Indeed it is possible that in these patients 4-hour intervals between treatment might be better than the originally chosen 6-hourly gaps.

Substitution of Inhaled for Oral Corticosteroids

Transfer to Inhaled 'Safe' Dosage when HPA Suppression Unlikely

Patients who have had oral prednisolone treatment for only a few days' or weeks can be assumed to have an intact HPA axis, and a change to an inhaled drug can be made rapidly. It is often convenient to have a few days overlap of the two treatments during which time the patient's inhalation technique can be checked, and he can get used to the regular use of a new inhalation device. The oral preparation is then stopped abruptly or tailed off rapidly over a few days. After a short course of an oral corticosteroid and sudden withdrawal of treatment, any HPA suppression is so transient that gradual tailing off is not necessary (Webb and Clark, 1981). In the corticosteroid assessment already described (p.169) the dose of 20 or 40mg prednisolone given for 7 to 10 days is immediately replaced by placebo tablets, and an inhaled corticosteroid. Many thousands of patients have had this kind of assessment with no recognised problems associated with the sudden withdrawal of prednisolone.

Transfer to Inhaled 'Safe' Dosage when HPA Suppression Likely

All patients who have been treated with an oral corticosteroid for many months, and certainly if treatment has been given continuously for years, must be assumed to have complete HPA suppression. It would, therefore, be dangerous to withdraw oral therapy from these patients rapidly, because of the risk of adrenal insufficiency. Fortunately, there is rarely any need to transfer from oral to inhaled treatment quickly and, therefore, this can usually be done gradually. When gradual reductions in oral prednisolone are made, for example, at a rate of 1mg per month, normal HPA function returns without there being any clinical evidence of hypoadrenalism in all but a minute number of patients. However, during the final stages of prednisolone withdrawal, and for some time afterwards, all patients should be assumed to have a less than adequate adrenal response to stress and appropriate replacement therapy should be given to cover operations etc. Once prednisolone has been withdrawn for a few months, provided the dose of the inhaled corticosteroid is not associated with systemic absorption, virtually all patients can be assumed to have recovered normal HPA function. There is usually no need to check the integrity of the HPA axis, if a patient is well and has a normal blood pressure. If, however, there is any clinical suspicion of hypoadrenalism appropriate tests of adrenal function should be performed (see Appendix 2). It must be emphasised, however, that normal plasma cortisol values, and a normal response to tetracosactrin, do not mean that HPA function has completely returned to normal. This can only be assessed accurately by measuring the plasma cortisol response to stress (e.g. insulin stress test), but this is an unpleasant and potentially dangerous test which fortunately is rarely necessary.

So far it has been assumed that the dose of inhaled corticosteroid substituted for oral treatment has been one which in itself is not capable of producing HPA suppression – i.e. a 'safe' dose.

Transfer to Inhaled 'High' Dosage when HPA Suppression Unlikely

HPA suppression occurs rapidly during treatment with prednisolone in a dose of 20 to 40mg daily, the dose usually needed to treat an acute episode of asthma or to gain control of chronic symptoms before maintaining control with an inhaled preparation. However, the effects on the HPA axis of a short course of prednisolone are transient and full recovery can be expected within a few days of treatment withdrawal (Webb and Clark, 1981). If, however, 'high' dose inhaled corticosteroid therapy (e.g. beclomethasone dipropionate 1600μg daily or more) is substituted for the oral drug it must be assumed that HPA suppression will persist as a result of absorption of the inhaled preparation, and appropriate safeguards taken. 'High' dose treatment could be used in this way for patients in whom substitution of low dose therapy has been shown to be incapable of maintaining control, in the hope that a higher dose will be effective and that gradual reductions in dose can be made in the future. However, unless it proves possible to reduce the dose of the inhaled drug to the 'low/safe' level, and to continue this for a prolonged period without any increases in dose (or supplemental oral corticosteroid therapy), it would be prudent to assume that the HPA axis is not functioning normally.

'High' dose inhalation therapy, following an initial short period of treatment with oral prednisolone, cannot be recommended unless it has been shown that 'low/safe' dose therapy does not control symptoms.

Transfer to Inhaled 'High' Dosage when HPA Suppression Likely

'High' dose inhalation therapy (e.g. beclomethasone dipropionate 1600μg daily or more) has been used in patients with severe chronic asthma in an attempt to withdraw oral prednisolone and to improve overall control of symptoms (Toogood et al., 1980a). It would seem logical to persist with high dose inhaled therapy if it allowed prednisolone to be withdrawn, or the dose to be substantially reduced. It could also be argued that this form of treatment should be continued, even if a significant reduction in prednisolone dosage could not be made, if control of asthmatic symptoms were substantially improved. However, there can be no justification for continuation of 'high' dose inhaled corticosteroids in patients who are no better, and who have not been able to reduce the dose of oral prednisolone. Some patients respond better to inhaled corticosteroid therapy than others and 'high' dose treatment is always worth trying in problem patients who have to take large doses of prednisolone.

Rapid Transfer to Inhaled 'Low/Safe' Dosage when HPA Suppression Likely

Occasionally, after many years of treatment with oral prednisolone, and resulting adrenal suppression, rapid withdrawal of the drug is desirable. For instance, this could be the case in patients who have developed side effects such as peptic ulceration or bone fractures due to osteoporosis. In these patients a 'low/safe' dose of the inhaled corticosteroid drug should be started and the dose of prednisolone quickly reduced to 5mg in a single dose in the morning and subsequently tailed off rapidly as soon as a normal morning plasma cortisol has been recorded. Blood for plasma cortisol estimation should be sampled before the morning prednisolone dose is taken. It can usually be assumed that completely normal HPA function will have returned after oral corticosteroid therapy has been discontinued for a few months. To confirm this, however, an insulin stress test would have to be performed.

Oral Corticosteroid Treatment Before Inhaled Therapy

There are a few patients who apparently respond to inhaled corticosteroids even though their asthma has not been controlled by quite large doses of prednisolone. However, most patients with asthma improve with both oral and inhaled therapies. In all patients with anything other than mild airflow obstruction it is important to give a course of oral prednisolone in an adequate dose, before inhalation treatment is started. This is to achieve maximum improvement with systemic treatment, since severe airflow obstruction itself can significantly decrease the effectiveness of inhaled therapy because it, and mucous plugging, prevent efficient distribution of any inhaled drug within the bronchi. In the treatment of moderate or severe asthma, therefore, there is more hope of success with inhaled corticosteroid therapy if a short course of prednisolone is given first. Similarly at times when symptoms are out of control in spite of inhaled therapy, it is necessary to achieve control again with short courses of oral prednisolone (see p.190). To maintain control it is also important that a bronchodilator inhaler is used appropriately (see p.189).

Other Problems Associated with Transfer to Inhaled Steroids

The great drawback of systemic corticosteroid therapy for asthma is that the drug, after being swallowed or injected, reaches all tissues of the body including the lungs although its therapeutic actions are only needed in the bronchi. The discovery that a corticosteroid with high topical, relative to systemic, activity could be used by inhalation in doses sufficient to exert the desired therapeutic effect in the lungs, yet small enough for that portion absorbed not to cause adrenal suppression and the side effects associated with it, was a major advance. However, when corticosteroids are withdrawn from body tissues as the systemic is replaced by inhaled therapy, symptoms which were previously controlled by the systemic treatment, by chance as it were, often recur. Eczema and allergic rhinitis are the most common conditions which flare-up after systemic therapy has been withdrawn. In the majority of cases it is known that these were a problem before systemic corticosteroid therapy was started and a warning can be given that there may be a recrudescence of symptoms which might require their own topical treatments. Warning patients to expect recurrence of eczema etc., and full explanation of the reason, is essential if they are to be expected to give full cooperation during the important conversion period from long term systemic to inhaled treatment. The nuisance of having to treat eczema and rhinitis/conjunctivitis with topical preparations is accepted by the informed patient who understands the risks of long term systemic corticosteroid treatment.

Occasionally mild depression and also joint pains can be experienced during and after withdrawal of systemic corticosteroid therapy. These symptoms are rarely anything other than a transient nuisance, but patients need explanation and reassurance.

Side Effects of Inhaled Corticosteroids

Systemic corticosteroid side effects do, of course, occur when large doses are inhaled for prolonged periods. However, the only recognised side effects of treatment with doses below those associated with systemic absorption are oropharyngeal candidiasis and huskiness of the voice.

Oral Candidiasis

With the conventional low doses of inhaled steroids (e.g. beclomethasone dipropionate 400 μg/24 hours) oropharyngeal candidiasis is uncommon and leads to clinical problems in only about 5% of patients (Milne and Crompton, 1974). When symptomatic thrush does occur it is usually easily dealt with by local treatment (e.g. amphotericin lozenges). In the few cases resistant to treatment, inhaled corticosteroid therapy can be withdrawn temporarily and a small dose of oral prednisolone substituted. It is usually possible to restart inhalation therapy after treatment of the oropharyngeal candidiasis. Fungal growth does not appear to occur below the larynx and in patients with allergic bronchopulmonary aspergillosis there is no evidence that inhaled corticosteroid therapy makes the condition worse (Research Committee of BTA, 1979).

A positive throat swab for Candida is often obtained from patients being treated with an inhaled corticosteroid, but this is usually of no importance (Milne and Crompton, 1974). Clinically relevant fungal overgrowth is somewhat more common with high dose treatment compared with conventional low dose therapy (Toogood et al., 1980b).

Hoarseness

Huskiness or hoarseness of the voice, without any evidence of oropharyngeal candidiasis, occurs in quite a large proportion of patients receiving long term inhaled corticosteroid therapy. The cause of this symptom is not understood, but it must be assumed to be a corticosteroid effect since it is not associated with excessive use of bronchodilator pressurised aerosols which, of course, employ the same propellant fluorocarbons. It has been suggested that the phenomenon results from a corticosteroid effect on the muscles of the larynx, but this is not proved; even if it were, a reassuring feature is that the symptoms do not appear to get worse with prolonged treatment. At the moment there is no known way of reversing or preventing voice symptoms, which are usually trivial, but patients should be warned that they may occur. Most patients are so impressed by the symptomatic relief of their asthma that they rarely bother to complain about minor voice symptoms occasioned by the treatment.

Table 11.3. Patients in whom continuous PEF monitoring should be considered

- Those with asthma severe enough to require treatment with a combination of an inhaled and an oral corticosteroid
- Those with asthma severe enough to require treatment with an inhaled corticosteroid in 'high' doses
- Those on 'low/safe' dose inhaled corticosteroid therapy, but who require frequent short courses of oral prednisolone for the treatment of acute episodes
- Those in whom the diagnosis of asthma is not in doubt, but in whom 'irreversible' airflow obstruction has developed
- Patients reluctant to accept that regular treatment is necessary for control of their asthmatic symptoms
- Any patient during periods of poor disease control
- During withdrawal of systemic corticosteroid therapy
- When an inhaled corticosteroid is given to a patient who has not had corticosteroid therapy previously, and in whom a formal corticosteroid assessment has not been performed

Monitoring Asthma Response and Symptom Control in Patients on Inhaled Corticosteroids

Ideally all patients being treated with an inhaled corticosteroid should have some form of continuous monitoring of disease control (table 11.3). This is particularly important, however, for those taking a combination of an inhaled and an oral corticosteroid, or an inhaled drug in a high dose. An intensive short corticosteroid assessment which uses objective measurements and is useful before starting corticosteroid therapy of any type has already been described (p.169). Following this assessment the patient can continue to record PEF twice daily to provide an objective assessment of long term control of airways obstruction. However, although this procedure can be extremely valuable, continuous objective monitoring of ventilatory function is not necessary in the majority of patients for whom an inhaled corticosteroid drug is prescribed.

Home Monitoring of Lung Function (PEF)

PEF Monitoring in Patients on Oral plus Inhaled Steroids

The fact that those with asthma severe enough to require treatment with both an inhaled and oral corticosteroid require this combination indicates that they are problem patients. They may have either severe chronic asthma, difficulty in using an inhaler properly or have other drug compliance difficulties, corticosteroid-resistant asthma, or been wrongly diagnosed as having chronic asthma. Inhaler technique can be checked easily and appropriate action taken if it is found to be deficient (Appendix 1). Compliance with oral drug regimens can be improved in most cases by sympathetic education or involving a relative or friend in a supervisory role.

Objective monitoring of PEF can be used to confirm that a combination of both treatments is necessary by revealing major fluctuations of airflow obstruction. Such measurements also provide objective confirmation that a temporary increase in the dose of prednisolone should be made to control an exacerbation. Retrospective assessment of PEF recordings may lead the clinician to suspect a diagnosis of chronic bronchitis rather than chronic asthma if there has been little or no variation in function for a considerable time. This can be very useful when a patient is not well known to the clinician and it is suspected that corticosteroids may have been started in the past without proper assessment. Under these circumstances a formal corticosteroid assessment with prednisolone in a dose of 40mg daily for at least 10 days, together with a bronchodilator reversibility test, should be performed. If a diagnosis of chronic bronchitis still seems likely attempts to withdraw oral treatment should be made immediately.

PEF Monitoring in Patients on 'High' Dose Inhalations

PEF monitoring can be helpful in patients with asthma severe enough to require treatment with an inhaled steroid in 'high' dose for all the reasons stated above. Furthermore, it is possible that acute severe episodes might be more troublesome in these patients (see p.177), and objective evidence of deterioration could be even more important, alerting the patient to the need to start treatment with prednisolone, or seek medical advice. Gradual deterioration of ventilatory function often occurs before a severe episode of asthma is recognised. Regular monitoring of PEF can be of tremendous value in allowing appropriate treatment of an exacerbation of asthma to be started early.

PEF Monitoring in Patients on 'Low/Safe' Dose Inhalations Needing Oral Courses for Acute Episodes

PEF monitoring is important in those on 'low/safe' dose inhaled corticosteroid therapy, but who require frequent short courses of oral prednisolone for the treatment of acute episodes. It records function when courses of prednisolone are necessary and confirms that the drug is not being taken unnecessarily. If regular PEF measurements confirm poor control of asthma a decision to add in regular oral prednisolone or to start 'high' dose inhalation therapy may be made. Such decisions are always easier when supported by objective evidence.

PEF Monitoring When Irreversibility is Present

There are some patients with genuine chronic asthma in whom gradual deterioration of ventilatory function occurs, resulting eventually in predominantly irreversible airflow obstruction. It is not known whether this deterioration can be prevented by early recognition and more intensive treatment, but this is certainly possible. It would, therefore, be appropriate to monitor regularly any patient found to be in this category. Home monitoring of PEF should, of course, be combined with regular assessments by a physician interested in asthma, so that bronchodilator reversibility tests and perhaps more sophisticated pulmonary function studies, can be performed at intervals. These patients may not have frequent episodes of acute severe asthma requiring medical intervention, and hence their condition may not be as obvious as that of those with repeated life threatening attacks of asthma. Careful monitoring and treatment of these patients at any early stage would be ideal.

PEF Monitoring for Patient Education

A proportion of patients with asthma refuse to accept they have a disease which requires regular treatment and often demand an instant cure. For these patients to see the results of PEF recordings is often a useful way of persuading them that they need to take treatment as recommended. Once the 'psychological barrier' has been overcome regular monitoring of PEF is rarely necessary.

PEF Monitoring at Times of Poor Symptom Control

Chronic asthma is a completely unpredictable disease and any patient may enter a phase during which control of symptoms is poor. If this occurs regular PEF monitoring often helps by providing objective confirmation of deterioration, which in turn allows rational therapeutic changes to be made.

PEF Monitoring During Systemic Steroid Withdrawal

During withdrawal of systemic corticosteroid therapy successful transfer from oral to inhaled corticosteroid therapy in doses not associated with systemic side effects must be the aim in all patients. This will not be possible in all, but objective assessment of ventilatory function during the time reductions are being made in the dose of the systemic preparation, can be of great value. Satisfactory PEF recordings can allow the withdrawal process to continue, and often the onset of inadequate control can be picked up earlier by objective measurements than by relying on symptoms. The early detection of breakthrough asthma can avert a potentially dangerous episode of acute severe disease.

PEF Monitoring when the Response to Steroids is Unknown

If a formal assessment has not been used to confirm corticosteroid responsiveness, it is always desirable to have objective confirmation of improvement on inhaled treatment. Improvement of ventilatory function is almost always accompanied by symptomatic change, but when there has been a less than complete subjective response, knowledge of the degree of objective improvement is always of value in deciding the next therapeutic move: discontinuation of corticosteroid treatment, 'high' dose inhaled treatment, assessment of response to a short course of oral prednisolone etc.

Subjective Monitoring of Response and Control

Most patients immediately appreciate response to treatment because of symptomatic relief and, therefore, the presence or absence of symptoms can be used to monitor treatment. Bronchodilator inhaler use and control of symptoms are obviously intimately related. Careful education of the patient about the significance of symptoms is vital, as is explanation of the actions and uses of all drugs being used. Recurrence of nocturnal symptoms is frequently an early sign that control of asthma is being lost.

A method of subjective assessment of symptoms can be included in a diary card together with a record of PEF measurements and bronchodilator inhaler use. If a subjective assessment of symptoms is made as well as a record of PEF, it is important that the symptom assessment is made before the measurement of lung function. This is to prevent the subjective symptom assessment being influenced by the PEF value. For instance, if a patient has been feeling well but sees a PEF reading which is lower than the expected this might influence his subjective assessment of symptoms. Conversely, a high PEF reading might persuade him to upgrade his symptom assessment without justification. All symptoms (cough, sputum, wheeze, breathlessness and chest tightness) can be assessed individually, but it is usually better to have one simple general assessment of asthmatic symptoms. The answer to a simple question such as: 'How has your asthma been in the last 12 (or 24) hours?' can be answered by using a simple symptom score or analogue scale (fig. 11.3).

Monitoring of Response and Control at the Clinic or Surgery

Most patients with chronic asthma are treated by general practitioners, but some patients with severe disease will attend hospital asthma clinics. Whether patients visit their general practitioners or the asthma clinic it is desirable that the following checks and investigations are made routinely:
1) Check of inhaler technique
2) Pulmonary function tests
3) Clinical assessment
4) Other investigations
5) Education check

Check of Inhaler Technique (see also Appendix 1)

This is obviously essential since the success of inhaled corticosteroid treatment is dependent upon patients being able to use their inhalers properly. Since patients often develop faulty inhalation techniques with time (Paterson and Crompton, 1976) it is important that regular checks are made. These can be done by asking the patient to demonstrate inhaler use with a placebo device and it is convenient to do this at the same time their ventilatory function is recorded. Indeed, it is more important for inhaler technique to be checked than it is to have an isolated measurement of ventilatory function.

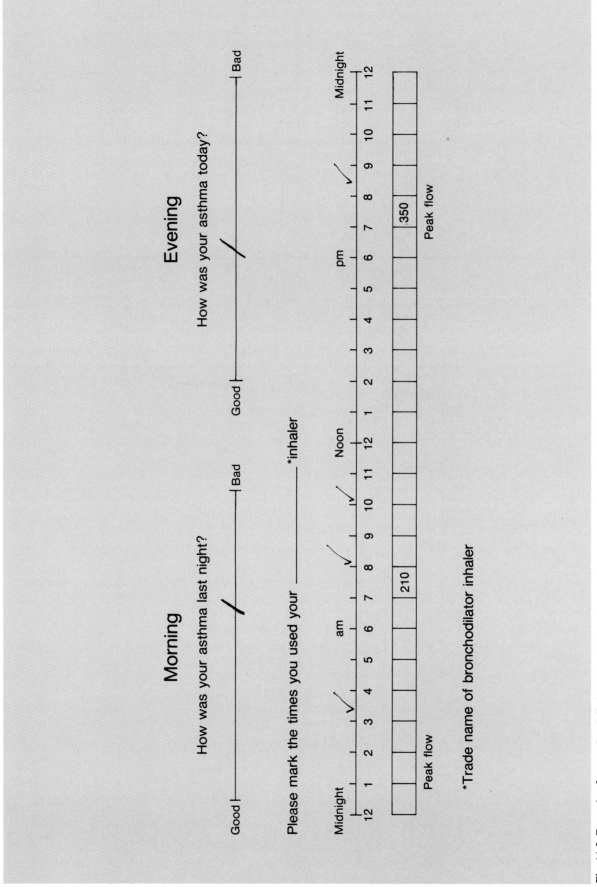

Fig. 11.3. Example of a completed diary card page showing symptom assessment preceding PEF recording. This type of record clearly shows the bronchodilator inhaler use in relation to PEF recordings. A separate sheet of instructions should be in front of each book of diary cards.

Pulmonary Function Tests
(see also Chapter III)

It is usual for PEF and/or FEV_1 and vital capacity (VC) to be measured at each visit to a hospital asthma clinic, but single recordings of these measurements, every few weeks or months, are of little value except in showing trends. For example, normal ventilatory function is often present during the day, especially in the afternoon, in patients who are wheezy and distressed at night. Conversely, a poor result may be a consequence of a recent cold, or simply hurrying to the clinic, in a patient whose long term overall control has been good.

Clinical Assessment

The most important part of clinical assessment is the history and specific questioning about nocturnal and exercise-induced symptoms. A full check on drug compliance should also be made at every visit, since even the most intelligent patients often take treatment incorrectly. A record of all extra drugs taken since the last visit should be made, with particular reference to prednisolone courses or 'booster' courses. However, enquiry about all treatments should be made since it is not uncommon for inappropriate concomitant therapy such as a β-adrenoceptor blocking drug, prescribed for angina or hypertension, to be responsible for a worsening of the control of asthmatic symptoms (p.65).

Auscultation of the chest rarely gives useful information, but some patients feel reassured by the auscultatory ritual.

Other Investigations

Urinalysis should be routine in all patients, but is of particular importance in those taking systemic corticosteroids or 'high' dose inhaled therapy, to detect glycosuria, which may be a manifestation of corticosteroid-induced diabetes mellitus. Also, a chest x-ray should be performed annually in these patients, because of the risk of tuberculosis, although such frequent x-ray examination is probably not necessary in patients on 'low/safe' dose inhaled corticosteroids. Patients with allergic bronchopulmonary aspergillosis may, of course, need x-rays more frequently (Research Committee of BTA, 1979). A chest radiograph is essential in all patients attending the clinic during an acute severe episode to exclude pneumothorax.

Throat swabs should be taken from patients with symptoms suggesting oropharyngeal candidiasis (p.181) and from those in whom there is clinical evidence of this. Swabs should not be taken routinely from asymptomatic patients, however, since many without clinical thrush and not requiring treatment will have a positive culture for *Candida albicans* (Milne and Crompton, 1974).

Education Check

An integral part of every visit to a hospital asthma clinic, or general practitioner's surgery, must be continuing education about asthma and its treatment, and a check that the patient has remembered what has been discussed previously. The minimum number of facts every patient should know about the disease and its management are:

- Correct use of the inhaler
- The difference between the bronchodilator and the corticosteroid inhaler, and a full understanding of how often each has to be used
- Diminished or lack of response to a bronchodilator inhaler means severe asthma which needs extra treatment

Self-monitoring and
Treatment

The patient who has been educated about his disease and its management can be allowed to make therapeutic decisions himself. In fact, the vast majority of patients can be taught when to take short courses of prednisolone, or to boost their dose if they are already on long term treatment, without seeking medical advice unless they are very sick. It is important for them to know that medical advice, or self-referral to hospital, is available should they need help (Crompton et al., 1979). Sympathetic education of the patient about his disease and its management should be undertaken as carefully with the asthmatic patient as it is with the diabetic. Asthma is a disease which fluctuates in severity rapidly, within short periods of time, therefore, fixed daily doses of all drugs are not appropriate. Patients should be taught how to adjust the dose of sympathomimetic bronchodilators and systemic corticosteroid therapy in response to symptoms and objective measurements of ventilatory function. The dose of an inhaled corticosteroid should, however, be constant in most patients.

Management of the
Severe Attack

Asthma is a totally unpredictable disease and all patients must be assumed to be at risk of developing a severe potentially fatal episode. They should be aware that a poor response to their bronchodilator inhaler is a reliable sign that a severe episode has developed, and that they then require systemic corticosteroids or an increase in dose immediately. Patients can be allowed to treat themselves with short courses of prednisolone, or make temporary increases in dose if they are on long term treatment, without necessarily seeking medical advice unless they are extremely ill. Other patients, perhaps because their disease pattern is one of rapid onset of severe episodes, or because they are less reliable for some reason, should be encouraged to seek medical advice as soon as possible after the onset of an acute episode. Those with a history of severe episodes of rapid onset should, of course, have their own supply of prednisolone to take in an initial loading dose of at least 20mg and at the same time calling for medical attention. Ideally, all patients with severe and poorly controlled symptoms, should have open access to local hospital facilities.

Are Patients on Inhaled
Corticosteroids More Likely
to Develop Acute Severe
Episodes?

In the early days of inhaled corticosteroid treatment one slight worry was the possibility that acute respiratory infections might be more common, and that these might trigger severe episodes of asthma. There is no evidence that this happens or that bronchial infections are more severe when they do occur in patients on inhaled corticosteroids (Toogood et al., 1980a). Theoretically, patients whose asthma is controlled by corticosteroids by inhalation are more at risk of developing a severe acute episode than patients being treated with systemic corticosteroids. The number of attacks should not be increased, but the severity of each could be worse in the patient on inhaled therapy. During an exacerbation bronchoconstriction may be responsible for the inhaled drug being less efficiently distributed in the bronchi, and if this is the case, it means that treatment in effect is being reduced during a stage of deterioration which could, therefore, make the attack worse. This does not apply to systemic corticosteroid therapy unless the patient deliberately reduces the dose. Therefore, patients on inhaled corticosteroid treatment and perhaps especially those who have been converted from systemic therapy, should have their own supplies of prednisolone to take immediately a break-through episode of asthma has been recognised, or they should be told to seek medical advice early.

Drug Treatment of a Severe Episode (see also Chapter VII)

Inhaled corticosteroids have no place whatsoever in the treatment of severe asthma, although some patients may, with benefit, temporarily increase their dose to combat a mild exacerbation. Inhaled corticosteroids should be replaced by systemic treatment in all severely ill patients: oral prednisolone in an initial loading dose of 20 to 40mg or an increase in dose by at least a factor of 4 for patients on long term treatment, together with intravenous hydrocortisone in an initial dose of at least 200mg. Ill patients should be admitted to hospital quickly and high concentration oxygen should be given at home whenever possible, and always during an ambulance journey to hospital. As a general guide a patient who is considered to be ill enough to require parenteral administration of a bronchodilator drug or nebulisation of a high dose of a β_2-receptor agonist, should also be given systemic corticosteroid therapy. Also, unless there is rapid and good response to this treatment admission to hospital should be arranged quickly.

Concomitant Therapy

Bronchodilators

Bronchodilator Inhalers

No patient requiring an inhaled corticosteroid should be on this treatment alone. Those with mild to moderate disease should have a bronchodilator inhaler and some may also be taking a sustained release methylxanthine preparation. All patients should have a bronchodilator inhaler to be used either regularly or whenever symptoms demand. This is the most flexible and rational way to use a bronchodilator, since the effective inhaled dose is minute compared to that of oral preparations and provides a much more rapid therapeutic response (Editorial, 1981). As a bonus, lack of response to the inhaled drug can be used as an indication of severe disease requiring extra treatment. The only disadvantage is that as many as 50% of patients cannot use the conventional pressurised aerosol properly if the only advice about its use is obtained from the manufacturer's instruction pamphlet.

It is rational to recommend the use of a bronchodilator inhaler a few minutes before the corticosteroid is inhaled in order to ensure that bronchoconstriction is at a minimum, in an attempt to improve inhalation and distribution of the corticosteroid. The patient can be told to use the bronchodilator before every dose of the corticosteroid or, if control of disease is very good, only if wheeze is present when inhaled corticosteroid treatment is due.

Bronchodilators by Nebuliser

In recent years there has been a growing tendency for doctors to prescribe high dose bronchodilator therapy, usually salbutamol or terbutaline by nebuliser, for the domiciliary treatment of some patients with troublesome asthma. The reasons for the increase in popularity of nebulisers are many, but include inability to use an inhaler, and the fact that high dose bronchodilator treatment by nebuliser is often used in hospital as a treatment of acute severe asthma. Young children are most often provided with nebulisers for home use because of their inability to use a pressurised or dry-powder inhaler and this is obviously very sensible and often very effective treatment. However, when adults are given nebulisers for home use it usually indicates that they have severe and poorly controlled disease, as most adults can be taught how to use a conventional inhaler, possibly with a spacer attachment, or a dry-powder inhaler. The potential danger of patients with poorly controlled disease having nebulisers at home is that they may have too much confidence in the efficacy of nebulised therapy and because of this may delay seeking medical advice during a severe attack. In the writer's view this form of treatment should only be given to patients who have the back-up of open access to hospital, so that if they are ill and do not respond to the nebulised bronchodilator, they can get to hospital as quickly as possible. If this back-up is not provided the widespread use of home nebulisers delivering high doses of bronchodilators could lead to the conditions which were in part, at least, responsible for the United Kingdom asthma deaths epidemic in the 1960s.

Oral β_2-Receptor Agonists
(see also Chapter VI)

There are numerous oral sympathomimetic bronchodilator preparations available and they are freely prescribed for patients with airways disease. However, for the reasons outlined above (p.189) it is much better that sympathomimetic bronchodilator treatment be prescribed by inhalation.

Methylxanthines
(see also Chapter VI)

These drugs cannot be given by inhalation and are usually prescribed in a slow-release form to be taken twice daily. They give rise to side effects more often than inhaled β_2-receptor agonists and treatment should be monitored by serum level estimation (see p.94).

Intravenous aminophylline is often used to treat patients with severe asthma, but should be avoided in those taking oral methylxanthines, because of the risk of catastrophic side effects (fig. 11.2).

Sodium Cromoglycate
(see also Chapter VI)

Some patients may be taking an inhaled corticosteroid and sodium cromoglycate, but this combination is unlikely to be helpful (p.147).

Oral Corticosteroids

Patients with severe disease who have to take prednisolone regularly as well as an inhaled corticosteroid will, of course, have their own supply of this drug by them. They should know that they must increase the dose of prednisolone by at least a factor of 4 to treat severe exacerbations of asthma. Patients who do not require regular treatment with oral prednisolone should be allowed to have a stock supply so that they can take a course of 20 to 40mg daily for 5 to 10 days for the treatment of an acute severe episode. They should be advised to seek medical attention if they are very distressed, but many episodes of asthma can be competently treated by the informed patient without recourse to his medical practitioner. A record of all prednisolone taken must, however, be kept by all patients and reported to their medical advisers at follow-up appointments, to allow strict retrospective supervision of self-treatment. When patients are taught about their disease and its management very few abuse the privilege of being allowed to take therapeutic decisions themselves. The vast majority are capable of doing this after proper education and with appropriate follow-up. Those who have to make frequent changes in prednisolone dose or take courses of treatment often, should be considered for PEF self-monitoring.

Antibiotics

Antibiotics are frequently prescribed unnecessarily in the treatment of asthma (p.168) but there are a few patients in whom bronchial infection triggers deterioration. Bronchial infection in these patients should be treated at the earliest possible stage, and often this is best achieved by providing them with a stock supply of a suitable wide spectrum antibiotic, and allowing them to start treatment as soon as they notice purulent sputum. There is, of course, no reason why they should not be allowed to treat themselves with an antibiotic and prednisolone.

In Conclusion

Inhaled steroids have transformed the management of chronic asthma. All initial promises have been fulfilled and there have been no serious side effects. Topical corticosteroids were justifiably prescribed with considerable caution in the first few years, but recently many clinicians have been using this effective and safe treatment much more freely. Continuous treatment of many thousands of patients has shown that efficacy does not decline with prolonged use, and more importantly side effects have proved to be even less than perhaps was anticipated. Oropharyngeal thrush is a problem in only a few patients, but trivial voice symptoms, which appear to be a specific effect of the corticosteroid on the vocal cords or their musculature, are quite common. Side effects associated with low dose treatment are trivial and confined to the mouth and throat. With a decade of experience we can now assume with confidence that this form of therapy is free from serious side effects, and if this is the case we should encourage a lowering of the prescription threshold to allow more patients to benefit. Twice-daily treatment is likely to be recommended for most patients in the future and this, together with the development of better and alternative delivery systems, will improve patient compliance. 'High' dose treatment is likely to be used more often in preference to the combination of an inhaled and an oral drug, but the long term effects of high dose topical therapy are unknown. Attempts to improve patient education must continue and our assessment of the individual patient should more often include objective measurement of ventilatory function. Inhaled corticosteroids used judiciously could improve the lives of untold numbers of asthmatic patients all over the world.

References

Brompton Hospital/Medical Research Council Collaborative Trial: Long term study of disodium cromoglycate in treatment of severe extrinsic or intrinsic bronchial asthma in adults. British Medical Journal 4: 383 (1972).

Brown, H. Morrow; Storey, G. and George, W.H.S.: Beclomethasone dipropionate; a new steroid aerosol for the treatment of allergic asthma. British Medical Journal 1: 585 (1972).

Cameron, S.J.; Cooper, E.J.; Crompton, G.K.; Hoare, M.V. and Grant, I.W.B.: Substitution of beclomethasone aerosol for oral prednisolone in the treatment of chronic asthma. British Medical Journal 4: 205 (1973).

Carmichael, J.; Paterson, I.C.; Diaz, P.; Crompton, G.K.; Kay, A.B. and Grant, I.W.B.: Corticosteroid resistance in chronic asthma. British Medical Journal 282: 1419 (1981).

Choo-Kang, Y.F.J. and Grant, I.W.B.: Comparison of two methods of administering bronchodilator aerosol to asthmatic patients. British Medical Journal 2: 119 (1975).

Clark, T.J.H.: Effect of beclomethasone dipropionate delivered by aerosol in patients with asthma. Lancet 1: 1361 (1972).

Crompton, G.K.; Grant, I.W.B. and Bloomfield, P.: Edinburgh Emergency Admission Service: report on 10 years' experience. British Medical Journal 2: 1199 (1979).

Editorial: The proper use of bronchodilator aerosols. Lancet 1: 23 (1981).

Gaddie, J.; Reid, I.W.; Skinner, C.; Petrie, G.R.; Sinclair, D.J.M. and Palmer, K.N.V.: Aerosol beclomethasone dipropionate: a dose-response study in chronic bronchial asthma. Lancet 2: 280 (1973).

Gwynn, C.M. and Smith, J. Morrison: A one year follow-up of children and adolescents receiving regular beclomethasone dipropionate. Clinical Allergy 4: 325 (1974).

McFadden, E.R. and Ingram, R.H.: Exercise-induced asthma. New England Journal of Medicine 301: 763 (1979).

Maberly, D.J.; Gibson, G.J. and Butler, A.G.: Recovery of adrenal function after substitution of beclomethasone dipropionate for oral corticosteroids. British Medical Journal 1: 778 (1973).

Milne, L.J.R. and Crompton, G.K.: Beclomethasone dipropionate and oropharyngeal candidiasis. British Medical Journal 3: 797 (1974).

Munch, E.P.; Taudorf, E. and Wecke, B.: Dose frequency in the treatment of asthmatics with inhaled topical steroid. European Journal of Respiratory Diseases 63: 143 (1982).

Paterson, I.C. and Crompton, G.K.: Use of pressurised aerosols by asthmatic patients. British Medical Journal 1: 76 (1976).

Research Committee of the British Thoracic Association: Inhaled beclomethasone dipropionate in allergic pulmonary aspergillosis. British Journal of Diseases of the Chest 73: 349 (1979).

Smith, M.J. and Hodson, M.E.: High dose beclomethasone inhaler in the treatment of asthma. Lancet 2: in press (1982).

Toogood, J.H.; Lefcoe, N.M.; Haines, D.S.M.; Jennings, B.; Errington, N.; Baksh, L. and Chuang, L.: A graded dose assessment of the efficacy of beclomethasone dipropionate aerosol for severe chronic asthma. Journal of Allergy and Clinical Immunology 59: 298 (1977).

Toogood, J.H.; Baskerville, J.C.; Jennings, B.H. and Lefcoe, N.M.: Optimal dosage in steroid-dependent asthma; in Mygind and Clark (Eds) Topical Steroid Treatment for Asthma and Rhinitis, p.107 (Baillière Tindall, London 1980a).

Toogood, J.H.; Jennings, B.; Greenway, R.W. and Chuang, L.: Candidiasis and dysphonia complicating beclomethasone treatment of asthma. Journal of Allergy and Clinical Immunology 65: 145 (1980b).

Tweeddale, P.M.; Godden, D.J. and Grant, I.W.B.: Hyperventilation or exercise to induce asthma? Thorax 36: 596 (1981).

Webb, J. and Clark, T.J.H.: Recovery of plasma corticotrophin and cortisol levels after a three-week course of prednisolone. Thorax 36: 22 (1981).

Willey, R.F.; Godden, D.J.; Carmichael, J.; Preston, P.; Frame, M. and Crompton, G.K.: Comparison of twice daily administration of a new corticosteroid budesonide with beclomethasone dipropionate four times daily in the treatment of chronic asthma. British Journal of Diseases of the Chest 76: 61 (1982).

Wyatt, R.; Waschek, J.; Weinberger, M. and Sherman, B.: Effects of inhaled beclomethasone dipropionate and alternate-day prednisone on pituitary-adrenal function in children with chronic asthma. New England Journal of Medicine 299: 1387 (1978).

Chapter XII

Inhaled Steroids in the Management of Childhood Asthma: including data from a longterm follow-up of a large, personal series

J. Morrison Smith

Early Trials

There can be little doubt that the introduction of corticosteroid treatment has done more than anything else to relieve the suffering of patients with asthma. In the early years of steroid use excessive caution probably contributed to many deaths and allowed many children and their families to continue to suffer distress and disruption of their lives because of fear of the side effects which might occur. Experience showed that the ill effects were greatly outweighed by the benefits of systemic steroid treatment in most children (Smith and Pizarro, 1973). Corticotrophin never proved a real alternative to oral prednisolone, although considerable interest was aroused by the work of Friedman and Strang (1966) showing less growth inhibition with corticotrophin. As long ago as 1958 serious efforts were being made to use inhaled steroid treatment in children (Smith, 1958). The only preparation then available was hydrocortisone hemisuccinate and in the absence of pressurised aerosols this was given by a hand-operated glass nebuliser. Not surprisingly clinical trials showed it to be ineffective.

The situation changed dramatically when the topically active steroid beclomethasone dipropionate became available as a pressurised aerosol (it had already been in use for some time in various forms as a local treatment for inflammatory skin disease). The first published trial by Morrow Brown et al. in 1972 described its use in a number of children and although not a double-blind controlled study it left little doubt that the preparation was effective and, in doses of 400μg daily, could in many cases replace prednisolone with good clinical evidence of recovery of adrenal function. Experimentally, Harris et al. (1973) showed that in human volunteers adrenal suppressive effects were unlikely at doses below 1mg daily (p.123).

A series of clinical trials of inhaled steroid treatment using beclomethasone dipropionate (Godfrey and Konig, 1973; Dickson et al., 1973; Smith, 1973) or betamethasone valerate (Frears et al., 1973) followed and these and other studies are discussed in Chapter IX. An early leading article in the Lancet (Editorial 1972) was not particularly enthusiastic about the new inhaled steroids, stating that 'whilst this new drug by aerosol is useful in mild asthma it seems to have no advantage over oral corticosteroids in the more severely steroid-dependent patients and caution should be exercised in transferring patients satisfactorily controlled on oral corticosteroids to aerosol beclomethasone'. While caution is always admirable, this luke-warm reception has hardly proved justified. Inhaled steroids are now widely used in moderate and severe asthma and although a few severe cases do not derive significant benefit and may be best managed entirely on oral steroid treatment (Herxheimer, 1981) this has proved to be the exception rather than the rule, particularly in children.

Initial trials are important but subsequent experience may be even more so, as the place of a new treatment becomes more accurately defined with time. Most of the early trials were concerned with children already having steroid treatment, long term, by mouth. Thus, Smith (1973) included 39 patients, average age 12 years, all receiving oral prednisolone, bronchodilators and sodium cromoglycate but still not symptom-free. Aerosol treatment with beclomethasone dipropionate 400μg daily, in 4 doses or a placebo was added to the treatment for 2 weeks, followed by a cross-over period of a further 2 weeks. Assessment was by way of daily symptom records and weekly clinical examination and ventilatory function tests. The advantage of the inhaled steroid was clearly significant symptomatically but less clear using the ventilatory function records. Results did not show any relationship to IgE levels and the emphasis placed on allergic asthma by Morrow Brown and colleagues was not substantiated. A further month on 'open' treatment with beclomethasone dipropionate suggested that the good effect was maintained. As stated, many of the patients in this initial clinical trial were either already having sodium cromoglycate or had been tried on this drug in the past. It seemed reasonable to expect the drugs to have a useful additive effect but in fact most patients who responded to inhaled steroid ceased to have sodium cromoglycate, probably for reasons of expense and because of the complexity of such dual treatment. However, subsequently Mitchell et al. (1976) studied the effect of combining these drugs in children previously untreated with either and concluded that there was no difference in efficacy using the combination compared with that of either drug given alone.

Long Term Results

A follow-up study of 66 children on beclomethasone dipropionate for at least one year (Gwynn and Smith, 1974) showed that 76% of the children were able to stop and remain off oral prednisolone. Those who responded well initially remained well throughout the year. No evidence of candidiasis was found. The death of one child, previously on oral steroids, but well controlled for some months on inhaled therapy, whose asthma rapidly worsened, reinforced the absolute necessity of providing patients with a reserve supply of prednisolone to use immediately, should their asthma deteriorate (p.190). Written instructions to take an immediate dose of at least 20mg and seek early medical advice is now, in some centres, allied to a system of self-admission to hospital (p.111). There is no doubt that children who have suffered from moderate or severe asthma during most of their lives may fail to complain when they deteriorate and their parents need to be warned to be vigilant. Daily records of symptoms (p.186) may help to demonstrate deterioration and, if available, twice daily records of peak flow rate measured with the cheap but adequate instruments now available (p.39) may also be of great value, quite apart from their use in clinical trials.

There have been a number of publications describing long term follow-up of patients on inhaled therapy (Francis, 1976; Brown et al., 1977; Godfrey et al., 1977). These are discussed further in Chapter IX. Data from the records of children treated with inhaled beclomethasone dipropionate in the 5 years subsequent to the Gwynn and Smith (1974) follow-up study are presented in the fol-

Table 12.1. Dose and dosage form of inhaled beclomethasone dipropionate used by asthmatic children 1975 to 1980 (author's personal series)

Year	Total no. of patients	Inhaled beclomethasone dipropionate		
		daily dose range (median) [μg]	aerosol (no. of pts.)	dry-powder inhaler (no. of pts.)
1975	49	100-600 (150)	49	0
1976	58	100-800 (200)	58	0
1977	69	100-900 (400)	60	9
1978	149	100-800 (400)	36	113
1979	222	150-800 (400)	4	218
1980	164	200-800 (400)	0	164

lowing section and provide a basis for the author's concluding views and recommendations.

Personal Series

A long term study of children on inhaled beclomethasone dipropionate was undertaken in Birmingham over many years in a group of 221 children about whom, in most cases, a considerable amount of information accumulated. Table 12.1 shows the numbers studied in each year and the dose and dosage form of inhaled steroid. It will be seen that the drug was given by aerosol up to 1977 but from 1978 to 1980 most children were using the dry-powder ('Rotahaler')[1] device. Cooperation is always difficult to estimate with accuracy but the change to the 'Rotahaler' was thought to be associated with a higher proportion of the children taking the treatment regularly and effectively. Bronchodilators were used regularly in most patients and from 1978 this too was usually administered via a dry-powder inhalation device[2].

Results

Figure 12.1 shows that continuous use of oral steroid fell steadily and fewer patients were in need of even temporary courses. By 1980, 91% of the children had required no oral steroid in the preceding year compared with 30% in 1975. Other forms of treatment, hospitalisation and special provision for education were also needed less frequently (table 12.2).

An attempt was made to assess the factors governing response to treatment by defining a group in whom response could be categorised as 'excellent' (table 12.3) and comparing them with the others who fell short of this ideal. By these criteria, of 218 children studied during 1979 to 1980, 38% had an 'excellent' response. Fewer of this 'excellent' group needed more than 400μg daily of beclomethasone dipropionate (fig. 12.2) but duration of treatment had

1 'Becotide Rotacaps' (Allen and Hanburys; Glaxo).
2 'Ventolin Rotacaps' (Allen and Hanburys; Glaxo).

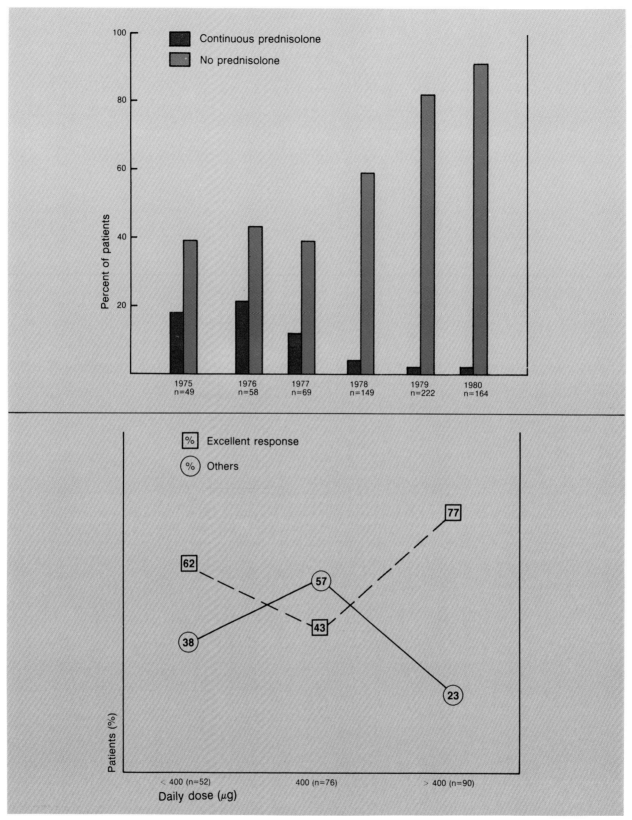

Fig. 12.1. Changes in oral prednisolone requirement in asthmatic children treated witn inhaled beclomethasone dipropionate (author's personal series).

Fig. 12.2. Response to treatment (excellent or otherwise)[1] of 218 asthmatic children, according to the daily dose of inhaled beclomethasone dipropionate (author's personal series).

1 See table 12.3.

Table 12.2. Percent of asthmatic children requiring a course of antibiotics, hospital admission or special education while on inhaled beclomethasone dipropionate (author's personal series)

Year	Total no. of patients	No. of patients (%)		
		antibiotics	hospital admission	special education
1975	49	7 (14)	2 (4)	12 (24)
1976	58	11 (19)	1 (2)	13 (22)
1977	69	11 (16)	7 (10)	11 (16)
1978	149	21 (14)	7 (5)	11 (7)
1979	222	20 (9)	3 (1)	14 (6)
1980	164	9 (5)	0	9 (5)

little effect on response (fig. 12.3). Higher daily salbutamol usage, as might be expected, was associated with a lower percentage of 'excellent' responses (fig. 12.4). The age when inhaled steroid was started probably had little effect on the likelihood of an 'excellent' response; the only age group with a markedly lower percentage of 'excellent' responders (> 15 years) being numerically small (fig. 12.5). There were fewer very stunted children among the 'excellent' group but little difference otherwise (fig. 12.6). Cooperation clearly had a bearing on response (fig 12.7) as might be expected.

As far as age of onset of asthma is concerned little difference in response was noted (fig. 12.8). The presence of eczema or hayfever was not associated with a greater likelihood of an 'excellent' response (fig. 12.9), although there was an indication of such an association in children with multiple positive skin tests; however, the numbers were smaller in this group (fig. 12.10). As far as sensitivity to particular skin test groups is concerned, there was little evidence that this was of importance. Contrary to earlier experience when only aerosol therapy was available the response pattern of the racial groups showed little difference (table 12.4).

Aspects of Management of Childhood Asthma

Reasons for Failure

Why do some children not respond to inhaled corticosteroids? Classified according to age, sex, duration of treatment, dosage and age on starting treatment it is not possible to predict those unlikely to respond (Gwynn and Smith, 1977). Similarly previous oral steroid therapy was not predictive of response. However, poor responders tended to belong to the more poorly educated families in the Registrar General's social classes IV and V, and a higher proportion of poor responders belonged to families where the parents had emigrated from Asia or from the West Indies. It was thus concluded that poor responses were probably largely related to poor compliance in taking treatment regularly and properly. This serves to emphasise the need for careful instruction of children and parents, constant checking of inhalation technique and constant encouragement. In countries where economic considerations might limit compliance with treatment regimens a further difficulty is likely to be experienced.

Techniques of administration of aerosols in children have been

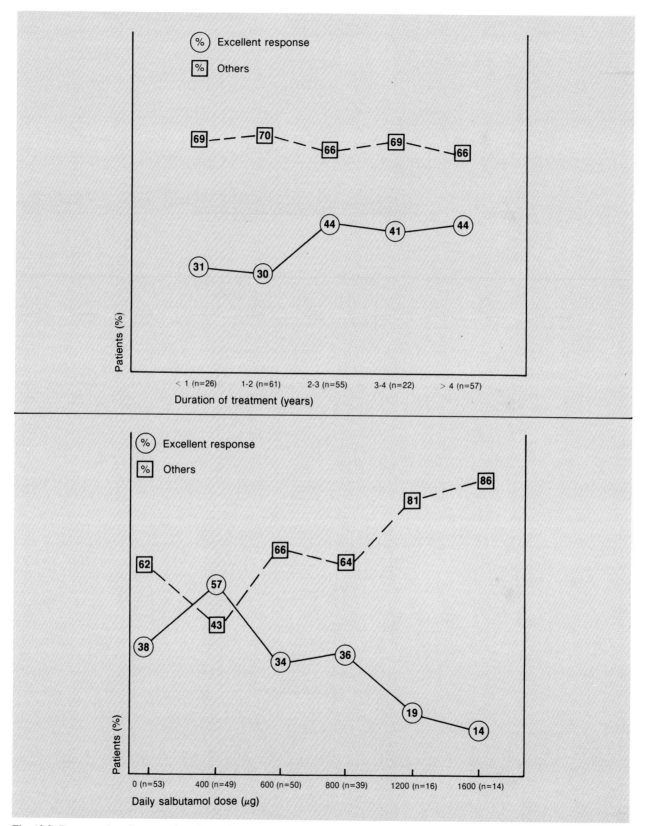

Fig. 12.3. Response (excellent or otherwise)[1] of 221 asthmatic children treated with inhaled beclomethasone dipropionate, according to the duration of treatment (author's personal series).

Fig. 12.4. Response (excellent or otherwise)[1] of 221 asthmatic children on inhaled beclomethasone dipropionate, according to daily use of additional therapy with salbutamol (as 'Rotacaps') [author's personal series].

1 See table 12.3.

Table 12.3. Criteria by which children were defined as having an 'excellent' response to inhaled beclomethasone dipropionate

In the past year:
1) No oral steroids
2) No antibiotics
3) No admission to hospital
4) No record of wheezing at any routine examination
5) $FEV_1 \geq 1$ litre (< 10 years) ≥ 1.5 litre (> 10 years)

discussed at length by Harper and Strunk (1981) and are further discussed in Appendix 1. However excellent the advice given it may well be a counsel of perfection for some children and certainly impossible to follow perfectly in the case of those with marked airways obstruction when treatment is initiated. Although much of this difficulty may be overcome by patient instruction and constant checking, some children require an initial period on high-dose oral steroid treatment to enable them to benefit from inhaled steroid.

Dry-powder Inhaler or Pressurised Aerosol?

Although used as recommended, fluorocarbon aerosol propellants are unlikely to be unsafe, there having been no recurrence of the high asthma death rates of the 1960's in spite of an increase in the continued use of pressurised aerosols (Editorial, 1975), it seems logical to deliver inhaled therapy for asthma by the simplest method and, if possible, without the need for additives. Clinical experience suggested a general improvement in cooperation in children, with an improvement in response (Smith and Gwynn, 1978), after the introduction of dry-powder inhalers. This has subsequently been confirmed. While there may be less advantage in using the device in adults (Lal et al., 1980; Campbell et al., 1980) there is no doubt that it is the best method of delivering the drug for children. The writer's view is that moderately severe asthma in children is best treated by giving twice-daily, supervised treatment with 200 to 400μg salbutamol followed by 200 to 400μg beclomethasone dipropionate – both given by dry-powder inhaler.

Concurrent Use of Bronchodilators

A leading article in the British Medical Journal (Editorial, 1975) noting the great improvement in the quality of life for many asthmatic children from the use of aerosol steroids was criticised by Phelan (1975) for failing to emphasise the important place that regular use of bronchodilators plays in management. In North America particularly, oral theophylline in full doses, controlled by monitoring theophylline blood levels, is popular but in the United Kingdom inhaled β_2-stimulants are more acceptable. In general their use in the moderate to severe asthmatic would be considered additional to rather than replacement therapy for inhaled steroid treatment. The writer could not accept Phelan's statement that no child should be started on corticosteroids, either by inhalation or orally, until it has been clearly demonstrated that a combination of regular sodium cromoglycate, oral theophylline and orciprenaline or salbutamol by inhalation has failed to give adequate control. Clark and Anderson (1978) reported that in adult patients the combination of regular dosage of β_2-stimulant and inhaled corticosteroid gave better control and although Mackay and Dyson

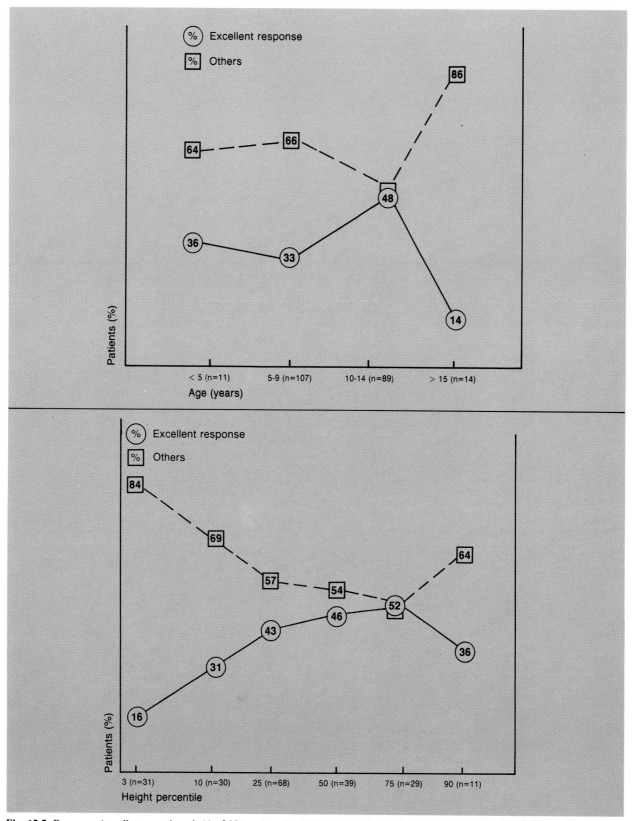

Fig. 12.5. Response (excellent or otherwise)[1] of 221 asthmatic children treated with inhaled beclomethasone dipropionate according to age at which treatment was begun (author's personal series).

Fig. 12.6. Response (excellent or otherwise)[1] of 217 asthmatic children treated with inhaled beclomethasone dipropionate, according to growth (height percentile) recorded at final assessment (1980) [author's personal series].

1 See table 12.3.

Table 12.4. Response ('excellent' or otherwise) of 218 asthmatic children treated with inhaled beclomethasone dipropionate, according to race (author's personal series)

Race	No. of patients	Response (%)	
		excellent	others
European	153	60 (39)	93 (61)
Negro	25	11 (44)	14 (66)
Asian	40	12 (30)	28 (70)

(1980), who also studied adults, did not find beclomethasone dipropionate more effective when preceded by salbutamol, the author's experience is that the overall control of asthma in children may be better when β_2-stimulants are used regularly in addition to inhaled steroids.

Exercise-induced Asthma

Exercise-induced asthma has been reviewed by Anderson et al. (1975). The phenomenon has been observed from early times and exists to some degree in most children with asthma. In some it is a particular problem and in a few it is the only manifestation of asthma. The effect of drugs on the prevention and treatment of exercise-induced asthma has been extensively studied. In general the sympathomimetic preparations give the best and most reliable inhibition. These drugs will not only relieve exercise-induced asthma but will also prevent it if given before exercise or very quickly afterwards. Sodium cromoglycate is a suitable preparation for children but is effective in most cases only when used immediately before exercise.

Corticosteroids are not effective in suppressing exercise-induced asthma acutely, the role of inhaled or oral steroids in this condition (p.121) being largely indirect. A child with uncontrolled asthma will usually be made worse by exercise, particularly in cold air. Better control of the asthma will reduce this tendency and often permit active participation in games without distress. Thus the study of exercise-induced asthma as an isolated phenomenon reveals little effect from inhaled corticosteroids, but when they are used in the general treatment of children with asthma they may well enable them to lead an active life, and participate in sports which would previously have led to acute attacks. There are, however, a proportion of children, generally well controlled on inhaled corticosteroids, who also need β_2-stimulants or cromoglycate to prevent attacks of exercise-induced asthma; prescription of these additional treatments, for use under appropriate circumstances, clearly, should not affect the important continued use of inhaled steroids for the general management of their asthma.

Undesirable Effects

There can be no doubt that the main object of introducing inhaled steroid therapy, in children in particular, was to avoid the ill effects of systemic steroids. The Cushingoid stunted child on systemic steroid treatment (fig. 12.11) was conspicuous in any paediatric asthma clinic and most paediatricians would agree that such children have become much less common since the introduction of inhaled steroids. Growth was always the main concern when systemic steroids were used in childhood asthma; such complications of corticosteroid treatment as uncontrolled infection, cataract

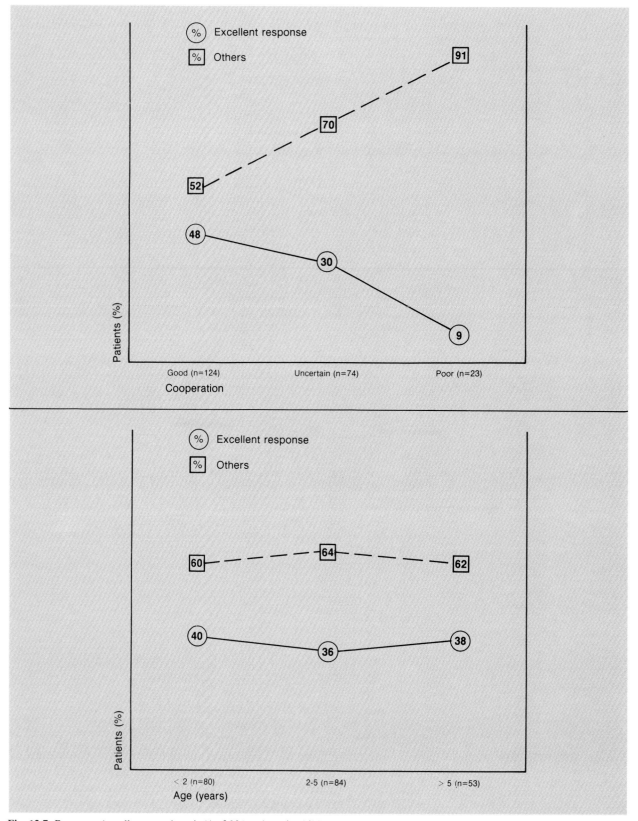

Fig. 12.7. Response (excellent or otherwise)[1] of 221 asthmatic children treated with inhaled beclomethasone dipropionate, according to quality of cooperation with medication instructions (author's personal series).

Fig. 12.8. Response (excellent or otherwise)[1] of 217 asthmatic children treated with inhaled beclomethasone dipropionate, according to age at the onset of asthma (author's personal series).

1   See table 12.3.

and osteoporosis were virtually unknown in the asthmatic and diabetes was very rare indeed. However, it is comforting to avoid any such risks.

Oral Thrush

Candidiasis has proved to be a fairly frequent occurrence in the adult asthmatic on corticosteroids by inhalation (p.159) but in children and teenagers it is virtually unknown and only a very few cases have been reported; clinical thrush is really not a practical problem (Kerrebijn, 1976) with this age group. One case of transient bilateral posterior subcapsular cataracts occurring in a child of 9 while on beclomethasone dipropionate was reported by Kewley (1980) but the association is uncertain.

Atrophy

The possible occurrence of mucosal atrophy in the respiratory tract has been studied in adults (Thiringer et al., 1975; Andersson, 1975) and experimentally in dogs (Poynter et al., 1975) without evidence of atrophic changes being noted (p.122).

Growth

There is no doubt that asthmatic children tend to be stunted to some degree, irrespective of treatment. Murray et al. (1976) showed that this was particularly so in those who started having asthma very early in life and that both chronic anorexia and chronic hypoxia may be factors responsible for poor growth. Daily or alternate-day oral steroids exaggerate this growth retardation (Chang et al., 1982). No significant difference in mean height growth of 30 children in the 12 months before and during treatment with beclomethasone dipropionate (Kerrebijn, 1976) was found and Kraepelien and Graff-Lonnivig (1979) did not find that beclomethasone dipropionate retarded growth or skeletal maturation in children.

HPA Function

The question of adrenal suppression is probably more controversial. Maberley et al. (1973) reported serial adrenal function tests with recovery of function in 2 months after changing from oral to inhaled steroid as judged by response to tetracosactrin. Most paediatricians have been satisfied that the change from prednisolone to inhaled beclomethasone dipropionate resulted in restoration of adrenal function to normal in due course (Kershnar et al., 1978), although response to stress might not fully recover for many years. Occasional unexpected deaths were reported (Mellis et al., 1976) but the children involved all had severe asthma, previously treated with systemic steroids, and postmortem evidence of mucous plugging (2 patients) or infection (1 patient), making the adrenal changes noted at postmortem difficult to interpret. In general, however, recovery of adrenal function was expected, and it was not considered that beclomethasone dipropionate impaired hypothalamic-pituitary-adrenal function in therapeutic doses (Spitzer et al., 1976). Thus the paper of Wyatt et al. (1978) concluding that alternate-day oral prednisone in doses of 20 to 40mg was no more likely to cause HPA depression than inhaled beclomethasone dipropionate in doses of 400 to 800µg daily was of interest. This paper considered 20 steroid-dependent children and 7 controls divided into 5 groups, studied over only 3 months (see Appendix 2). Bhan et al. (1980) studied 43 patients, in 3 groups (one having had previous oral steroid but been on inhaled beclomethasone dipropionate for an average of more than 3 years, and

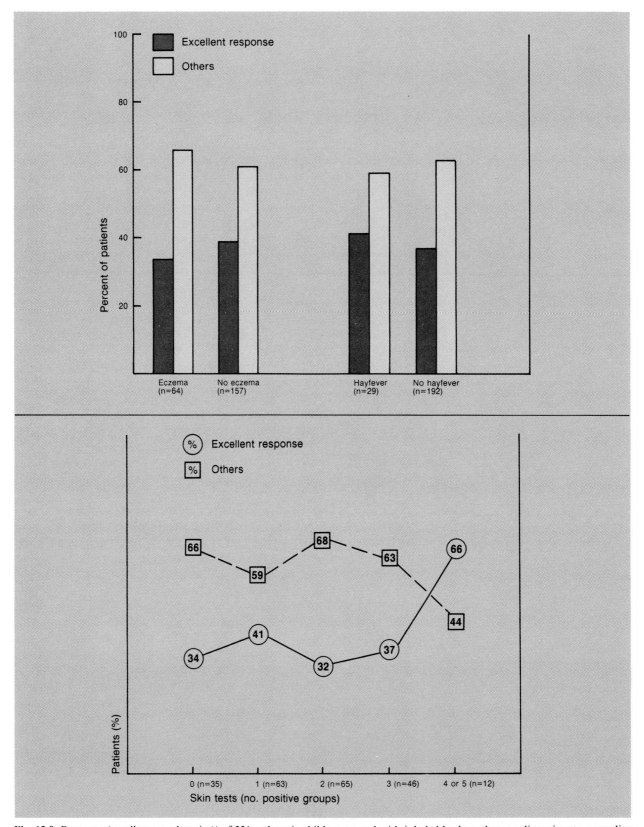

Fig. 12.9. Response (excellent or otherwise)[1] of 221 asthmatic children treated with inhaled beclomethasone dipropionate, according to the presence or absence of atopy (author's personal series).

Fig. 12.10. Response (excellent or otherwise)[1] of 221 asthmatic children treated with inhaled beclomethasone dipropionate, according to the number of skin test allergen groups to which there was a positive response > 5mm diameter (author's personal series).

1   See table 12.3.

a second group who had had no previous oral steroid but inhaled steroids for a similar period; a third group had never had any steroid) and their results did not suggest any clinically significant adrenal suppression as a consequence of long term inhalations of this corticosteroid.

In the course of a decade's experience of using corticosteroids by inhalation in asthmatic children we have not seen any of the Cushingoid side effects common in oral steroid-treated children or even the less florid manifestations sometimes seen with alternate-day regimens (Wyatt et al., 1978; Siegal et al., 1979).

Therapeutic Groups in Childhood Asthma

Childhood asthma may be classified into several therapeutic groups:

1) Mild intermittent cases and those with purely exercise-induced attacks who are probably best treated with β_2-stimulants alone.

2) Mild but persistent cases suitable for sodium cromoglycate and only changed to inhaled corticosteroids if this fails.

3 Most moderate and severe cases for whom inhaled corticosteroids with or without regular use of a β_2-stimulant is the most suitable treatment.

4) Rarely, apparently very severe, inhaled steroid-resistant cases are encountered; oral steroids and bronchodilators may have to be given in high dosage. Even in these difficult patients inhaled steroids should be used to allow a lower oral maintenance dose than might otherwise be necessary.

In Summary

The lessons learned from our experience of treating childhood asthma with inhaled corticosteroids can be summarised thus:

1) Inhaled corticosteroids (beclomethasone dipropionate $400\mu g$ daily, or equivalent) can be considered at least equivalent to 5mg of prednisolone and can be safely given to children from 3 years upwards.

2) The dose can be increased (beclomethasone dipropionate $800\mu g$ daily or equivalent), certainly after 10 years of age, without significant risk of adverse effect.

3) There is no convincing evidence that, in these doses, there is clinically significant impairment of function of the hypothalamic-pituitary-adrenal axis.

4) There is no evidence that either beclomethasone dipropionate or betamethasone valerate (the 2 inhaled steroids most studied), in therapeutic doses, impair growth, and some evidence that, as a group at least, children who are changed from oral to inhaled steroids with good control of their asthma show an improvement in growth.

5) After many years' experience with inhaled steroids it can be concluded that in children and adolescents oral candidiasis is so rare as to be of no importance.

6) A high proportion of treatment failures are due to poor patient compliance rather than failure of the treatment itself. Thus all the following methods of improving adult patient cooperation (most of which are dealt with in detail elsewhere in this book) should also be considered for children:

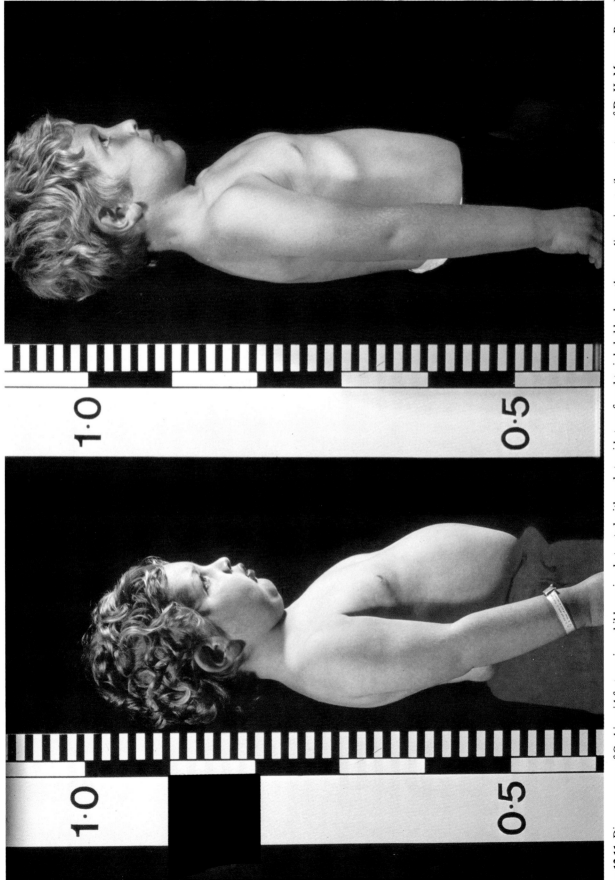

Fig. 12.11. Disappearance of Cushingoid features in a child previously treated with oral steroids transferred to inhaled beclomethasone dipropionate (by courtesy of Dr H. Morrow Brown).

- Initial, and regular follow-up checks of inhalation technique Appendix 1)
- Education of the parent, and the child as soon as old enough, about asthma and its treatment
- Special instruction on the difference between bronchodilator and steroid inhalations (p.178)
- Clear instructions on what to do if the asthma gets worse
- Home monitoring of symptoms (p.43, p.186)
- Home monitoring of lung function (p.39, 186)
- Recording of daily drug usage (p.44, 186)

In addition, with children, special consideration should be given to the device chosen:

- Use dry-powder inhalers for young children and in any patient who has difficulty with a pressurised aerosol.

[Children down to 3 years of age can generally manage to inhale from a dry-powder device, and a solution for use with a nebuliser, at present under investigation, holds promise for use in infants (p.149)]

7) Atopic status does not appear to have any direct bearing on success or failure of inhaled corticosteroids.

8) Combination with sodium cromoglycate has not usually proved successful in improving response but some patients may be more suitably managed on cromoglycate than on inhaled steroid (category 2 above).

9) The regular use of β_2-stimulant and corticosteroid, both by inhalation, has proved useful in many children, particularly when administered from a dry-powder inhalation device (see Appendix 1).

10) Exercise-induced asthma will in most cases respond best to β_2-stimulants or prevention with sodium cromoglycate. Children whose asthma is well controlled with inhaled steroids improve their ability to exercise without getting asthma and may need no additional treatment.

11) No particular group of asthmatics need be excluded from treatment with inhaled steroids except those temporarily or permanently suffering from such severe airways obstruction that systemic steroid treatment is mandatory.

12) Patients with severe airways obstruction may require a short period of systemic steroid treatment when inhaled therapy is first started.

13) Where severe attacks have occurred in the past, and when patients have previously been on oral steroids for long periods, the need to re-introduce systemic steroids promptly in any acute deterioration must be fully appreciated by those concerned. Parents may be supplied with emergency doses of prednisolone and instructions to use a fully adequate dose promptly and seek further medical advice. In this connection holidays and weekends need special mention.

In Conclusion

Martin et al. (1982) recently reported that a great many young people who suffer from asthma from before the age of 7, even at 21, have little understanding of their condition and its treatment. People with asthma need to have an understanding of their disease and need to have adequate treatment; many have neither. In the majority of cases their childhood can be made free, or almost free, of distress and asthmatic children can achieve adult life without serious impairment of their educational and career prospects. We have the means to help them and we must do so. Inhaled steroids are among the most useful therapeutic agents, highly effective in most cases with minimal risk of unwanted effects yet they are almost certainly underused, even in countries where they have been available for 10 years.

Acknowledgements

The follow-up study of patients in Birmingham was carried out with the help of computer facilities provided by Glaxo Research Ltd. I would like to express my thanks to the Medical Director, Dr David Harris, and to Mr A.G. Butler and Mr W.D. Robinson who made it possible to collect and analyse the information, and to my wife who also took part.

References

Anderson, S.D.; Silverman, M.; Konig, P. and Godfrey, S.: Exercise induced asthma. British Journal of Diseases of the Chest 69: 1 (1975).

Andersson, E.: An investigation of the bronchial mucous membrane after long-term treatment with beclomethasone dipropionate. Postgraduate Medical Journal 51 (Suppl. 4): 32 (1975).

Bhan, G.L.; Gwynn, C.M. and Morrison Smith, J. Morrison: Growth and adrenal function of children on prolonged beclomethasone dipropionate treatment. Lancet 1: 96 (1980).

Brown, H. Morrow; Storey, G. and George, W.H.S.: Beclomethasone dipropionate: a new steroid aerosol for the treatment of allergic asthma. British Medical Journal 1: 585 (1972).

Brown, H. Morrow; Storey, G. and Jackson, F.A.: Beclomethasone dipropionate aerosol in long-term treatment of perennial and seasonal asthma in children and adults: a report of five and a half years experience in 600 asthmatic patients. British Journal of Clinical Pharmacology 4(Suppl. 4): 2595 (1977).

Campbell, I.A.; Finnegan, O.C.; Todd, J. and Smith, D.: A comparison of aerosol and powder inhalation of beclomethasone. British Journal of Diseases of the Chest 74: 419 (1980).

Chang, K.C.; Miklich, D.R.; Barwise, G.; Chai, H. and Miles-Lawrence, R.: Linear growth in chronic asthmatic children: the effects of the disease and various forms of steroid therapy. Clinical Allergy 12: 369 (1982).

Clark, R.A. and Anderson, P.B.: Combined therapy with salbutamol and beclomethasone inhalers in chronic asthma. Lancet 3: 70 (1978).

Dickson, W.; Hall, C.E.; Ellis, M. and Horrocks, R.H.: Beclomethasone dipropionate aerosol in childhood asthma. Archives of Disease in Childhood 48: 671 (1973).

Editorial: Beclomethasone dipropionate aerosol in asthma. Lancet 2: 1239 (1972).

Editorial: Fluorocarbon aerosol propellants. Lancet 1: 1073 (1975).

Editorial: Treatment of asthmatic children with steroids. British Medical Journal 1: 413 (1975).

Francis, R.S.: Long-term beclomethasone dipropionate aerosol therapy in juvenile asthma. Thorax 31: 309 (1976).

Frears, J.F.; Wilson, L.C. and Friedman, M.: Betamethasone 17-valerate by aerosol in childhood asthma. Archives of Disease in Childhood 48: 856 (1973).

Friedman, M. and Strang, L.B.: Effect of long-term corticosteroids and corticotrophin on the growth of children. Lancet 2: 568 (1966).

Godfrey, S.; Balfour Lynn, L. and Tooley, M.: Beclomethasone dipropionate aerosol in childhood asthma: a three to five year follow up. British Journal of Clinical Pharmacology 4(Suppl. 4): 2735 (1977).

Godfrey, S. and Konig, P.: Beclomethasone aerosol in childhood asthma. Archives of Disease in Childhood 48: 665 (1973).

Gwynn, C.M. and Smith, J. Morrison: A one year follow-up of children and adolescents receiving regular beclomethasone dipropionate. Clinical Allergy 4: 325 (1974).

Gwynn, C.M. and Smith, J. Morrison: Long-term results with beclomethasone dipropionate aerosol in children with bronchial asthma: Why does it sometimes fail? British Journal of Clinical Pharmacology 4(Suppl. 4): 2695 (1977).

Harper, T.B. and Strunk, R.C.: Techniques of administration of metered-dose aerosolised drugs in asthmatic children. American Journal of Diseases in Childhood 135: 218 (1981).

Harris, D.M.; Martin, L.E.; Harrison, C. and Jack, D.: The effect of oral and inhaled beclomethasone dipropionate on adrenal function. Clinical Allergy 3: 243 (1973).

Herxheimer, H.: Should corticosteroid aerosols be used in severe chronic asthma? (Editorial) Thorax 36: 401 (1981).

Kerrebijn, K.F.: Beclomethasone dipropionate in long-term treatment of asthma in children. Journal of Paediatrics 89: 821 (1976).

Kershnar, H.; Klein, R.; Waldman, D.; Berger, W.; Rachelefsky, G.; Katz, R. and Siegel, S.: Treatment of chronic childhood asthma with beclomethasone dipropionate aerosols: II. Effect on pituitary-adrenal function after substitution for oral corticosteroids. Paediatrics 62: 189 (1978).

Kewley, G.D.: Possible association between beclomethasone dipropionate aerosol and cataracts. Australian Paediatric Journal 16: 117 (1980).

Kraepelien, S. and Graff-Lonnivig, V.: Long-term treatment with beclomethasone dipropionate aerosol in asthmatic children with special reference to growth. Allergy 34: 57 (1979).

Lal, S.; Malhotra, S.M.; Gribben, M.D. and Butler, A.C.: Beclomethasone dipropionate aerosol compared with dry powder in the treatment of asthma. Clinical Allergy 10: 259 (1980).

Maberly, D.J.; Gibson, G.J. and Butler, A.G.: Recovery of adrenal function after substitution of beclomethasone dipropionate for oral corticosteroids. British Medical Journal 1: 778 (1973).

Mackay, A.D. and Dyson, A.J.: BTA study of beclomethasone dipropionate plus salbutamol. British Journal of Diseases of the Chest 74: 321 (1980).

Martin, A.J.; Landau, L.I. and Phelan, P.D.: Asthma from childhood at age 21: the patient and his disease. British Medical Journal 1: 380 (1982).

Mellis, C.M.; Steiner, N. and Phelan, P.D.: Beclomethasone dipropionate aerosol for asthmatic children requiring maintenance oral steroid therapy. Medical Journal of Australia 1: 957 (1976).

Mitchell, I.; Paterson, I.C.; Cameron, S.J. and Grant, I.W.B.: Treatment of childhood asthma with sodium cromoglycate and beclomethasone dipropionate aerosol singly and in combination. British Medical Journal 3: 457 (1976).

Murray, A.B.; Fraser, B.M.; Hardwick, D.F. and Pirie, G.E.: Chronic asthma and growth failure in children. Lancet 2: 197 (1976).

Phelan, P.D.: Treatment of asthmatic children with steroids. British Medical Journal 3: 227 (1975).

Poynter, D.; Spurley, N.W. and Ainge, G.: A toxicity study with beclomethasone dipropionate in the dog with particular reference to the respiratory tract. Postgraduate Medical Journal 551(Suppl. 4): 27 (1975).

Siegel, S.C.; Katz, R.M. and Rachelefsky, G.S.: Prednisolone and beclomethasone for treatment of asthma. New England Journal of Medicine 300: 986 (1979).

Smith, J. Morrison: Hydrocortisone hemisuccinate by inhalation in children with asthma. Lancet 2: 1248 (1958).

Smith, J. Morrison: A clinical trial of beclomethasone dipropionate aerosol in children and adolescents with asthma. Clinical Allergy 3: 249 (1973).

Smith, J. Morrison and Gwynn, C.M.: Clinical comparison of aerosol and powder administration of beclomethasone dipropionate in asthma. Clinical Allergy 8: 479 (1978).

Smith, J. Morrison and Pizarro, Y.A.: Evaluation of systemic steroid treatment in children with asthma. Practitioner 211: 664 (1973).

Spitzer, S.A.; Kaufman, H.; Koplovitz, A.; Topilsky, M. and Blum, I.: Beclomethasone dipropionate and chronic asthma. Chest 70: 38 (1976).

Thiringer, G.; Eriksson, N.; Malmberg, R. and Svedmyr, N.: Bronchoscopic biopsies of bronchial mucosa before and after beclomethasone dipropionate therapy. Postgraduate Medical Journal 51(Suppl. 4): 30 (1975).

Wyatt, R.; Waschek, J.; Weinberger, M. and Sherman, B.: Effects of inhaled beclomethasone dipropionate and alternate-day prednisone in pituitary-adrenal function in children with chronic asthma. New England Journal of Medicine 299: 1387 (1978).

Appendix 1   The Correct Use of Inhalers

S.P. Newman

Techniques for Using Metered Dose Aerosols

Since their introduction in the early 1960s, metered dose inhalers have been very widely prescribed. These devices have the merits of being unobtrusive, compact and apparently simple to use. The benefits of the inhaled route for delivering therapeutic aerosols to the lungs are well recognised, in the case of corticosteroids for example, where administration of appropriate compounds by aerosol can produce the desired therapeutic effect with a greatly reduced incidence of systemic side effects compared to oral ingestion.

The use of a metered dose inhaler is, however, much more difficult than swallowing a tablet, and requires a fair degree of skill on the patient's part as well as time and effort spent on tuition by doctors. The manufacturers of metered dose aerosols try to assist in this by issuing an instruction sheet to patients describing how, in their opinion, the inhaler should be used. These instructions vary widely from brand to brand. Regrettably, considerable controversy also exists in the literature as to the 'correct' technique for using metered dose aerosols, in that no two review papers seem to recommend exactly the same technique. Instructions published in 5 review articles over the last decade are summarised in table 1. Patients are generally advised to take deep (vital capacity) inhalations, but apart from this, instructions differ. The inhaled flow rate is often unspecified, although a 'slow' inhalation may be recommended. The users of one popular brand of steroid aerosol are advised to inhale 'suddenly', implying rapid inhalation. Patients are often not told the lung volume at which the aerosol should be actuated (that is: early in the breath, in the middle of the breath or late in the breath). Instructions about breath-holding are usually vague and vary widely. If more than one dose is to be taken, then an interval of 1 to 2 minutes is generally specified on manufacturers' leaflets.

It is unclear how these instructions have been derived, since only very recently has any experimental evidence for the correct use of metered dose inhalers been published. Uncertainty as to the proper technique for using inhalers may cause confusion for both doctors and patients, and this might partly explain why many patients are said to misuse their inhalers. Paterson and Crompton (1976) found that 14% of patients attending their asthma clinic were 'doubtfully efficient' or 'inefficient' users of metered dose inhalers. Saunders (1965) found that 14 of 46 patients studied were not using their inhalers correctly; 11 were not obtaining full benefit as a consequence. Aerosol administered by a physician may sometimes be more effective than aerosol administered by the patient himself (Orehek et al., 1976).

This appendix reviews the evidence for the correct use of metered dose aerosols, with particular reference to inhaled cortico-

Table I. Published techniques for using pressurised aerosol bronchodilators

Reference	Inhaled volume	Inhaled flow rate	Lung vol. at actuation	Breath-holding pause
Butler (1973)	Vital capacity	Unspecified	Unspecified	A few seconds
Miller (1973)	Vital capacity	Slow	Unspecified	Several seconds
Pain (1973)	Vital capacity	Unspecified	At beginning of inhalation	As long as possible
Grainger (1977)	Vital capacity	Slow	At beginning or inhalation	As long as possible
CLAB[1] (1979)	Vital capacity	Slow	One third of way through inhalation	5-10 seconds

1 Canadian Lung Association Bulletin

steroids. However, published clinical studies which have compared therapeutic responses following various inhalation manoeuvres have involved bronchodilator aerosols and not corticosteroids. No definitive studies to find the best inhalation technique for corticosteroid metered dose aerosols have yet been described, and it is necessary therefore to extrapolate the findings from bronchodilator studies. Obviously bronchodilators with their almost immediate and easily measurable response lend themselves to this type of therapeutic experiment; however, evidence about corticosteroids can be gained from studies of pressurised aerosol deposition, since the technique which delivers the greatest quantity of aerosol to the airways may also give rise to the greatest therapeutic effect.

Elementary Problems

Some very trivial errors may bedevil the use of metered dose inhalers. For instance, it seems obvious that the cap should be removed from the inhaler mouthpiece before use. However, 3 patients out of a group of 130 asked to demonstrate the use of their inhalers failed to do this (Epstein et al., 1979). The inhaler must be held upright, or else the metering chamber will not refill properly after actuation. Again, this might seem obvious, but 13 of 130 patients observed by Epstein et al. (1979) were unaware of this. Language difficulties may cause further confusion. At a recent symposium, a set of instructions given in English, but by a German speaker, advised patients to hold the canister 'upright down'. The canister should be shaken several times before use, in order to disperse the drug uniformly throughout the propellants. The drug substance may have a different density from the propellants and may therefore tend to rise to the top or sink to the bottom of the canister. If the canister is not shaken, then an incorrect or variable quantity of drug may be released in each metered dose; 41 of 130 patients studied by Epstein et al. (1979) did not follow this simple rule.

The occasional patient seems to be totally unaware of the most basic facts about inhalation devices, and when asked to demonstrate the use of an inhaler may place the actuator mouthpiece under the nose or in an ear. The importance of adequate tuition by doctors, in order to eliminate such elementary errors, cannot be over-stressed.

Position of Actuator with Respect to Mouth

Having decided that metered dose aerosols must be directed into the mouth and not elsewhere, how should the canister be positioned? Should it be held tightly between the lips as most manufacturers recommend? Should it be placed between the lips but with the mouth wide open? Or should it be held away from the mouth (fig. 1)?

It has been accepted for some years that the great majority (> 90%) of the dose from a pressurised canister is deposited in the oropharynx and subsequently swallowed, and that only about 10% reaches the lungs directly (Davies, 1975). It is believed to be the local action of the small percentage of the dose delivered to the lungs that exerts the therapeutic effect. Since only small amounts of corticosteroid are released in each metered dose (typically 50μg), the swallowed portion is insufficient to cause a significant therapeutic effect – oral doses are many times greater than this. Furthermore, with beclomethasone dipropionate for instance, much of the swallowed drug is metabolised as it passes through the gut, and enters the circulation in an inactive form. High oropharyngeal deposition and low bronchial deposition are inevitable consequences of the pressurised delivery system. The correct inhalation technique is likely to deliver as much aerosol as possible to the required site of action within the bronchial tree, and this might depend, at least in part, upon reducing losses in the oropharynx.

Lips Open or Closed?

Patients are usually instructed to hold the inhaler mouthpiece firmly between the lips (fig. 1a). However, holding the mouth wide open, but with the actuator mouthpiece placed between the lips (fig. 1b) is sometimes recommended (Tuttle and Sidorov, 1977; Canadian Lung Association Bulletin, 1979). This has the effect of enlarging the oral cavity so that the cone-shaped spray might less readily deposit on the buccal mucosa. Dolovich et al. (1981) found an enhanced lung deposition of an inert radiolabelled aerosol, generated from a pressurised inhaler, using this technique.

The quantity of aerosol which impacts in the oropharynx must depend at least in part upon the position of the tongue at the moment the aerosol is released. If the tongue obstructs the aerosol spray (fig. 1c), then few particles are likely to reach the lungs. Care should be taken to keep the tongue on the floor of the mouth when the aerosol is actuated. Variability in tongue position may partly explain the wide inter-subject variability that is observed in pressurised aerosol deposition (Newman et al., 1981a).

Connolly (1975) compared the effects of the orthodox (lips closed round mouthpiece) technique for using a bronchodilator aerosol with that of holding the actuator a few centimetres from the open mouth (fig. 1d). The latter technique was significantly more effective in raising peak expiratory flow rate. Time and distance are created, over which the propellants may evaporate and be slowed down by air resistance. A smaller and more slowly moving aerosol arrives at the back of the mouth, and is less susceptible to deposition in the oropharynx. Dolovich et al. (1981) found a progressive increase in drug delivery to the lungs as the aerosol was moved to 4cm from the open mouth. However, when the actuator is held away from the mouth, there is a danger of spraying the aerosol accidentally onto the face, and the benefits of reduced oropharyngeal deposition may be lost. This problem may be overcome by using a dry-powder inhaler (p.224) or a 'spacer' device.

Spacer Devices

A 'spacer' or 'extension' device is placed between the actuator and the lips (figs. 1e and 1f). It may take the form of a tube or cone of 10 to 25cm length, which creates distance between the actuator and the mouth, but which at the same time guides the aerosol in the right direction. Studies carried out with a variety of designs of spacer have shown a marked reduction in oropharyngeal deposition (Morén, 1978; Corr et al., 1980; Newman et al., 1981a), and in some cases an increase in the amount of aerosol reaching the lungs (Newman et al., 1981a). Studies with bronchodilator aerosols have shown an enhanced therapeutic effect when a spacer is used, presumably because of enhanced drug delivery to the lungs (Ellul-Micallef et al., 1980; Lindgren et al., 1980). Spacer devices may be size-selective, in that they may allow smaller particles to pass into the lungs, while trapping some of the larger particles which would otherwise be deposited in the oropharynx. Such a reduction in oropharyngeal deposition may be particularly valuable in the case of corticosteroid aerosols, since the incidence of oropharyngeal candidiasis is raised in asthmatic patients using steroid aerosols, compared with patients taking oral steroids or no steroids at all (Hodson et al., 1974). Positive yeast cultures may be obtained from the throats of many asymptomatic patients using corticosteroid aerosols (Milne and Crompton, 1974). The use of spacer attachments to metered dose aerosols might well reduce the incidence of oropharyngeal candidiasis in patients using corticosteroid aerosols.

Actuating the Aerosol

Synchronisation

Synchronisation between inhalation and aerosol release is of paramount importance if a metered dose inhaler is to be used correctly. Actuation must coincide with a supporting airstream to carry the drug into the lungs, if an adequate number of drug particles are to reach their receptor sites. Failure to synchronise is sometimes termed rather curiously a 'hand-lung' problem. Estimates of the proportion of patients who have this trouble vary, but published figures range up to 38% (Earis and Bernstein, 1978; Epstein et al., 1979). Coady et al. (1976a) found that out of 103 patients, 33 (32%) failed to synchronise inhalation with aerosol release. Nine patients failed to release the dose, 14 did not inspire significantly, and 10 actuated the aerosol either before inhalation had started or after it had finished (fig. 2). Delivery of bronchodilator aerosol which is not synchronised with inhalation leads to a reduced therapeutic effect (Newman et al., 1981b). Failure to synchronise may well be the most important form of misuse of metered dose aerosols, and furthermore, patients undergoing an acute asthma attack might find synchronisation particularly difficult.

Several techniques have been proposed to help those patients who cannot adequately synchronise inhalation and aerosol release, some of which are highly ingenious. A light or sound attachment may be placed on an inhaler, to signify to the user that inhalation is occurring and that the time is ripe for firing the aerosol. Breath-actuated pressurised aerosols are also used (D'Arcy and Kirk, 1971). The patient's inspiratory effort triggers a spring mechanism which releases the aerosol. Spacer devices may have a particularly valuable role to play in the delivery of metered dose aerosols in patients with synchronisation problems. Bloomfield et al. (1979) found that the bronchodilator response to terbutaline aerosol was reduced when there was a brief pause between aerosol actuation

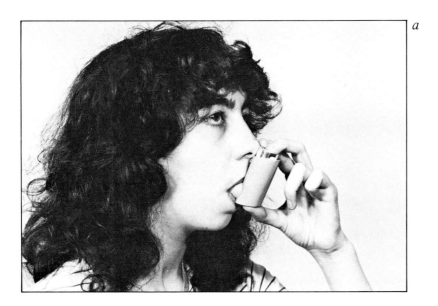

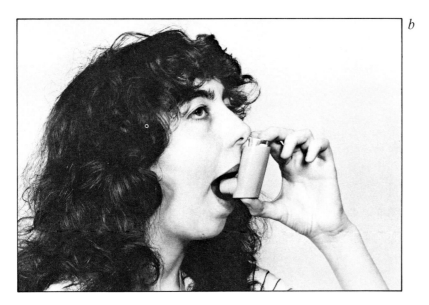

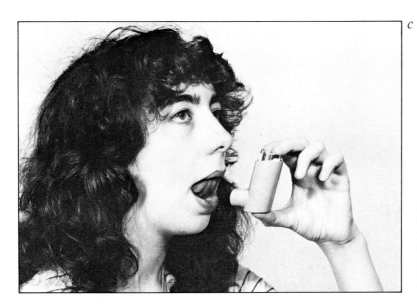

Fig. 1. Positioning the actuator in relation to the mouth (a) 'orthodox' position – mouthpiece held firmly between the lips, (b) mouthpiece placed between the lips, but with the mouth open, (c) the tongue may obstruct the aerosol spray, (d) actuator held away from the mouth, (e and f) use of spacer devices.

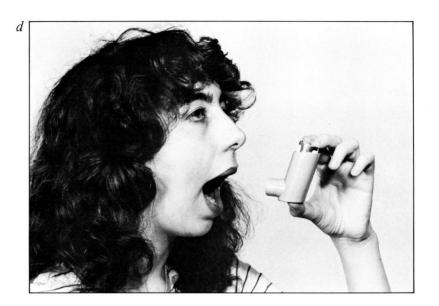

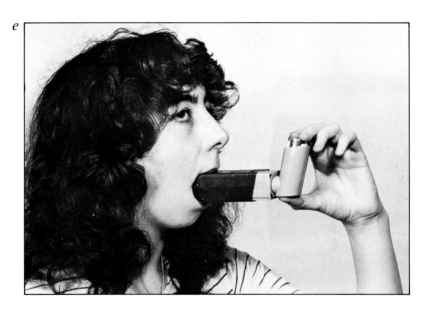

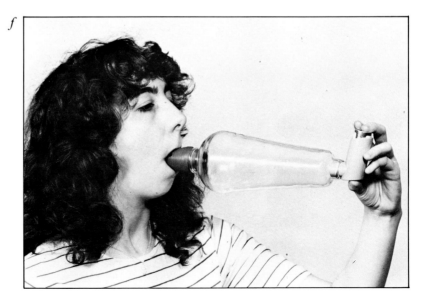

and inhalation. However, when inhalation was performed via a 10cm tube spacer device, this loss of response no longer occurred, even though the pause after actuation was maintained. Further studies showed that spacers gave an enhanced bronchodilator effect in patients specially selected for their failure to synchronise inhalation and aerosol release (Godden and Crompton, 1981). Under these circumstances, the aerosol is temporarily 'stored' in the spacer device for a few seconds before inhalation, so that synchronisation is no longer important. Some large 'reservoir bag' spacers (fig. 1f), usually equipped with one-way valves to control inhalation and exhalation, are specifically designed with this in mind (Freigang, 1977; Sackner et al., 1981; Corr et al., 1982), and may be very valuable for children, old people and those with arthritis, who may have particular difficulty with synchronisation.

'Cold-Freon' Effect

Another form of misuse of metered dose aerosols may be almost as common as poor synchronisation. This is sometimes called the 'cold-Freon' effect; in other words releasing the aerosol into the mouth causes cessation of inhalation (fig. 2e). In practice, about two-thirds of the patients who have this problem stop inhaling altogether, whilst in the remaining third, inhalation continues via the nose (Crompton, 1982). As in the case of poor synchronisation, there is no supporting airstream to carry the aerosol into the lungs. It is important to impress upon patients the need to continue inhaling after actuation so that the drug particles may penetrate into the lower respiratory tract.

Multiple Actuation

Some patients fire the aerosol twice during a single inhalation (fig. 2f). However, an interval of at least 30 seconds between the release of successive metered doses is essential. When the aerosol is actuated, there is an immediate temperature drop of about 15°C in the vicinity of the actuator orifice, owing to rapid evaporation of some of the propellants, and ambient temperature is not restored for about 30 seconds. The characteristics of the aerosol spray may be adversely affected at low temperatures. Furthermore, there may be inadequate time for the metering chamber to refill after the first actuation, so that a reduced amount of drug may be released during the second actuation. The practice of multiple actuation should be discouraged, therefore.

Position of the Head

It is occasionally recommended that the head should be tilted back when the aerosol is actuated, so that the drug particles may follow a straighter path en route to the trachea. The probability of impaction in the oropharynx depends partly upon the angle around which the particles must pass, and a reduction in the acuteness of this angle ought theoretically to reduce losses in this region of the respiratory tract.

Inhalation Mode

Inhaled Flow Rate

Changes in inhaled flow rate, breath-holding and lung volume all give rise to marked changes in the pattern of aerosol deposition in the respiratory tract. Since aerosol therapy depends upon delivery of drug to receptor sites within the bronchial tree, it seems reasonable that changes in the mode of inhalation of therapeutic aerosols should influence clinical response.

Several studies have been carried out in the last few years on both the clinical efficacy and the deposition of metered dose aerosols inhaled under systematically varied conditions. In studies carried out at the Royal Free Hospital, we have found a combination of two factors – a slow inhaled flow rate (30 L/min) and 10 seconds breath holding – to give both the greatest bronchodilator response to terbutaline sulphate pressurised aerosol and the greatest deposition in the lungs (Newman et al., 1981b, c, 1982).

Breath-holding Interval

Both deposition and bronchodilator response were reduced at a higher inhaled flow rate (80 L/min) or with only 4 seconds breath-holding (fig. 3). The faster flow rate causes an enhancement of deposition in the oropharynx by inertial impaction, while the

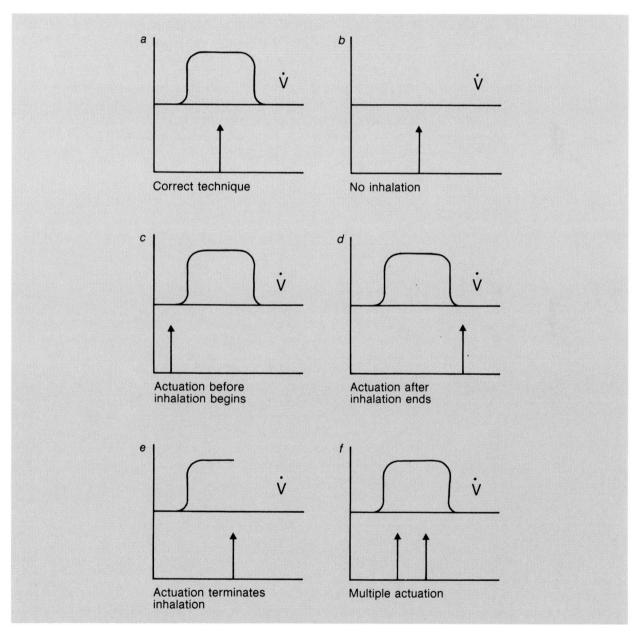

Fig. 2. Actuating the aerosol. Inhaled flow rate (V, upper traces) and aerosol release (lower traces) are shown under 6 conditions. In (a) the aerosol is used correctly, since actuation and inhalation are synchronised. Figs. 2 (b-f) show incorrect use; in (b) no inhalation has taken place; in (c) and (d) actuation and inhalation do not coincide; in (e) actuation terminates inhalation; in (f) the aerosol has been actuated more than once in a single inspiratory manoeuvre.

short breath-holding pause allows insufficient time for particles to settle onto the airways under gravity. These findings are supported by other recent studies. Dolovich et al. (1981) noted that the amount of pressurised aerosol deposited in the lungs was greater for inhaled flow rates < 60 L/min than for flow rates > 60 L/min. The bronchodilator response to fenoterol aerosol was greater following inhalation at 64 L/min than at 192 L/min (Lawford and McKenzie, 1981a).

Slow inhalation combined with 10 seconds breath-holding seems to be the inhalation mode of choice, but regrettably it is not adopted by the majority of patients. The average peak inspiratory flow rate of a group of asthmatic patients using their metered dose inhalers was found to be 207 L/min (Coady, 1976b). In the patients observed by Epstein et al. (1979) while using their aerosols, only 42% (55 of 130 patients) inhaled slowly and deeply, and only 44% (57 of 130) held the breath for 10 seconds. Patients could be encouraged to inhale slowly if the width of the annulus between the actuator and the canister, through which the inhaled air passes were reduced. However, this would increase the resistance of air flow through the device, and many patients might find this unacceptable. An interesting suggestion, made by one of our patients, was a removable cap with fine holes drilled in it, to fit over the top of the actuator. This could be used to ensure a slow steady

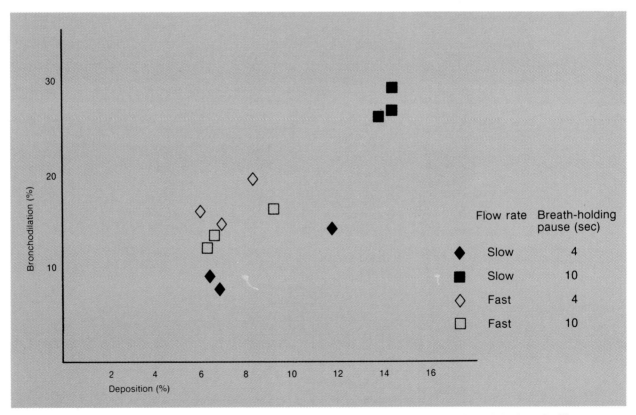

Fig. 3. Effect of inhalation mode. Both pressurised aerosol deposition in the lungs (horizontal-axis) and the bronchodilator response to terbutaline sulphate aerosol (vertical-axis) depend critically upon the inhaled flow rate and the subsequent duration of breath-holding. The greatest deposition (approx. 14% of the dose) and the greatest bronchodilator response (approx. 30% increase in forced expiratory volume in one second) occurred with a combination of slow inhaled flow rate (≈ 30 L/min) and 10 seconds breath-holding. For each combination of flow rate and breath-holding, the aerosol was released at 3 different lung volumes. Data taken from Newman et al. (1981b,c, 1982).

rate of air flow through the device, but could be removed by patients finding the increase in resistance uncomfortable.

Lung Volume

There is controversy concerning the lung volume during the course of inhalation at which aerosol should be actuated. In our studies with terbutaline aerosol we found that bronchodilatation was independent of the lung volume at actuation when the optimal inhaled flow rate and breath-holding pause were used. Under other circumstances, actuation at a low lung volume gave better bronchodilatation than actuation at a high lung volume (Newman et al., 1981b). In contrast, Riley et al. (1976, 1979) found that isoproterenol was more effective when actuated at a high lung volume. The airways are wider at high lung volumes, and the enhanced therapeutic effect was attributed to more even distribution of aerosol within the lungs. The reason for the differing findings between our own studies and those of Riley are not clear. There were differences between the studies in the type of patient studied, the inhaled flow rate, the duration of breath-holding and the type of aerosol used, and one or more of these factors may explain the discrepancies.

Exhalation Before Inhalation?

Patients are generally advised to exhale to residual volume before inhalation, and then inhale fully to total lung capacity. However, Lawford and McKenzie (1981b) found that inhalation commencing at functional residual capacity (normal resting level) gave a bronchodilator response to fenoterol aerosol equal to that achieved by commencing inhalation at residual volume. Starting to inhale from functional residual capacity would have the merit of simplifying the inhalation manoeuvre, since patients could 'fire and inhale' without the need for preliminary exhalation.

Repeat Doses

The standard treatment of inhaled therapeutic agents from metered dose devices often consists of 2 puffs taken several times daily. The manufacturers generally advocate an interval of 1 to 2 minutes between puffs, in order to allow the canister to return to thermal equilibrium and for the metering chamber to refill, as previously described.

Several authors have recommended 'sequential inhalations' for bronchodilator aerosols, in other words maintaining a 10 to 20 minute interval between puffs so that the first dose may open partially obstructed airways into which the second dose may then penetrate. The second dose may then reach bronchi inaccessible to the first dose. This technique may produce greater bronchodilatation than that achieved by the same quantity of drug given as a large single dose (Heimer et al., 1980; Ullah et al., 1981). It is doubtful whether the same considerations apply to corticosteroid aerosols, since these substances do not cause an immediate change in airway calibre. Furthermore, the technique of 'sequential inhalation' is inconvenient and introduces a further complication into the use of metered dose inhalers, as many patients might simply forget to take their second dose. Successive doses of corticosteroid aerosol should therefore be taken about 1 minute apart, as suggested by the manufacturers. 'Sequential dosing' might have a different role to play in steroid aerosol therapy, however. A bronchodilator aerosol is often prescribed to pretreat patients taking corticosteroid aerosols. The bronchodilator aerosol is given a few minutes prior

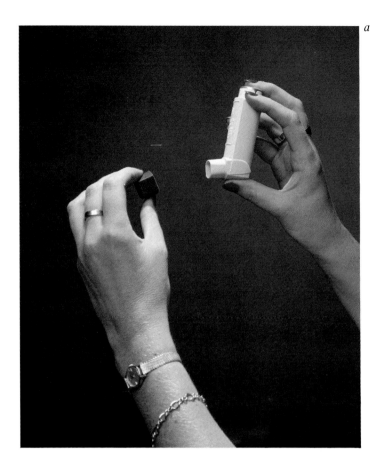

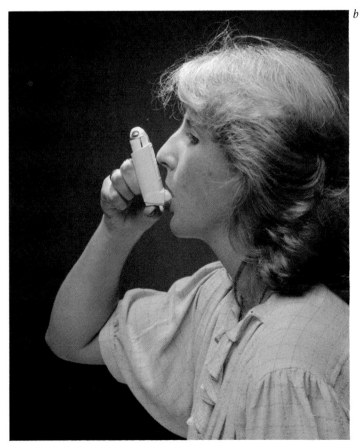

Fig. 4. Rules for using a metered dose aerosol: a) remove cap and shake canister thoroughly; b) actuate aerosol while inhaling slowly and deeply; c) hold breath for 10 seconds or longer; d) wait about 1 minute if the dose is to be repeated.

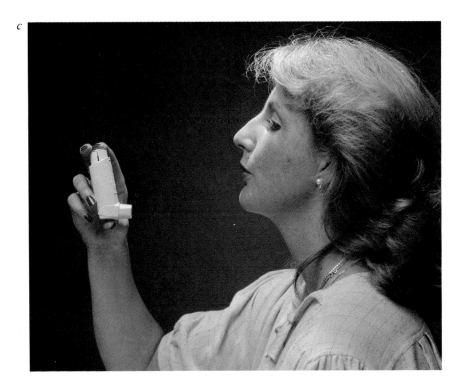

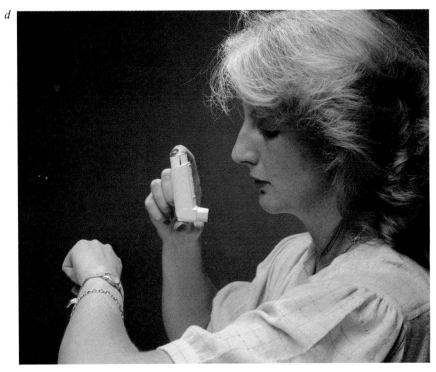

to the steroid aerosol in order to enlarge the airways, so that the latter may penetrate more distally into the bronchial tree.

Correct Inhalation Technique for Metered Dose Aerosols

The evidence for the correct use of metered dose aerosols here reviewed comes largely from tests of clinical efficacy carried out with β-adrenergic bronchodilators and from measurements of pressurised aerosol deposition. The inhalation technique which deposits the greatest quantity of aerosol in the lungs also gives rise to the greatest response to an inhaled bronchodilator. It seems reasonable that this consideration should also apply to inhaled corticosteroids, so that the optimal inhalation technique may be the same for all types of metered dose aerosol, irrespective of the drug involved. Systematic clinical trials with corticosteroid aerosols ought ideally to be carried out to verify this, although they would be very tedious to perform. From the point of view of regional deposition, the optimum inhalation mode (slow inhalation with 10 seconds breath-holding) seems to be sensible, as it is a recognised technique for delivering aerosol to peripheral airways.

Bearing in mind these factors, it is possible to set out the following rules for using metered dose aerosols (fig.4):
• Remove the cap and hold the inhaler upright
• Shake the canister thoroughly
• Actuate the aerosol while inhaling slowly and deeply
• Hold the breath for 10 seconds, or for as long as possible
• If the dose is to be repeated, wait about 1 minute.

This technique, recently dubbed the 'ten second rule' (Mohan, 1981), may be used with the lips closed round the actuator, or with the mouth open. A spacer attachment may be particularly useful for steroid inhalation, reducing the quantity of aerosol deposited in the oropharynx. The simple rules listed above are within the capabilities of the majority of patients, and should result not only in more efficient delivery of aerosol to the lungs, but also in enhanced patient compliance. There is no evidence to suggest that these rules do not apply both to patients with asthma and those with bronchitis, and to those with mild and severe airway obstruction.

Importance of Tuition

It is vitally important that patients using metered dose devices should be instructed carefully and correctly in their use when first prescribed. All patients should be assumed to be unable to use a metered dose inhaler unless proved otherwise (Crompton, 1982). It is equally important that periodic checks be made at frequent intervals, preferably with placebo aerosols, on a patient's technique, to detect any errors that have developed. Many patients adopt a faulty technique if the manufacturer's instruction sheet is the only guidance they are given before starting treatment with an aerosol, and this form of instruction alone is inadequate.

Patients should be instructed not only *how* to use a metered dose aerosol, but also *when* to do so. In a recent study, 47 of 100 patients admitted to varying their dose of steroid aerosol according to their symptoms on a particular day, even though they knew that they should use the inhalers regularly (MacFarlane and Lane, 1980). Regular users of metered dose aerosols tend to have a better technique than occasional users (Epstein et al., 1979). Furthermore some patients may use the wrong type of aerosol unless carefully instructed. For instance, a proportion of patients are known on oc-

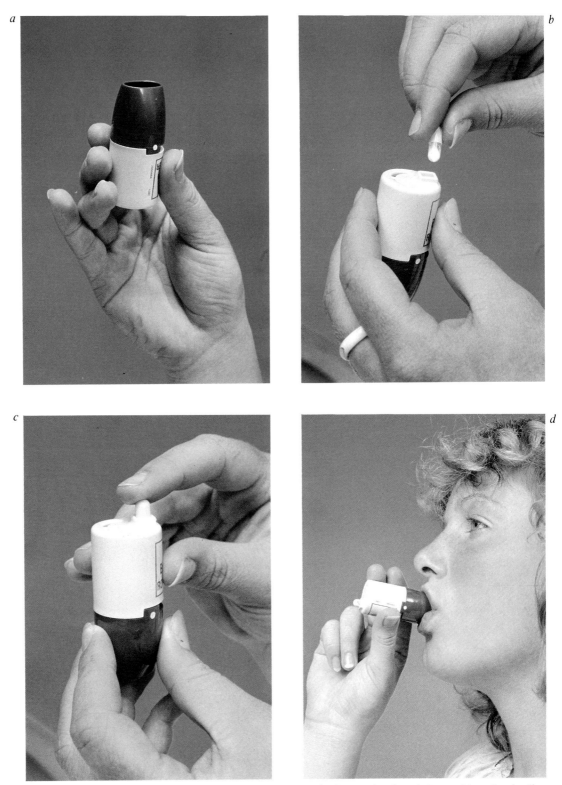

Fig. 5. A dry-powder inhaler (a). A gelatin capsule of the drug in dry powder form is inserted into the loading orifice (b). A half-turn to the device cuts the capsule (c) and breathing in draws the drug down into the lungs (d).

casion to use steroid or sodium cromoglycate aerosols in the mistaken belief that they will control acute wheezing attacks (MacFarlane and Lane, 1980). Proper tuition, repeated at regular intervals, helps to eliminate errors of this type.

Dry-powder Inhalers

For children, old people and all patients who continue to be inefficient users of metered dose aerosols even after repeated tuition, breath-actuated dry-powder inhalers may well be the solution (fig. 5). Dry-powder inhalers were introduced originally for delivery of the prophylactic agent sodium cromoglycate, but are now available for use with bronchodilators and corticosteroids (Hallworth, 1977). In these devices, the drug is provided as a finely milled powder in a gelatin capsule, which the patient mounts inside the inhaler. The capsule is either pierced by a set of needles, separated into two halves or cut in half by rotating the device. As the patient inhales through the device, the drug powder is drawn out of the capsule by the turbulent airstream, and is taken down into the lungs. Unlike pressurised aerosols it is not necessary for the patient to synchronise dose release with inhalation, since actuation is brought about by the inspiratory effort. An additional, theoretical advantage is that no chlorofluorocarbon propellants are required in dry-powder inhalers.

Dry-powder inhalers resemble metered dose inhalers in their inefficient delivery of drug to the lungs. Lactose carrier is generally added to the capsules in order to facilitate emptying, but much of this consists of particles too large to be inhaled into the lungs. Drug and lactose particles tend to form large agglomerates and consequently most of the drug itself is lost in the oropharynx. Although there have been no direct estimates of deposition of corticosteroids using dry-powder inhalers, pharmacokinetic studies (Walker et al., 1972) estimated that as little as 5% of a dose of sodium cromoglycate reaches the bronchial tree. The mode of inhalation presumably plays a role in determining clinical efficacy, but this has yet to be determined experimentally. The drug capsules may empty erratically at low inhaled flow rates. In practice this type of device has proved very successful, especially in children (chapter XII).

In some ways, dry-powder inhalers are less simple and convenient to operate than metered dose aerosols, since patients must understand the internal construction of the devices in order to load the capsules and deliver the drug powder to the lungs successfully. Some patients may find the concept of inhaling a powder – albeit a non-toxic one – less acceptable than inhaling a 'mist' from an aerosol or nebuliser. Nevertheless dry-powder inhalers undoubtedly have a role to play in corticosteroid aerosol therapy in those who by reason of age or lack of dexterity, have difficulty using conventional pressurised aerosols.

References

Bloomfield, P.; Crompton, G.K. and Winsey, N.J.P.: A tube spacer to improve inhalation of drugs from pressurised aerosols. British Medical Journal 2: 1479 (1979).
Butler, J.: Bronchodilator treatment of obstructive airway disease. Drug Therapy 3: 69 (1973).
Canadian Lung Association Bulletin: Technique for using an inhaled pressurised aerosol. Canadian Lung Association Bulletin 58: 1 (1979).
Coady, T.J.; Stewart, C.J. and Davies, H.J.: Synchronization of bronchodilator release. Practitioner 217: 273 (1976a).

Coady, T.J.; Davies, H.J. and Barnes, P.: Evaluation of a breath-actuated pressurised aerosol. Clinical Allergy 6: 1 (1976b).

Connolly, C.K.: Methods of using pressurized aerosols. British Medical Journal 3: 21 (1975).

Corr, D.; Dolovich, M.; McCormack, D.; Ruffin, R.E.; Obminski, G. and Newhouse M.: The Aerochamber: A new demand-inhalation device for delivery of aerosolized drugs. American Review of Respiratory Disease 121: 123 (1980).

Corr, D.; Dolovich, M.; McCormack, D.; Ruffin, R.E.; Obminski, G. and Newhouse M.: Design and characteristics of a portable breath-actuated, particle size selective medical aerosol inhaler. Journal of Aerosol Science 13: 1 (1982).

Crompton, G.K.: Problems patients have using pressurized aerosol inhalers. European Journal of Respiratory Diseases 63 (Suppl.): 101 (1982).

D'Arcy, P.F. and Kirk, W.F.: Development of a new device for inhalation therapy. Pharmaceutical Journal 206: 306 (1971).

Davies, D.S.: Pharmacokinetics of inhaled substances. Postgraduate Medical Journal 51 (Suppl. 7): 69 (1975).

Dolovich, M.; Ruffin, R.E.; Roberts, R. and Newhouse, M.T.: Optimal delivery of aerosols from metered dose inhalers. Chest 80 (Suppl.): 911 (1981).

Earis, J.E. and Bernstein, A.: Misuse of pressurized nebulizers. British Medical Journal 1: 1554 (1978).

Ellul-Micallef, R.; Morén, F.; Wetterlin, K. and Hidinger, K.G.: Use of a special inhaler attachment in asthmatic children. Thorax 35: 620 (1980).

Epstein, S.W.; Manning, C.P.R.; Ashley, M.J. and Corey, P.N.: Survey of the clinical use of pressurized aerosol inhalers. Canadian Medical Association Journal 120: 813 (1979).

Freigang, B.: A new method of beclomethasone aerosol administration to children under 4 years of age. Canadian Medical Association Journal 117: 1308 (1977).

Godden, D.J. and Crompton, G.K.: An objective assessment of the tube spacer in patients unable to use a conventional pressurized aerosol efficiently. British Journal of Diseases of the Chest 75: 165 (1981).

Grainger, J.R.: Correct use of aerosol inhalers. Canadian Medical Association Journal 117: 584 (1977).

Hallworth, G.W.: An improved design of powder inhaler. British Journal of Clinical Pharmacology 4: 689 (1977).

Heimer, D.; Shim, C. and Williams, M.H.: The effects of sequential inhalations of metaproterenol aerosol in asthma. Journal of Allergy and Clinical Immunology 66: 75 (1980).

Hodson, M.E.; Batten, J.C.; Clarke, S.W. and Gregg, I.: Beclomethasone dipropionate aerosol in asthma: Transfer of steroid-dependent asthmatic patients from oral prednisone to beclomethasone dipropionate aerosol. American Review of Respiratory Disease 110: 403 (1974).

Lawford, P. and McKenzie, D.: Does inspiratory flow rate affect bronchodilator response to an aerosol β_2-agonist? Thorax 36: 714 (1981a).

Lawford, P. and McKenzie, D.: Pressurized aerosol technique. Lancet 2: 1003 (1981b).

Lindgren, S.B.; Formgren, H. and Morén, F.: Improved aerosol therapy of asthma: effect of actuator tube size on drug availability. European Journal of Respiratory Diseases 61: 56 (1980).

MacFarlane, J.T. and Lane, D.J.: Irregularities in the use of regular aerosol inhalers. Thorax 35: 477 (1980).

Miller, W.F.: Aerosol therapy in acute and chronic respiratory disease. Archives of Internal Medicine 131: 148 (1973).

Milne, L.J.R. and Crompton, G.K.: Beclomethasone dipropionate and oropharyngeal candidiasis. British Medical Journal 3: 797 (1974).

Mohan, G.: The effective use of aerosol bronchodilators. Modern Medicine 26: 38 (1981).

Morén, F.: Drug deposition of pressurized inhalation aerosols. I. Influence of actuator tube design. International Journal of Pharmaceutics 1: 205 (1978).

Newman, S.P.; Morén, F.; Pavia, D.; Little, F. and Clarke, S.W.: Deposition of pressurized suspension aerosols inhaled through extension devices. American Review of Respiratory Disease 124: 317 (1981a).

Newman, S.P.; Pavia, D. and Clarke, S.W.: How should a pressurized β-adrenergic bronchodilator be inhaled? European Journal of Respiratory Diseases 62: 3 (1981b).

Newman, S.P.; Pavia, D. and Clarke, S.W.: Improving the bronchial deposition of pressurized aerosols. Chest 80 (Suppl.): 909 (1981c).

Newman, S.P.; Pavia, D.; Garland, N. and Clarke, S.W.: Effects of various inhalation modes on the deposition of radioactive pressurised aerosols. European Journal of Respiratory Diseases 63 (Suppl.): 57 (1982).

Orehek, J.; Gayrard, P.; Grimaud, C. and Charpin, J.: Patient error in the use of bronchodilator metered aerosols. British Medical Journal 1: 76 (1976).

Pain, M.C.F.: The treatment of asthma. Drugs 6: 118 (1973).

Paterson, I.C. and Crompton, G.K.: Use of pressurized aerosols by asthmatic patients. British Medical Journal 1: 76 (1976).

Riley, D.J.; Weitz, B.W. and Edelman, N.H.: The responses of asthmatic subjects to isoproterenol inhaled at differing lung volumes. American Review of Respiratory Disease 114: 509 (1976).

Riley, D.J.; Liu, R.T. and Edelman, N.H.: Enhanced responses to aerosolized bronchodilator therapy in asthma using respiratory manoeuvres. Chest 76: 501 (1979).

Sackner, M.A.; Brown, L.K. and Kim, C.S.: Basis of an improved metered aerosol delivery system. Chest 80 (Suppl.): 915 (1981).

Saunders, K.B.: Misuse of inhaled bronchodilator agents. British Medical Journal 1: 1037 (1965).

Tuttle, C.B. and Sidorov, J.: Correct use of aerosol inhalers. Canadian Medical Association Journal 117: 21 (1977).

Ullah, M.I.; Newman, G.B. and Saunders, K.B.: Influence of age on response to ipratropium and salbutamol in asthma. Thorax 36: 523 (1981).

Walker, S.R.; Evans, M.E.; Richards, A.J. and Paterson, J.W.: The fate of (^{14}C) sodium cromoglycate in man. Journal of Pharmacy and Pharmacology 24: 525 (1972).

Appendix 2

Some Tests of Pituitary Adrenal Function and Their Application to the Management of Steroid-treated Asthma Patients

Jonathan Webb

Treatment with corticosteroids will cause hypothalamic-pituitary-adrenal (HPA) suppression by reducing corticotrophin (adrenocorticotrophic hormone, ACTH) production which in turn leads to a reduced secretion by the adrenal gland of cortisol. If this sequence of events continues, atrophy of the adrenal gland follows. The degree of HPA suppression is dependent on the dose, duration, frequency, time of day, and route of administration of the steroid. The higher the plasma corticosteroid level the greater the HPA suppression until a certain critical level is reached when maximum suppression occurs. The duration of treatment is very important, a single dose will cause suppression of ACTH production but recovery of production is rapid; however, when repeated doses are given recovery of ACTH production is less rapid and with prolonged therapy, recovery of HPA function in some individuals may take months. There is a natural rhythm of cortisol production during each 24-hour cycle with the lowest levels occurring about midnight and highest levels between 7 and 10 am. A negative feedback system exists whereby a low plasma cortisol will stimulate ACTH production. Steroid administration at midnight when plasma cortisol levels are low will suppress ACTH production more than if given at 8 am when endogenous cortisol levels are at their peak. There is less HPA axis suppression if daily oral steroids are given as a morning dose. Oral steroids given in divided doses throughout the day will suppress HPA function more than the same total dose given in the morning on alternate days, as the short half-life of the commonly used steroids (e.g. prednisolone 2.1-3.5h), allows the ensuing low plasma level to stimulate ACTH production. Regular divided doses through the day maintain continuously high plasma levels thus continuously inhibiting ACTH production.

Steroids are very well absorbed from the gut so that oral and intravenous steroids are probably equally liable to suppress HPA function. Inhaled steroids are deposited mainly in the mouth and most of the dose is swallowed and inactivated, only a relatively small proportion reaching the lower respiratory tract. Although a large proportion of an inhaled steroid dose is probably absorbed the high topical potency of the compounds used by this route means that comparatively low doses are needed and this means that marked HPA suppression is unlikely.

Tests of HPA Function

The HPA system secretes ACTH and cortisol at basal rates which vary during the day (circadian variation). Stress will increase the rates of secretion and low levels of circulating cortisol will stimulate an increase in ACTH secretion. These different aspects of HPA function can be assessed separately (fig. 1).

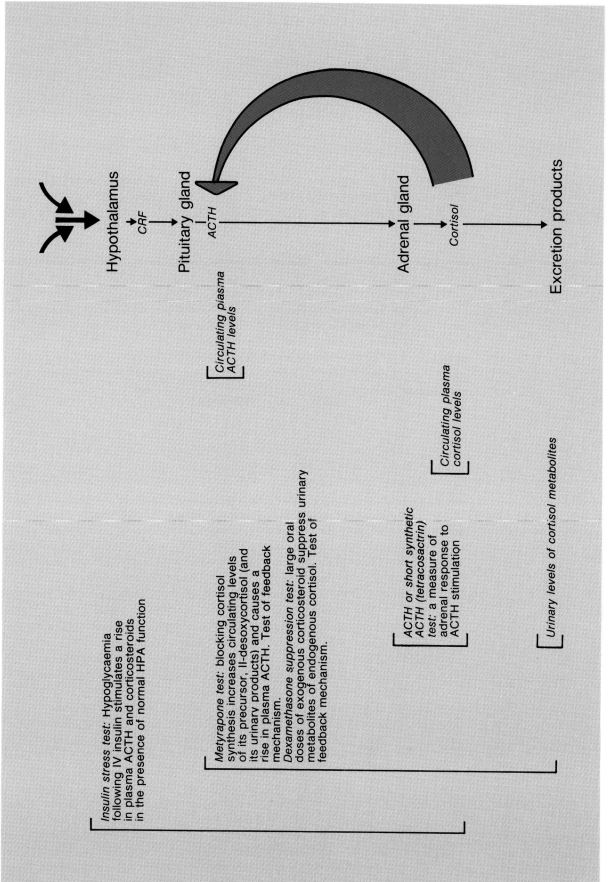

Fig. 1. Schematic representation of the hypothalamic-pituitary-adrenal axis showing those parts of the axis tested by the biochemical tests referred to in the text.

The basal secretion rates of ACTH and cortisol can be estimated by measuring basal serum ACTH and cortisol levels and 24-hour urinary excretion of corticosteroid metabolites.

The ability of the HPA axis to respond to stress is more difficult to assess. The ability of the adrenal gland to respond to ACTH can be tested by giving an injection of synthetic ACTH (tetracosactrin). Insulin-induced hypoglycaemia will cause ACTH secretion and a rise in serum cortisol levels and this is thought to mimic 'physiological' stress. The negative feedback system can be tested by giving a high dose of exogenous corticosteroid e.g. dexamethasone, and demonstrating an appropriate fall in urinary excretion of endogenous corticosteroid metabolites or by blocking the formation of cortisol from 11-desoxycortisol (substance S) by giving metyrapone and demonstrating a rise in either serum levels of substance S or urinary corticosteroid metabolites.

Circadian variation can be tested by measuring cortisol levels at 8 am and midnight and demonstrating a circadian variation.

The majority of these tests are time consuming and therefore of little value in routine clinical practice. The most useful tests in asthmatic patients are the basal cortisol levels and the ability of the adrenal gland to respond to synthetic ACTH. A more detailed account of these tests will follow after a discussion of the different methods of corticosteroid administration in asthma and their relative effects on the HPA axis.

HPA Function in Asthmatic Patients on Corticosteroids

The use of steroids in asthma falls broadly into 4 categories, inhaled maintenance treatment, short high-dose systemic courses during exacerbations, continuous oral maintenance therapy and injections of depot ACTH.

Inhaled Steroids

Beclomethasone dipropionate is the inhaled corticosteroid most studied in respect of its effect on hypothalamic-pituitary-adrenal function. Considerable HPA suppression occurs with high doses of beclomethasone dipropionate ($2000\mu g$ per day) [Choo-Kang et al., 1972]. There is debate concerning the degree and clinical significance of HPA suppression with the more usually used beclomethasone dipropionate dose ($400\mu g$/day). HPA suppression was demonstrated in children treated with inhaled beclomethasone dipropionate (Wyatt et al., 1979). In this study serum cortisol, urinary free cortisol, and the 11-desoxycortisol (substance S) response to metyrapone were significantly decreased to a similar degree in patients receiving either alternate-day oral steroids (range 20-40mg prednisolone) or inhaled beclomethasone dipropionate (400 to $800\mu g$ per day) when compared with a control group, and were lowest when alternate-day oral and inhaled steroids were given together (see figs. 8.3, 8.4). These findings were at variance with those of other workers (Godfrey and König, 1974; Klein et al., 1977) and it has been suggested (Siegel et al., 1979; p.126) that the design of this study may have contributed to this disparity.

These contradictory findings illustrate the difficulties of interpreting the results of tests of HPA function. While biochemically there are unresolved aspects, clinically it is widely held that an absence of signs of hypercorticism (and the resolution of such signs in patients on alternate-day oral steroids when transferred to inhaled steroids [Weinberger and Sherman, 1979]) supports the view that any HPA suppression from normally used doses of in-haled corticosteroids is minimal.

The same difficulties of interpretation apply to a report of the deaths of 3 asthmatic children (Mellis and Phelan, 1977) in whom postmortem examinations demonstrated atrophic adrenal glands. These children had been converted from daily oral prednisolone to inhaled beclomethasone dipropionate 5 months before death and short ACTH-stimulation tests were in the normal range one month before their deaths.

Short Course High-dose Corticosteroids

Short term high-dose steroid courses can arbitrarily be de-fined as a dose of 20mg prednisolone or more, daily for up to one month's duration. HPA suppression has been demonstrated bio-chemically after such courses (Spiegel et al., 1979; Webb and Clark, 1981). Figure 2 shows the results of plasma cortisol and ACTH levels on the 5 days after stopping the steroid in 7 patients given 40mg (20mg twice daily) of prednisolone for 3 weeks. Although biochemical suppression has been demonstrated there are no re-ports of failure to respond to stress after such short courses of treatment and many physicians do not think it necessary to 'tail off' a dose of steroids after short high-dose courses (p.109).

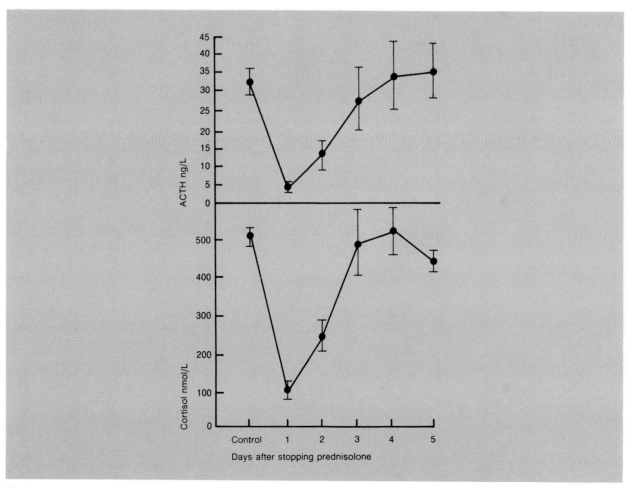

Fig.2. Recovery of ACTH and cortisol levels in 7 patients with asthma after a 3-week course of prednisolone (40mg/day) From Webb and Clark, 1981.

Continuous Oral
Maintenance Therapy

Following long term continuous steroid therapy there are a number of steroid withdrawal syndromes (Dixon and Christy, 1980) which have been subdivided into 4 types:

1) Symptomatic and biochemical evidence of HPA suppression
2) Recrudescence of the disease for which the drug was originally prescribed
3) Dependence upon steroids, either physical or psychological, with demonstrably normal HPA function and no recrudescence of underlying disease
4) Biochemical evidence of HPA suppression without symptoms or recurrence of the underlying disease.

Recovery of HPA function after long term corticosteroids is extremely variable and may take up to 9 months (Graber et al., 1965). The most dangerous but very rare complication following long term steroid treatment is failure to respond to stress, particularly surgical stress. Reports of postoperative death associated with irreversible shock and adrenal atrophy following long term steroid treatment first appeared in the early 1950s (Salassa et al., 1953). It was pointed out then that HPA function suppression was entirely due to suppression of endogenous ACTH production and that inability to cope with the stress of surgery was probably infrequent. Jasani et al. (1968) have shown that the rise in plasma 11-hydroxycorticosteroids during operation was reduced in a group of patients with rheumatoid arthritis on a mean dose of 6.5mg of prednisolone per day (mean duration 42 months) when compared with a control group. One patient developed hypotension but, although cortisol levels failed to rise in many of the remaining patients operated on, they did not develop hypotension postoperatively. This implies that other factors must also be involved in the development of postoperative shock in these patients. Cope (1966) has pointed out that most cases of 'post steroid-therapy collapse' are due to medical diagnostic failure rather than adrenal failure and that evidence of low cortisol levels occurring in this widely suspected phenomenon was remarkably scanty.

ACTH

Injections of depot ACTH are now rarely used in the treatment of chronic asthma. This method of administration is inconvenient, does not produce pharmacological levels of cortisol, and suppresses hypothalamic-pituitary function. Although overall HPA function is less suppressed, weight for weight, than with oral corticosteroids (Carter and James, 1970; Daly et al., 1974), ACTH injections given during attempts to 'tail off' oral steroids are dangerous as this further depresses the hypothalamic-pituitary end of the HPA axis (Donald and Espiner, 1975).

Tests of HPA Function in Asthmatic Patients

In routine clinical practice there are only a very limited number of tests which are of value. In asthmatic patients who have depressed HPA function secondary to treatment with corticosteroids it is important to know if the basal levels and response to stress have returned to normal. Basal rates can be assessed by measuring serum cortisol levels, however, the choice of test to assess the stress axis is more controversial. The insulin hypoglycaemia test is often quoted as the most reliable test of this aspect of

HPA function; although it is probably the most rigorous test used in research studies (p.123) it is potentially dangerous and time-consuming. The need for evidence about the recovery of the HPA axis after treatment with corticosteroids in routine clinical practice is best served by the short ACTH (tetracosactrin) test. The rise in plasma cortisol has been shown to be very similar following tetracosactrin injection or insulin-induced hypoglycaemia (Lindholm et al., 1978). Jasani et al. (1968) showed that the increase in cortisol during surgery in a group of corticosteroid treated patients was more reliably predicted by the short ACTH test than the insulin hypoglycaemia test. For these reasons it has been suggested that the only tests required for assessment of the return of HPA function are basal cortisol levels and a short synacthen test (Byyny, 1976).

Practical Details

Measurement of Plasma Cortisol[1]

The two methods of measurement used most commonly are a fluorometric method which is relatively simple and cheap and a more complex and rather more specific method using displacement analysis (binding assay).

Fluorometric method: Cortisol and corticosterone dissolved in sulphuric acid have a fairly specific fluorescence and although this method is not specific for cortisol, in practice this fact can usually be ignored. Certain drugs e.g. spironolactone, mepacrine and fusidic acid will also fluoresce at similar wave lengths and increase the apparent levels of cortisol 5- to 20-fold. Normal value: 8 am to 10 am 170-600 nmol per litre (6-22μg per 100ml).

Binding assay: Labelled cortisol and a cortisol-binding protein from plasma (transcortin) or an antibody against cortisol are required for this method (analogous to the T3 resin-uptake method in thyroid function testing). The binding assay is more specific than the fluorometric method and requires only a very small volume of blood. Its chief disadvantage is that prednisolone or prednisone affect the result – posing a problem when assessing HPA axis recovery in patients with asthma who are being 'tailed off' their dose of oral corticosteroid. Normal value: 8 am to 10 am 80-550 nmol per litre (3-20μg per 100ml).

Short ACTH (Tetracosactrin) Test[1]

A basal blood sample is taken between 8 and 10 am and 250μg of tetracosactrin, a synthetic ACTH, injected either intramuscularly or intravenously. Exactly 30 minutes later a repeat blood sample is taken. Normal response: 30 minutes after tetracosactrin injection plasma corticosteroid level should reach a minimum of 500 nmol per litre (20μg) with an increment of at least 200 nmol (7μg).

1 Conversion table
5μg per 100 mls =   138 nmol per litre
10   =   276
15   =   414
20   =   552
25   =   690
30   =   828
35   =   966
40   = 1104

References

Byyny, R.L.: Withdrawal from glucocorticoid therapy. New England Journal of Medicine 295: 30 (1976).

Carter, M.E. and James, V.H.T.: Comparison of effects of corticotrophin and corticosteroids on pituitary function. Annals of Rheumatic Diseases 29: 91 (1970).

Choo-Kang, Y.F.J.; Cooper, J.E. and Grant, I.W.B.: Beclomethasone dipropionate by inhalation in the treatment of airway obstruction. British Journal of Diseases of the Chest 66: 101 (1972).

Cope, C.L.: The adrenal cortex in internal medicine. British Medical Journal 2: 847 (1966).

Daly, J.R.; Fletcher, M.R.; Glass, D.; Chambers, D.J.; Bitensky, L. and Chayen, J.: Comparison of effects of long-term corticotrophin and corticosteroid treatment on responses of plasma growth hormone, ACTH, and corticosteroid to hypoglycaemia. British Medical Journal 2: 521 (1974).

Dixon, R.B. and Christy, N.P.: On the various forms of corticosteroid withdrawal syndrome. American Journal of Medicine 68: 224 (1980).

Donald, R.A. and Espiner, E.A.: The plasma cortisol and corticotrophin response to hypoglycaemia following adrenal steroid and ACTH administration. Journal of Clinical Endocrinology and Metabolism 41: 1 (1975).

Godfrey, S. and König, P.: Treatment of childhood asthma for 13 months and longer with beclomethasone dipropionate aerosol. Archives of Disease in Childhood 49: 591 (1974).

Graber, A.L.; Ney, R.L.; Nicholson, W.E.; Island, D.F. and Liddle, G.W.: Natural history of pituitary-adrenal recovery following long-term suppression with corticosteroids. Journal of Clinical Endocrinology 25: 11 (1965).

Jasani, M.K.; Freeman, P.A.; Boyle, J.A.; Reid, A.M.; Driver, M.J. and Buchanan, W.W.: Studies of the rise in plasma 11-hydroxycorticosteroids (11-OHCS) in corticosteroid-treated patients with rheumatoid arthritis during surgery: correlations with the functional integrity of the hypothalamo-pituitary adrenal axis. Quarterly Journal of Medicine 37: 407 (1968).

Klein, R.; Waldman, D.; Kershnar, H. et al.: Treatment of chronic childhood asthma with beclomethasone dipropionate aerosols. I. A double-blind crossover trial in nonsteroid-dependent patients. Pediatrics 60: 7 (1977).

Lindholm, J.; Kehlet, H.; Blichert-Toft, M.; Dinesen, B. and Riishede, J.: Reliability of the 30-minute ACTH test in assessing hypothalamic-pituitary-adrenal function. Journal of Clinical Endocrinology and Metabolism 47: 272 (1978).

Mellis, C.M. and Phelan, P.D.: Asthma deaths in children – a continuing problem. Thorax 32: 29 (1977).

Salassa, R.M.; Bennett, W.A.; Keating, F.R. and Sprague, R.G.: Postoperative adrenal cortical insufficiency. Occurrence in patients previously treated with cortisone. Journal of the American Medical Association 152: 1509 (1953).

Siegel, S.C.; Katz, R.M. and Rachelefsky, G.S.: Letter. New England Journal of Medicine 300: 986 (1979).

Spiegel, R.J.; Oliff, A.I.; Bruton, J.; Vigersky, R.A.; Echelberger, C.K. and Poplack, D.G.: Adrenal suppression after short-term corticosteroid therapy. Lancet 1: 630 (1979).

Webb, J.R. and Clark, T.J.H.: Recovery of plasma corticotrophin and cortisol levels after a three-week course of prednisolone. Thorax 36: 22 (1981).

Weinberger, M. and Sherman, B.: Letter. New England Journal of Medicine 300: 987 (1979).

Wyatt, R.; Washek, M.S.; Weinberger, M. and Sherman, B.: Effects of inhaled beclomethasone dipropionate and alternate-day prednisolone on pituitary-adrenal function in children with chronic asthma. New England Journal of Medicine 299: 1387 (1979).

index